W9-BGH-093

ESSENTIALS OF NUTRITION AND DIET THERAPY

ESSENTIALS OF NUTRITION AND DIET THERAPY

SUE RODWELL WILLIAMS, M.R.Ed., M.P.H.

Instructor in Nutrition and Clinical Dietetics, Kaiser
Foundation School of Nursing; Nutrition Consultant and
Program Coordinator, Health Education Research Center,
Kaiser-Permanente Medical Center, Oakland, California;
Lecturer, Nutritional Science and Community Nutrition,
College of Alameda, Alameda, California; Lecturer,
Nutrition Education, School of Human Development and
Education, California State Polytechnic University,
San Luis Obispo, California; Field Faculty, M.P.H.–
Dietetic Internship Program, University of California,
Berkeley, California

Illustrated

THE C. V. MOSBY COMPANY

Saint Louis   1974

Library of Congress Cataloging in Publication Data

Williams, Sue Rodwell, 1922-
     Essentials of nutrition and diet therapy.

     Includes bibliographical references.
     1. Nutrition.   2.   Diet in disease.   I.   Title.
[DNLM: 1. Diet therapy.   2.   Nutrition.   QU145   W727e
1974]
RA784.W643   612′.3   73-23018
ISBN   0-8016-5568-4

GW/M/M   9   8   7   6   5   4

TO

MY STUDENTS

*whose "whys" and "hows" and "so whats"
keep my feet to the fire of knowledge and
make the learning process exciting
and ever new to me*

PREFACE

Change is the essence of life. If anything is to remain viable and relevant, it too must change to meet changing needs. Two basic areas of profound change in the field of health care demand a new approach, a strengthening and broadening of the material: (1) changes in nutritional science and practice to match a rapidly changing food environment and (2) changes in society and basic technology that have created an increasing number of new health workers and demand consequent changes in methods of delivering health care and dealing with new problems.

As a result of these pressing needs, the guiding purpose throughout the design of this book has been twofold: (1) to strengthen and broaden the base of knowledge, skills, and insights required for realistic function as a health worker in today's changing world and (2) to relate this knowledge to social needs and to the increasing number of health care assistants who share various responsibilities for the quality of person-centered care necessary to meet these needs. This team of health workers involves many persons who are concerned with the nutritional base of health—not only nurses, dietitians, and physicians but also their many assistants, including practical and licensed vocational nurses, diet technicians, medical and dental assistants, dental hygienists, and other therapists.

This underlying philosophy of change and human need is discussed in Chapter 1. An understanding of today's social issues and needs is essential for such person-centered health care.

To fulfill this basic purpose, the book has been divided into three sections. Part One, An Introduction to Human Nutrition, develops the basic concepts of nutritional science by means of a problem-solving approach. It provides a background of sound nutritional principles and includes clinical applications to relate these principles to human health. Part Two, Community Nutrition: The Life Cycle, applies nutritional concepts to community and family needs, relating psychologic, social, economic, and cultural influences to serious individual and community nutritional problems and their solutions. It underscores the nutritional basis for positive health throughout the growth and development continuum of life. Part Three, An Introduction to Diet Therapy, provides a basic manual of clinical nutrition, basing therapeutic needs firmly on a normal nutritional framework.

I am grateful to many colleagues and friends for helping to stimulate and develop my thinking. I am especially grateful to my students, who always teach me a great deal and whose constantly inquiring minds make the learning process exciting and ever new to me. Also I am grateful for the constant support and encouragement of my loving family, without whom I would never be able to accomplish such projects as this. For specific technical assistance I am grateful to George Straus, whose clear and beautiful illustrations have greatly enhanced the learning value of this book. Especially do I thank my excellent typist, Helen McGrath, who stayed with me to the end and provided both concise typescript and much personal support.

Sue Rodwell Williams

CONTENTS

APPENDIXES

PART

ONE

AN INTRODUCTION TO HUMAN NUTRITION

CHAPTER 1 NUTRITION AND HEALTH

Questions about nutrition and the changing food environment are of increasing public concern. Thoughtful students in allied fields of health care are also asking basic questions concerning the role of nutrition in their work and rightly so. Why should persons working in health care fields be concerned about nutrition? What is health and how is nutrition related to it? What is nutrition? What does it *do*? How does one discover the definition of nutrition?

Answers to questions such as these are important to any student in a health-related course of study; they help set realistic personal learning goals related to life experiences and personal career objectives.

First of all, to answer such questions and to meet realistic and practical needs in today's world, a study of nutrition and health care must focus on *change*. Our physical bodies are constantly changing—this is the basis of life. Personalities are changing; scientific knowledge is changing; society is changing. Second, to maintain health these constant changes must be in some kind of *positive balance* to produce an integrated whole. Thus the learning concepts of *change* and *balance* will provide the fundamental framework for this study of basic nutrition.

To provide a beginning background for study, consider how far reaching the effects of change in today's world are on nutrition and health, how persons view and define health and disease, ways of providing health care, and the role of nutrition in health care.

CHANGING CONCEPTS OF HEALTH AND DISEASE

In the past, health has usually been defined simply as the absence of disease. Thus the basic approach to care was curative. The education and training of hospital and community workers centered primarily on learning certain skills for treatment of illness or for crisis intervention. To a large extent this is still true.

Increasingly, however, health is coming to be viewed in broader positive terms of maintaining health, including mental and social as well as physical health. In fact, in 1946 such a view was written into the preamble of the new World Health Organization constitution: "Health is a state of complete physical, mental and social well-being, and not merely the absence of disease or infirmity." Perhaps the word "complete" used concerning health is unrealistic. However, the idea of a positive approach to maintaining health and preventing illness is present. This more positive concept of health has as its goal providing human beings with the opportunity to achieve a sense of personal productivity and self-fulfillment. To meet such goals, today's education for work in the health care fields must involve an integrated study of the whole person, his community, and his health needs. This approach incorporates the idea of "the abundant life." It values quality of life beyond mere physical survival.

Causes of change in the concepts of health and disease

Two basic factors that have contributed to changes in health values and practices are the rapid increases in scientific knowledge and in population.

Scientific knowledge explosion. The rate of expansion of present scientific knowledge is almost incomprehensible. About 95% of all the scientists who have ever lived are alive today. Knowledge of nutrition, the body's intricate chemistry, and its interaction with the environment is constantly increasing. Also, technology for applying this basic knowledge is rapidly advancing. To integrate and use this knowledge challenges and taxes health care facilities. Cures for specific diseases and a wide variety of treatment techniques, drugs, and electronic instruments have all become a regular part of medical care.

Although lifesaving and extending in many ways, such rapidly expanding scientific knowledge has created problems. With increased specialization has come more fragmentation of care and removal of patients still further from their physicians and other allied health workers, sometimes creating feelings of being lost in the system. Also, with this increasing complexity of care have come increasing costs.

Population explosion. In many parts of the world, alarming threats of famine are appearing as population increases compete with decreasing food supplies. Although so critical a point seems distant in North America, the increasing concentration of poorer population groups in crowded city ghettos has increased the extent of general malnutrition. The population has not only increased in total numbers but has also changed markedly in its age distribution. With the control of childhood diseases, life expectancy is greatly increased. A larger number of persons live to older ages and develop chronic illnesses. Also, increased mobility and transfer of workers in industry have produced a more transient population; this has caused changing family patterns, life-styles, and social values and has brought attendant problems in providing continuing health care to meet changing needs.

CHANGES IN METHODS OF PROVIDING HEALTH CARE

These rapid changes in attitudes toward health and disease, life styles and society, and general scientific knowledge and technology are producing changes in the health care system. Four basic changes seem certain:

1. Change from a *focus* mainly on the physical symptoms of disease to a focus on the social issues involved in its cause. This change is based on the more positive approach of preventing illness. It recognizes that the root causes of much disease are social problems such as poverty; race; war; inadequate housing, food, and sanitation; prejudice; ignorance; and alienation. Thus to treat only the symptoms of such disease without attacking its roots is futile. In the future, health workers at all levels will be more involved in community and legislative action, family and community health projects, and primary family care and health education.

2. Changes in *systems of delivery* of health care. These changes are based on two concepts:

a. *The health team.* A group of health care specialists and assistants team their various skills and resources to provide primary care. This team approach not only uses the family physician, nurse practitioner, and nutritionist but also requires more primary care assistants, such as licensed vocational or practical nurses, diet technicians, home health aides, clinic aides, and community street workers.

b. *Variety of settings for service.* In addition to the central-core medical center, or hospital, the number of various satellite clinics or health centers will increase. This means more extended-care facilities based on degree of care needed; more community health centers and special clinics such as those for nutrition, home-management counseling, and maternity and child care; and more outreach clinics in remote rural areas.

3. Changes in *consumer relations*. Patients, or health clients, must increasingly be recognized as members of the health team. They must be involved in planning and decision making concerning their own health needs. They must have more opportunity, therefore, for better education in nutrition and general health to help them toward more positive health behavior, wiser use of health care facilities, and self-care. More health care assistants and peer group workers will be needed for such an ongoing educational service.

4. Changes in *payment for services*. The traditional fee-for-service practice of American medicine and the rapidly rising costs of medical care often place such care beyond the reach of many persons who need it most. Thus some kind of prepaid group health insurance or some program of national health insurance will have to be provided. This also means a greater involvement of patients or clients in their own health care.

NUTRITION IN HEALTH CARE

In the midst of such significant changes in society and in approaches to health care, nutrition can no longer be viewed in the narrow, isolated sense that may have been common in the past: it is intimately involved in these broader changes and in total health care.

Changing concepts of nutrition

Several interrelated areas of social and scientific change are reflected in changing nutritional needs, problems, and priorities.

Rapidly changing food environment. Advancing knowledge of food science and technology is being applied by the growing food industry to produce an infinite number of new food products. These include a wide variety of processed, combination, "convenience," synthetic and textured foods. Two basic problem areas result:

1. Primary single foods of generally known nutrient composition tend to be used less. This means that guidelines referring only to primary foods (such as the basic four food groups) require qualification and extension and have limited value in planning meals for nutrient adequacy. A practical guide related more to nutrient contribution of foods needs to be developed.

2. The need for nutrition education in schools, homes, clinics, hospitals, and the marketplace has increased. Confusing claims and counterclaims and misleading advertising increase the difficulty of buying wisely. Increased knowledge of buying behavior and market research could be applied to nutrition education and product-identification programs supported by food store chains. Some food chains have made such a beginning using a staff of home economists and consumer specialists to produce nutrition education materials and buying guides. The new nutrient labeling regulations recently established by the FDA should be a helpful beginning step in this direction. (See p. 109.)

Increased consumer awareness and action. The development of broad communication media, especially television, and the national attention given to nutritional problems of the poor and the aged and questionable food additives have increased public awareness of the role of nutrition in health. Questions are being raised, and consumers are seeking information on nutrition. Too often, however, commercial television advertising has conveyed misinformation and promoted nonnutritious food habits, such as the use of excessive sweet snacks by young children. More responsible nutrition education action by consumers and concerned professional nutrition groups is a necessity.

Changing socioeconomic and population trends. Shifts in population patterns and the increasing number of older persons have focused attention on nutrition problems in two basic areas:

1. Malnutrition in poverty areas of large cities, especially among minority groups, in migrant working populations, in rural areas throughout the South, and on Indian reservations.

2. Malnutrition and chronic health problems in the aging population. Attitudes of the youth- and action-oriented society in this country toward the aged, compounded by problems of health and economic security, often isolate and bring despair to elderly persons. Realistic programs are needed for nutrition education, food assistance related to better nutrition, and care of chronic conditions such as heart disease and diabetes.

DEFINITION OF NUTRITION

It is evident, then, that nutrition has to be defined in terms of its function in meeting human needs. Two background tools, a framework for identifying human needs and a functional statement of basic nutrition concepts, may provide helpful guides.

Identifying personal health needs

Human needs may be identified using four basic frames of reference: age group needs, stress factors, health status, and basic human needs.

Age group needs. Human beings progress through normal growth and development from the prenatal period, birth, infancy, and childhood stages of growth through adulthood in the continuous aging process to death. In each of these stages specific physical growth patterns and psychosocial development occur. Each age group has its special needs and nutritional requirements. Food habits are specifically related to the growth and development process.

Stress factors. The stresses in an individual life situation may be caused by physical or emotional problems. Depending on his personal strength, reserves, and resources available, the stress may be well handled or unmanageable. The degree of adjustment or method of coping will have to be considered in determining needs.

Health status. An individual's degree of health or disease, not only his real situation but also his situation as *he* perceives it, determines nutritional needs or food modifications required.

Basic human needs. Such physiologic survival needs as food and water and safety and comfort, respectively, must be met before the higher needs for love, self-esteem, and creative growth can be met. Basic nutrition and health needs are related to each of these general human needs for personal integrity.

Basic concepts of nutrition

The statement of basic concepts of nutrition, according to essential function and need (p. 7), has been developed by the Inter-Agency Committee on Nutrition Education of the USDA Agricultural Research Service. It may serve as a useful guide in relating nutrition to human life and health needs.

Relation of nutrition to health

Nutrition is specifically related to health in two basic ways—physically and emotionally.

Physical health. Life in its most fundamental sense—survival—depends on air, water, and food. These basic life-support materials supply the body with certain essential chemicals that enable it to do its work. Oxygen from the air combines with chemical materials —nutrients—in food and water to enable the body to carry on all its functions: (1) the production of energy, (2) the building and maintenance of body tissue, and (3) the control of the various body processes involved in producing energy and building tissue. We must have energy for work and physical activities, and we must build body cells and tissues. The essential nutrients supply the fuel and building blocks for carrying on these activities. In a biologic sense, people literally are what they eat.

Some general evidences of good nutrition

Basic concepts of nutrition*

1. Nutrition is the food you eat and how the body uses it. We eat food to live, to grow, to keep healthy and well, and to get energy for work and play.
2. Food is made up of different nutrients needed for growth and health.
   a. All nutrients needed by the body are available through food.
   b. Many kinds and combinations of food can lead to a well-balanced diet.
   c. No food, by itself, has all the nutrients needed for full growth and health.
   d. Each nutrient has specific uses in the body.
   e. Most nutrients do their best work in the body when teamed with other nutrients.
3. All persons, throughout life, have need for the same nutrients, but in varying amounts.
   a. The amounts of nutrients needed are influenced by age, sex, size, activity, and the state of health.
   b. Suggestions for the kinds and amounts of food needed are made by trained scientists.
4. The way food is handled influences the amount of nutrients in food, its safety, appearance, and taste.
   a. Handling means everything that happens to food while it is being grown, processed, stored, and prepared for eating.

*From Inter-Agency Committee on Nutrition Education, Agricultural Research Service, U. S. Department of Agriculture, Nutrition Program News, Sept.-Oct., 1964.

Table 1-1. Clinical signs of nutritional status

	GOOD	POOR
General appearance	Alert, responsive	Listless, apathetic; cachexia
Hair	Shiny, lustrous; healthy scalp	Stringy, dull, brittle, dry, depigmented
Neck glands	No enlargement	Thyroid enlarged
Skin, face and neck	Smooth, slightly moist; good color, reddish pink mucous membranes	Greasy, discolored, scaly
Eyes	Bright, clear; no fatigue circles	Dryness, signs of infection, increased vascularity, glassiness, thickened conjunctiva
Lips	Good color, moist	Dry, scaly, swollen; angular lesions (stomatitis)
Tongue	Good pink color, surface papillae present, no lesions	Papillary atrophy, smooth appearance; swollen, red, beefy (glossitis)
Gums	Good pink color; no swelling or bleeding; firm	Marginal redness or swelling; receding, spongy
Teeth	Straight, no crowding; well-shaped jaw; clean, no discoloration	Unfilled caries, absent teeth, worn surfaces, mottled, malpositioned
Skin, general	Smooth, slightly moist, good color	Rough, dry, scaly, pale, pigmented, irritated; petechiae, bruises

Continued.

Table 1-1. Clinical signs of nutritional status—cont'd

	GOOD	POOR
Abdomen	Flat	Swollen
Legs, feet	No tenderness, weakness, or swelling; good color	Edema, tender calf; tingling, weakness
Skeleton	No malformations	Bowlegs, knock-knee, chest deformity at diaphragm, beaded ribs, prominent scapulae
Weight	Normal for height, age, body build	Overweight or underweight
Posture	Erect, arms and legs straight, abdomen in, chest out	Sagging shoulders, sunken chest, hump back
Muscles	Well developed, firm	Flaccid, poor tone; undeveloped, tender
Nervous control	Good attention span for age; does not cry easily; not irritable or restless	Inattentive, irritable
Gastrointestinal function	Good appetite and digestion; normal, regular elimination	Anorexia, indigestion, constipation, diarrhea
General vitality	Endurance; energetic, vigorous; sleeps well at night	Easily fatigued, no energy, falls asleep in school, looks tired, apathetic

are a well-developed body, average weight for body size, and good muscles. The skin is smooth and clear, the hair is glossy, and the eyes are clear and bright; posture is good and facial expression alert. Appetite, digestion, and elimination are good. Compare the more detailed evidences of good and poor states of nutrition given in Table 1-1.

Human personal needs. Although food and water are essential for survival, man does not eat to sustain his physical body alone. Food has many meanings and helps to meet a number of personal, social, and cultural needs. Unmet personal needs may contribute to actual physical illness. Nutrition and food, therefore, are related to both physical and emotional health.

Practical application. Nutrition should be applied by health workers in everyday practice in three basic ways:

1. *Developing a sound basic working knowledge of nutrition.* This includes a knowledge of nutrients and their functions and the ability to distinguish between sound and unreliable references and resources.

2. *Using the human approach.* In dealing with individuals, personal life style and situation must be considered. Practical problems related to meeting nutritional needs are important.

3. *Applying principles of nutrition education in every situation.* Nutrition education is necessary to improve individual nutritional status, combat malnutrition and misinformation in needy areas, and motivate persons toward desired food behavior changes. All this has to be accomplished through a recharged and sensitized *person-centered* approach.

PLAN OF STUDY

To meet these basic objectives, the plan of study used here will concentrate on two basic areas: content, including basic science principles, community resources, and patient care; and reference tools.

Content

Part I, "An Introduction to Human Nutrition," will introduce the basic elements of nutrition, the nutrients and their functions in the body. These functions will be developed around three fundamental problems: energy, building and rebuilding tissue, and regulation and control. Part II, "Community Nutrition: the Life Cycle," will consider the food environment and the web of factors that control it; factors that influence individual choices from available foods, development of cultural food patterns and habits, and nutrition educa-

tion; and various age group needs of the life cycle. Part III, "An Introduction to Diet Therapy," will discuss the hospitalized patient and the principles of diet therapy in various disease situations.

Reference tools

Finally, tools for reference will be included in the Appendixes. Food value reference tables will provide a background for simple calculations. Finally, an index is provided for quick location or cross referencing of desired topics for study.

Recognizing the importance of food will deepen and facilitate patient care. Nutrition as a science and an art is applicable not merely to the patient on a special diet: it is a constant vital part of *person-centered* care for every patient.

CHAPTER 2 CARBOHYDRATES: THE PROBLEM OF ENERGY

For a basic understanding of nutrition, the human body should be considered in terms of the three most basic physiologic problems it must solve to survive and remain healthy. Then the question arises, "How does nutrition meet these survival needs?"

First, we must have *energy* to move about, work, play, and run our bodies. How do we get it?

Second, we must *build* our bodies from a small single cell and grow from a baby into an adult, all the while constantly rebuilding and repairing our changing tissues. How do we do it?

Third, if all this is going on, some type of regulation must be needed to *control* these changes and maintain the whole system in balance. What are the control agents and how do they operate? All three of these problems are interrelated but will be studied one at a time; then it can be seen how they fit together.

THE PROBLEM OF ENERGY

Energy is necessary for life to go on. It is the power of an organism or a machine to perform its work. Any energy system, to be successful, must provide four basic components:

1. A raw fuel
2. A means of changing the raw fuel to a refined fuel that the machine can use

3. A means of getting this refined fuel to the site of energy production
4. A means of burning the fuel at the production site to produce energy

These necessary parts of an energy system can be applied to the human energy system to see how the body solves this basic problem of existence. First of all, the two major fuels the body uses for energy are *carbohydrates* and *fats*.

CARBOHYDRATES AS RAW FUEL

The raw fuel forms of carbohydrates are starches and sugars as they occur naturally. Plants are the main sources of carbohydrates in the human diet. Since energy on this planet comes ultimately from the sun and its nuclear reactions, plants in the presence of sunlight transform the sun's energy into plant food. They use carbon dioxide from the air and water in the soil, along with chlorophyll in green leaves as a chemical catalyst, to manufacture starches and sugars. Since the body can rapidly break down these sugars and starches to yield energy, carbohydrates are called "quick energy" foods. They provide our major source of energy.

Several practical reasons have contributed to the large quantities of carbohydrates in diets all over the world. First, they are widely available; they are easily grown in plants such as grains, vegetables, and fruits. In some countries carbohydrate foods make up almost the entire diet of the people. In the American diet, about 50% of the total calories is in the form of carbohydrates. Second, they are relatively low in cost. As income lowers, the proportion of carbohydrate foods in the diet rises. This becomes a special concern with low-income families. Third, carbohydrates are practical because they may be stored easily. Compared with other types of foods, carbohydrate foods can be kept in dry storage for relatively long periods of time without spoilage. Modern processing and packaging have further extended the shelf life of carbohydrate products almost indefinitely.

The name *carbohydrate* comes from the chemical nature of this substance. It is composed of carbon, hydrogen, and oxygen. The hydrogen and oxygen occur in the same $2:1$ ratio as that found in water (2 hydrogen atoms to 1 oxygen atom: H_2O). Thus the name *carbohydrate* indicates its basic chemical composition.

CLASSIFICATION OF CARBOHYDRATES

The three major groups of carbohydrate foods are monosaccharides, disaccharides, and polysaccharides.

Monosaccharides. The simplest form of carbohydrate is the *monosaccharide*, often called *simple sugar*. Following are the three main monosaccharides important in human nutrition:

1. *Glucose.* A moderately sweet sugar, glucose is found naturally preformed in a few foods, but mainly it is created in the body from starch digestion. In human metabolism, all other types of sugar are converted by the body into glucose. It is the form in which sugar circulates in the bloodstream and is oxidized to give energy. It is found in some foods such as corn syrup.

2. *Fructose.* The sweetest of the simple sugars, fructose is found in fruits and honey. In human metabolism, it is converted to glucose for energy.

3. *Galactose.* The simple sugar galactose is not found free in foods but is produced in human digestion from lactose (milk sugar) and is then changed to glucose for energy. This reaction is reversible and, during lactation, glucose may be reconverted to galactose, since the lactose component in breast milk is produced from galactose.

Disaccharides. Disaccharides are double sugars made of two monosaccharides. The three main disaccharides with their two components are (1) sucrose = glucose + fructose; (2) lactose = glucose + galactose; and (3) maltose = glucose + glucose. In each of these disaccharides, glucose is one of the two components.

1. *Sucrose.* Sucrose is common table sugar. It is the most prevalent disaccharide in the diet, contributing about 25% of the total carbohydrate calories. It is found in many food sources, including cane and beet sugar, brown sugar, sorghum cane and molasses, maple syrup, pineapple, and carrot roots.

2. *Lactose.* Lactose is the sugar in milk. During lactation it is formed in the body from glucose to supply the carbohydrate component of milk. It is the least sweet of the disaccharides, about one sixth as sweet as sucrose. Thus it is often used in high-carbohydrate, high-calorie liquid feedings when the necessary quantity of sucrose would be too sweet to be tolerated. When milk sours, as in the initial stages of cheese making, the lactose is changed to lactic acid and separates in the liquid whey from the remaining solid curd. The curd is then processed for cheese. Therefore, although milk has a relatively high carbohydrate content (lactose), one of its main products—cheese—has none.

3. *Maltose.* Maltose occurs in malt products and in germinating cereals. As such, it is a negligible dietary carbohydrate. However, it is important as an intermediate product of starch digestion.

Polysaccharides. Polysaccharides are even more complex carbohydrates made up of many units of one monosaccharide. The most important polysaccharides in human nutrition include starch, dextrins, cellulose, pectins, and glycogen.

1. *Starch.* Starch is the most significant polysaccharide in human nutrition. It is a compound made up of glucose chains; hence it yields only glucose on digestion. Starch granules vary in size and shape according to the source. Potato granules, for example, are relatively large, whereas rice granules are small. Grinding or cooking helps make the starch available for use by breaking down the cell walls.

Starch is by far the most important source of carbohydrate and accounts for about 50% of the total carbohydrate intake in the American diet. In other countries where it is the staple food substance, it makes up an even higher proportion of the total diet. Major food sources include cereal grains, potatoes and other root vegetables, and legumes.

2. *Dextrins.* Dextrins are polysaccharide compounds that are intermediate products of starch breakdown and the formation of maltose during digestion. Dextri-Maltose, an infant formula preparation, is a combination of dextrins and maltose.

3. *Cellulose.* Cellulose is a polysaccharide that human beings cannot digest because they lack the necessary digestive enzymes. Therefore it remains in the digestive tract and contributes important bulk to the diet. This bulk helps move the digestive food mass along and stimulates peristalsis. (See p. 86.) Cellulose forms the supporting framework of plants. The main sources are stems and leaves of vegetables, seed and grain coverings, skins, and hulls.

4. *Pectins.* Pectins are also nondigestible polysaccharides. They are found mostly in fruits and possess a gel-like thickening quality. They are often used as a base for jellies. This ability to solidify to a gel also makes them useful in cosmetics and drugs.

5. *Glycogen.* Glycogen, often called *animal starch,* is formed in the body from glucose and is stored in relatively small amounts in the liver and muscle tissues.

FUNCTIONS OF CARBOHYDRATES

Energy. As previously discussed, the primary overall function of carbohydrate in human nutrition is to provide a main energy source. Although fat also is a fuel, it is primarily a storage form, and the body may function without it in the diet. However, the body tissues require a constant dietary supply of carbohydrates to exist. The amount of carbohydrate held in the body is relatively small. A total of approximately 365 gm. is stored in the liver and the muscle tissues and is present in circulating blood sugar. Following is the breakdown of carbohydrate storage in the body of a man weighing 70 kg:

Liver glycogen	110 gm.
Muscle glycogen	245 gm.
Extracellular blood sugar	10 gm.
Total	365 gm. (1,460 calories)

These 365 gm. of glucose provide energy sufficient for only about 13 hours of moderate activity. Therefore carbohydrates must be ingested regularly and at moderately frequent intervals to meet the energy demands of the body.

Protein-sparing action. Carbohydrate has a regulating influence on protein metabolism. The presence of sufficient carbohydrate for energy demands prevents using up too much of the protein supply for energy purposes. This *protein-sparing action* of carbohydrate allows a major portion of protein to be used for its basic structural purpose of building tissue.

Antiketogenic effect. The amount of carbohydrate present also determines how much fat will be broken down. Therefore it affects the formation and disposal rates of *ketones.* Ketones are intermediate products of fat metabolism, which normally are broken down to fatty acids. However, in extreme conditions such as starvation or uncontrolled diabetes in which carbohydrate is inadequate or unavailable, these ketones accumulate and produce a condition called *ketosis,* or *acidosis* (p. 22). Thus the *antiketogenic effect* of carbohydrates prevents a damaging excess of ketone formation and accumulation.

Special functions of carbohydrates in vital organs. The action of the heart is a life-sustaining muscular exercise. The glycogen stored in cardiac muscle is an important emergency source of energy. In a damaged heart, poor glycogen stores of a low-carbohydrate intake may cause cardiac symptoms or angina.

A constant amount of carbohydrate is necessary for proper functioning of the central nervous system. Its regulatory center, the brain, contains no stored supply of glucose. Therefore it is especially dependent on a minute-to-minute supply of glucose from the blood. Sustained and profound hypoglycemic shock may cause irreversible brain damage. In all nerve tissue, carbohydrate is indispensable for functional integrity.

CHANGING RAW FUEL TO USABLE REFINED FUEL

The form of refined fuel that the body must have for energy from carbohydrates is *glucose*. The process by which the body changes these raw fuel carbohydrate foods (starches and sugars) to glucose for use in the body is *digestion*. Digestion is accomplished by two basic actions: a mechanical one in which the food is chewed, broken up into smaller particles, swallowed, and moved along the gastrointestinal tract by various muscle actions and a chemical one in which enzymes and other helping substances are secreted by glands in the mouth, stomach, and intestines. Accessory organs next to the digestive system, the liver, pancreas, and gallbladder, produce and store additional enzymes and helping materials. These enzymes break the food particles down into simpler and simpler forms, until the final refined form of fuel that the body can use—glucose—is produced. In the following discussion these processes are traced through the successive parts of the gastrointestinal tract.

Mouth. Mastication, the chewing of food, breaks it into fine particles and mixes it with saliva. During this process, *ptyalin*, an enzyme of the saliva secreted by the parotid gland, acts on starch to begin its breakdown into dextrins and maltose. Usually, however, the food does not stay in the mouth long enough for much of this change to be completed, so that it is conveyed into the stomach still mostly in starch form.

Stomach. Mechanical digestion is continued in the stomach by successive wavelike contractions of the muscle fibers of the stomach wall. This action is called *peristalsis*, which further mixes food particles with gastric secretions to allow the chemical activity of digestion to take place more easily. The gastric juice contains no specific enzyme for the breakdown of carbohydrate. Hydrochloric acid in the stomach counteracts the alkaline activity of ptyalin. Mechanical digestion continues to bring the carbohydrate to the pyloric valve at the bottom of the stomach as part of the food mass, now a thick, creamy *chyme*. This food mass is then ready for emptying into the duodenum, the first portion of the small intestine.

Small intestine. Peristalsis continues to aid digestion in the small intestine by mixing and moving the food mass along the length of the tube. Chemical digestion of carbohydrate is completed in the small intestine by enzymes from two sources: (1) the *pancreatic juice*, which enters the duodenum through the common bile duct and contains an amylase called *amylopsin*, an enzyme that continues the breakdown of starch to maltose, and (2) the *intestinal juice*, which contains three disaccharidases—*sucrase, lactase,* and *maltase.* These three enzymes act on their respective disaccharides—sucrose, lactose, and maltose —to produce the monosaccharides glucose, galactose, and fructose. Now these simple sugars are ready for absorption. Interestingly enough, these disaccharidases are almost exclusively *intracellular,* that is, they are located and act mainly within the cells of the mucosa (the inner layer of the intestinal wall). Thus the main digestion of disaccharides takes place not in the lumen of the intestine as one would think but within the intestinal mucosal cells.

These processes of carbohydrate digestion

Table 2-1. Summary of carbohydrate digestion

ORGAN	ENZYME	ACTION
Mouth	Ptyalin	Starch → Dextrins → Maltose
Stomach	None	(Above action continued to minor degree)
Small intestine	Pancreatic amylopsin	Starch → Dextrins → Maltose
	Intestinal sucrase	Sucrose → Glucose + Fructose
	lactase	Lactose → Glucose + Galactose
	maltase	Maltose → Glucose + Glucose

by which the refined fuel form of glucose is produced are summarized in Table 2-1.

CARRYING REFINED FUEL TO "PRODUCTION SITES"—CELLS

The refined fuel glucose is now ready to be carried to the cells to produce energy. The process by which the body transports this basic end product of carbohydrate digestion to the cells in the body is called *absorption*.

Absorbing structures. The structure of the mucosal membrane of the small intestine greatly enhances the absorption process (see Fig. 8-4, p. 89). First, *mucosal folds* in the surface tissue (much like the folds in an accordion) enlarge the surface area. Second, millions of tiny fingerlike projections called *villi* are on the surface of these folds of the mucous membrane. These small projections further increase the surface area. Third, on the surface of each villus are still smaller projections, called *microvilli*. Together, these three structures provide a greatly increased absorbing surface, which allows 90% of the digested food material to be absorbed in the small intestine. Only water absorption remains to be accomplished in the large intestine.

Route of absorption. The simple sugars glucose, galactose, and fructose are absorbed through the intestinal wall and carried into the portal circulation by means of the blood capillaries in the villi. They are carried directly through the portal circulation to the liver. Here the fructose and galactose are

converted to glucose, which, in turn, is converted to glycogen for storage. The glycogen is reconverted to glucose as needed by the body. Stored liver glycogen is available for use as a quick energy source, especially in times of stress.

BURNING THE REFINED FUEL AT PRODUCTION SITES TO PRODUCE ENERGY
Cell metabolism

Cells are the functional units of life in the human body. In individual cells glucose is burned to produce energy through a series of chemical reactions involving specific cell enzymes. The final energy produced is then available to the cell to do its work. Extra glucose not immediately needed for energy may also be changed to fat and stored as a reserve supply of energy.

These processes by which energy is produced by the body are called *metabolism*. Metabolism may be defined as the sum of the physical and chemical processes in a living organism by which energy is made available for the functioning of the organism and by which protoplasm, the basic substance of cells and tissues, is produced, maintained, or broken down. A *metabolite* is a product of a specific metabolic process.

Hormones controlling glucose metabolism

A number of hormones directly and indirectly influence the metabolism of glucose and thereby regulate the blood sugar level according to the body's need. These hormones may be classified according to whether they lower or raise the blood sugar level. Hormones are specific chemical substances produced by endocrine glands in the body. They act as control agents to regulate and integrate the various metabolic processes of the body.

Hormone that lowers blood sugar level. *Insulin* is the only hormone that lowers the blood sugar level. This hormone is perhaps more widely known than all the others. It is produced by beta cells of the pancreas, which are specialized for this purpose. The beta cells form "islands" of endocrine tissue within the pancreatic tissue. They are called the *islets of Langerhans*, named for the scientist who discovered and studied them.

FUNCTION OF INSULIN. Insulin promotes the use of blood sugar and hence prevents it from reaching too high a level in the blood— a condition called *hyperglycemia*. It does this in three ways:

1. By converting glucose to glycogen in the liver, where the glycogen is then stored
2. By converting glucose to fat for storage in adipose tissue
3. By increasing cell wall permeability to glucose—this process allows glucose to pass from the fluids outside the cell through the cell wall into the cell to be burned to supply needed energy

Hormones that raise blood sugar level. A number of hormones effectively raise the blood sugar level:

1. *Glucagon* is also produced by the islets of Langerhans in the pancreas. However, it is produced by neighboring cells called *alpha cells* and has an opposite effect to that of insulin. Glucagon raises the blood sugar level by increasing the breakdown of stored liver glycogen and its conversion to glucose.

2. *Steroid hormones* of the adrenal cortex raise the blood sugar level by stimulating the breakdown of protein to release glucose-forming units. The steroids also act as insulin antagonists and block the sugar-lowering effect of insulin.

3. *Epinephrine*, which is secreted by the adrenal medulla, also raises the blood sugar level by stimulating the breakdown of liver glycogen to produce glucose. Epinephrine is sometimes administered to diabetic patients in insulin shock to counteract the severe hypoglycemia. Epinephrine causes a quick release of readily available glucose from the stored glycogen for immediate use.

4. *Growth hormone (GH) and adrenocorticotrophic hormone (ACTH)* are hormones secreted by the anterior pituitary gland. They raise the blood sugar level by acting as insulin antagonists.

5. *Thyroxin* is the principal hormone secreted by the thyroid gland. It raises blood sugar because it influences the rate of insulin destruction and that of glucose absorption from the intestine and liberates epinephrine.

Energy production from glucose

Once in the cell, glucose must undergo a series of chemical reactions to produce energy for the body's various demands. This energy is produced through three basic stages:

STAGE I. *Production of a common molecule.* Through the action of a series of enzymes in the cytoplasm of the cell, the glucose is successively broken down to a small common molecule, a 2-carbon fragment of the original 6-carbon glucose. This common molecule is called *active acetate*. It is the final basic fuel that the cell burns for energy.

STAGE II. *Common energy cycle.* The 2-carbon fragment moves into the small organelle in the cell where energy is finally produced. This intracellular structure, the *mitochondrion*, is frequently called the "powerhouse" of the cell. Here, through another series of enzymatic activities, the 2-carbon fragment is converted into energy compounds. This series of reactions is commonly called the *Krebs cycle*.

STAGE III. *Production of a chemical compound for binding and storing energy.* An additional series of enzymes in the mitochondria provides a means of trapping the energy produced and storing it in a special chemical compound ready to be broken down and released for energy as needed. This special energy compound, unique for binding energy, is ATP (adenosine triphosphate).

SIGNIFICANCE OF CARBOHYDRATE METABOLISM

What is the significance of this overall picture of carbohydrate metabolism for students in nutrition, nursing, dentistry, and other allied health care fields? At least two basic concepts can be gained from this general background knowledge: (1) the close interrelatedness of nutrients and (2) the relation of the separate chemical reactions of the body to the total process of metabolism. An intimate metabolic relationship exists between the basic nutrients and their metabolites. No one substance exists or operates alone during metabolism; rather there is a tremendously significant interdependence among them all.

All nutrients do their best work in partnership with other nutrients. From this fact two practical conclusions may be drawn:

1. The emphasis in health teaching and nutrition education should be on achieving a sound balanced nutritional basis for any dietary program.

2. Some deficiency states may be *iatrogenic*, that is, induced by medical treatment, they may have their origin in a fad, or they may be caused by long-term, overzealous emphasis on one particular nutrient to the exclusion of other equally essential ones.

As a serious student, you will translate this general background information clearly and in simple terms to individual partients. Because you understand the relationship of the part to the whole, you will be able to help patients understand their basic health needs and to accept and follow through with whatever treatment is indicated in specific situations.

CHAPTER 3 FATS: THE PROBLEM OF ENERGY

To further solve its energy problem, the body turns to fat in addition to carbohydrate as another major fuel source. Fat is a valuable fuel because it is a highly concentrated source of energy, having about twice the energy value of carbohydrate. Also fat has an almost unlimited storage capacity in the body as adipose fat tissue.

FATS AS RAW FUEL

Fats are substances such as fat, oil, waxes, and related compounds that are greasy to the touch and insoluble in water. Substances of this class are called *lipids*. Some raw fuel food forms of fat are easily seen as fat and are called *visible fats*. These include butter, margarine, oil, salad dressings, bacon, and cream. Other food forms of fat are more hidden and less visible. These include egg yolk, meat fats, olives, avocados, and nuts. For example, even when all the visible fat has been removed from meat, an average of 6% of the fat surrounding the muscle fibers will still remain.

Margarine and shortenings are made from relatively less expensive vegetable oils such as cottonseed, soybean, corn, or coconut oil. They are produced by the introduction of hydrogen into the fat molecule under carefully controlled conditions. Margarine is then further processed by churning with cultured milk to give the flavor of butter. It is usually also fortified with vitamin A—15,000 units per pound (p. 44)—and vitamin D. Nutritionally,

fortified margarine is the equivalent of butter and has the same caloric value.

Americans eat a relatively large amount of fat, about 40% of the total calories in their diet. This means that the average American eats approximately 100 pounds of fat a year. This is somewhat excessive, since about 25% of that total is sufficient for need. The Food and Nutrition Board of the National Research Council reports that an adequate intake of fat is about 25% of the total calories, with 1% to 2% as the essential fatty acid, linoleic acid. However, agreement on the required level of fat is limited, and the human body appears to be able to function on a relatively wide range of fat intake.

Like carbohydrate, fat is composed of the basic structural elements of carbon, hydrogen, and oxygen. However, in fat the relative hydrogen content is higher. Fat is therefore a much more concentrated form of fuel. It provides more than twice the number of calories as the same amount of carbohydrate would. However, fat has to go through more changes to produce energy, so that it is not such a quick form of energy as carbohydrate. It is therefore considered more as a storage form of energy to be utilized as needed by the body.

CLASSIFICATION OF FATS (LIPIDS)

Fats may be divided into three main groups: simple, compound, and derived lipids.

Simple lipids. The simple lipids are called

neutral fats. The chemical name for these basic fats is *triglycerides.* This name indicates their chemical structure: a glycerol base with three fatty acids attached.

Compound lipids. Compound lipids are various combinations of fat with other components. Three types of compound lipids are important in human nutrition: phospholipids, glycolipids, and lipoproteins. Of these, the health worker should be most aware of *lipoproteins.* This type of compound, fat combined with protein, provides the main transport form of fat substances in the bloodstream. These plasma lipoproteins contain cholesterol, neutral fat or triglycerides, and fatty acids. Fats always must travel in the blood bound with protein in varying ratios because fat alone is insoluble in water, the base of blood. The lipoprotein compound again illustrates the intimate interrelationships in the body among the various nutrients. Recently the lipoproteins associated with atherosclerosis (heart disease) have been typed for better identification. Types II and IV (p. 251) are the most commonly encountered types of lipid disorders, associated with elevated blood levels of liproproteins and triglycerides.

Derived lipids. Derived lipids are fat substances produced from fats and fat compounds during digestive breakdown. Three important members of this group are glycerol, steroids, and fatty acids.

GLYCEROL. Glycerol is the water-soluble base of triglycerides, or neutral fats. It forms about 10% of the fat. After it is broken off in digestion, it is available for the formation of glucose in the diet.

STEROIDS. Steroids are a class of fat-related substances that contain sterols. A main member of this group is *cholesterol,* a complex fat-related compound found in practically all body tissues, especially in brain and nerve tissues, bile, blood, and the liver, where most of the cholesterol is synthesized. Cholesterol is synthesized within the body independently of the dietary intake. It has been estimated that the human body normally synthesizes about 2 gm. of cholesterol daily.

Although cholesterol may be synthesized in the liver, as well as in the intestinal wall, alteration of dietary cholesterol *does* seem to affect serum cholesterol more than was previously thought. Radioactive-tagged cholesterol in the diet has been recovered in large quantities from the atheromatous plaques in blood vessel walls in atherosclerosis. Hence treatment for elevated blood cholesterol or elevated blood lipids and atherosclerosis may include a therapeutic restriction of cholesterol-rich foods (see Appendix B). These foods include egg yolk, organ meats, shellfish, and dairy fat. The blood level of cholesterol is normally maintained at about 150 to 300 mg./ 100 ml of blood. Cholesterol is a vital substance in the body. It is a component of the bile salts and also a precursor of vitamin D. On exposure to sunlight, cholesterol in the skin is converted to *7-dehydrocholesterol,* one of the main D vitamins in the body. Cholesterol is also closely associated chemically with the sex and adrenal hormones.

FATTY ACIDS. The fatty acids are the key refined fuel forms of fat that the cell burns for energy; thus it is important to focus attention on them. They are the basic structural units of fat and may be saturated or unsaturated in nature.

Saturated and unsaturated fatty acids. The state of saturation or unsaturation of fatty acids is an important chemical characteristic. This state results from the ratio of hydrogen atoms to carbon atoms in the basic carbon chain that forms the individual fatty acid. If a given fatty acid is filled with as much hydrogen as it can take, the fatty acid is said to be completely *saturated* with hydrogen. Food fats composed mainly of such saturated fatty acids are called *saturated fats.* These fats are mostly of animal origin.

However, if the fatty acid has fewer hydrogen atoms, it is obviously less saturated. If it has only one place where there are fewer hydrogen atoms, the fatty acid is called a *monounsaturated* fatty acid. If two or more places along the carbon chain of the fatty acid have less hydrogen attached, with a resulting double bond between the carbon atoms involved, it is called a *polyunsaturated* fatty acid. Food fats composed mainly of unsaturated fatty acids are usually from plant sources.

Food fats. From the preceding facts, the concept of degrees of saturation and unsaturation of fatty acids in food fats can be derived. The general saturated-unsaturated spectrum of food fats is shown below. One would expect the more saturated food fats to be the more solid hard ones. Usually this is the case. The saturated food fats are animal fats, and the fat toward the center of the spectrum is softer in texture. The fats on the unsaturated end of the spectrum, of plant origin, are usually free-flowing oils that do not solidify even at low temperatures. This classification is helpful in explaining to patients on modified fat diets the correct choices of food fats.

Essential fatty acids. The term *essential* or *nonessential* when applied to fatty acids refers to their necessity in the diet because the body does not produce them. *Linoleic acid* in particular meets this criterion, and has several important functions in the body:

1. Strengthening capillary and cell membrane structure
2. Combining with cholesterol to help transport it in the blood
3. Helping to lower serum cholesterol, probably as a result of its role in transporting cholesterol
4. Prolonging blood-clotting time.

Chain lengths of fatty acids. Another characteristic of fatty acids that is important in their absorption is the length of the carbon chain composing their structure. They are constructed of chains of carbon atoms filled with hydrogen and some oxygen. These chains may vary in length from short chains of 4-carbon atoms upward to medium-chain lengths of 10- to 12-carbon atoms and on to long-chain fatty acids, composed of as many as 24-carbon atoms. The long-chain fatty acids are more difficult to absorb and require a helping carrier. The medium- and short-chain fatty acids are more soluble in water and hence can be absorbed more easily directly into the bloodstream. Therefore in malabsorptive diseases of the intestine when the absorbing surface is inflamed or infected, the short- or medium-chain fat products may be the indicated form to use. A commercial product called MCT (medium-chain triglycerides) has been produced; it is an oil made up of medium- and short-chain fatty acids that can be used in the diet in the same fashion as any ordinary vegetable oil.

FUNCTION OF FATS

In addition to its basic function as a primary source of energy, fat also serves a structural function. It generally provides padding for vital organs and nerves, holding them in place and helping to absorb shocks. Further protection for the entire body is provided by the subcutaneous layer of fat. This not only protects the body but also insulates it against rapid temperature changes or excessive heat loss; hence it is an important aid in maintaining body temperature. In colder climates and seasons, therefore, fat generally assumes

								Vegetable oils peanut soybean	
Beef suet	Mutton tallow	Red meats	Poultry	Seafood	Egg yolk	Dairy fat	Olives, olive oil	cottonseed corn safflower
		SATURATED						UNSATURATED	
		Animal fat						Plant fat	

a greater role in the diet to supply needed body heat.

CHANGING RAW FUEL TO USABLE REFINED FUEL

The raw fuel, various animal and plant fats (triglycerides) naturally occurring in foods, is taken into the body with the diet. Then the task is to change these raw fuel fats into a refined fuel form of fat that the cells can burn for energy. These key refined fuel forms are the fatty acids. The body accomplishes this task through the process of fat digestion.

Mouth. No fat digestion takes place in the mouth. In this first portion of the gastrointestinal tract, fat is simply broken up into smaller particles through chewing and moistened for passage into the stomach with the general food mass.

Stomach. Little if any fat digestion takes place in the stomach. General peristalsis continues the mechanical mixing of fats with the stomach contents. A small amount of the gastric lipase *tributyrinase* begins the chemical breakdown of the *tributyrin* in butterfat. However, as the other gastric enzymes act on their specific nutrients in the food mix, fat is separated out and made more readily accessible to its own chemical breakdown, which follows in the small intestine.

Small intestine. Not until fat reaches the small intestine do the chemical changes nec-essary for fat digestion take place. Agents from two major sources accomplish this task.

BILE SALTS FROM THE LIVER AND GALL-BLADDER. The presence of fat in the duodenum (first section of the small intestine) stimulates the gallbladder to release bile, which has been produced in the liver. The gallbladder serves to concentrate and store bile until it is needed to help digest fat. Bile accomplishes two tasks: (1) it emulsifies the fat by breaking it into small particles or globules, thus greatly enlarging the surface area available for action of the enzymes, and (2) it lowers the surface tension of the finely dispersed fat globules, thus allowing the enzymes to penetrate more easily. This is similar to the wetting action of detergents.

LIPASE FROM THE PANCREAS. The pancreatic juice contains a powerful enzyme for digesting fat. This *pancreatic lipase* is called *steapsin*. In a gradual stepwise fashion this pancreatic lipase breaks off one fatty acid at a time from the glycerol base of the neutral fats (triglycerides). Each succeeding step of this breakdown is accomplished with increasing difficulty. In fact, only a relatively small amount, less than one third of the total fat present, actually reaches complete breakdown. Thus the final products of fat digestion are some fatty acids, some glycerol, and the still-remaining diglycerides and monoglycerides: these are the products that remain to be

Table 3-1. Summary of fat digestion

ORGAN	ENZYME	ACTIVITY
Mouth	None	Mechanical, mastication
Stomach	No major enzyme	Mechanical separation of fats as protein and starch digested out
	Small amount of gastric lipase tributyrinase	Tributyrin (butter fat) to fatty acids and glycerol
Small intestine	Gallbladder bile salts (emulsifier)	Emulsifies fats
	Pancreatic lipase (steapsin)	Triglycerides to diglycerides and monoglycerides in turn, then fatty acids and glycerol

absorbed. Some remaining fat may be carried on into the large intestine and eliminated as fecal fat. A summary of fat digestion is given in Table 3-1.

CARRYING REFINED FUEL TO PRODUCTION SITES—CELLS

In the small intestine the products of fat digestion thus far must be absorbed. These products are glycerol and fatty acids, along with fats not completely broken down (glycerides) and some cholesterol. All these must be absorbed into the intestinal wall; however, this is not an easy task. The problem is that fats are not soluble in water and the blood is basically water; hence fat always requires some type of solvent carrier. To accomplish this task of transporting fat from the intestine into the bloodstream, the body has three basic stages of operation:

STAGE I. *Initial absorption.* Bile combines with products of fat digestion in a bile-fat complex and carries the fat into the intestinal wall.

STAGE II. *Absorption in mucosal cells of intestinal wall.* Inside the intestinal wall, bile separates again from the fat complex and is returned to circulation to accomplish its tasks over and over again. Two important operations are accomplished on the fat products inside the intestinal wall:
1. The digestion of the remaining glycerides is completed with the help of another enzyme, an *enteric lipase.*
2. With the resulting fatty acids and glycerol, new triglycerides are re-formed for use by the body as fat.

STAGE III. *Final absorption.* These newly formed human fats—triglycerides—and other fat materials present are combined with a small amount of protein as a carrier (albumin) to form lipoproteins. These lipoproteins formed from dietary fat are called *chylomicrons.* Thus protein at this point is the significant carrier for fat. These lipoproteins are absorbed first into the lymphatic system and then eventually into the portal blood. Through this system the fats are carried first to the liver for conversion to other lipoprotein transport forms and then to the tissue cells to be burned for energy.

Thus these important transport forms of fat in the blood, the lipoproteins, are produced in two places—the intestinal wall immediately after fat digestion and the liver during continued fat metabolism.

BURNING REFINED FUEL AT PRODUCTION SITES TO PRODUCE ENERGY

In the cells, fatty acids are used as concentrated fuel to produce energy. These derived units of fat have about twice the energy value of glucose products; therefore fat has a little more than twice the calorie value of carbohydrate.

Stages of fat metabolism

The production of energy from fat follows the same general pattern as that of carbohydrate:

STAGE I. *Production of a common molecule.* The fatty acids are gradually broken down into the same common molecule as glucose: the small 2-carbon fragment called active acetate.

STAGE II. *Common energy cycle.* As with glucose, this small fragment enters the mitochondria and is burned for energy through a series of special enzyme changes. This action takes place in the Krebs cycle.

STAGE III. *Binding and storing energy.* ATP (adenosine triphosphate) is the chemical compound in which the energy formed is trapped and stored ready for use as needed.

Balance of fat and carbohydrate metabolism

Thus fatty acids are burned (oxidized) in balance with glucose. When there is sufficient glucose to keep refueling the Krebs cycle to run it properly, the fatty acid fragments can be oxidized normally. When there is insufficient glucose entering the system to keep the Krebs cycle going, these products of fat metabolism cannot be burned properly, and intermediate products called ketones are formed. When this occurs, a state of ketosis, or acidosis, is caused. Such a situation would occur in uncontrolled diabetes or with the use of fad reducing diets that contain little or no carbohydrate to keep refueling the Krebs cycle from glucose. The excess fatty acids not used for energy are reconverted to tissue fat and stored as adipose fat tissue for use as needed.

Hormones controlling fat metabolism

Since fat and carbohydrate metabolism are so closely interrelated, the same hormones that affect carbohydrate metabolism also affect fat metabolism.

1. *Growth hormone (GH), adrenocorticotrophic hormone (ACTH),* and *thyroid-stimulating hormone (TSH),* which are all secreted by the pituitary gland, increase the release of free fatty acids from adipose tissue by imposing energy demands on the body.

2. *Cortisone* and *hydrocortisone,* which are secreted by the adrenal gland, cause the release of free fatty acids. Epinephrine stimulates the breakdown of stored triglycerides.

3. The important fat-forming (lipogenetic) activity of *insulin,* which is secreted by the pancreas, has been described (p. 15). *Glucagon,* also secreted by the pancreas, has an opposite effect by increasing the release of free fatty acids from adipose tissue.

4. *Thyroxine,* which is secreted by the thyroid gland, affects fat metabolism by stimulating adipose tissue release of free fatty acids. It also lowers blood cholesterol.

Effect of body temperature on fat metabolism

Lowering of body temperature stimulates the release of fatty acids, which then supply fuel to return the body temperature to normal.

CHAPTER 4 ENERGY REQUIREMENTS

Energy is a primary necessity for ongoing life. In human nutrition carbohydrates and fats provide the major fuel supply for power in the human energy system. *Energy metabolism* deals with the real and dynamic fact underlying all life—*change*. These constant, multiple changes in the forms of the body's physiologic constituents—its nutrients and their metabolites—produce energy for the body's work.

Several additional interrelated concepts are involved in the study of energy metabolism. These deal with such basic questions as (1) How is energy measured? (2) How does the human body get its different forms of energy? (3) How is energy controlled in the human system? and (4) How are basal and total energy requirements determined?

MEASUREMENT OF ENERGY
Calories

Since the body can perform work only as energy is released and since all work takes the form of heat production, energy may be measured in terms of heat equivalents. Such a heat measure is the *calorie*. A kilocalorie (1,000 small calories) is the amount of heat required to raise one kilogram of water 1° C.

The calorie values of various foods have been determined by the use of instruments called *calorimeters*. These various food values may be found in Appendix A. The average calorie value of each of the three major nutrients is known as its respective *fuel factor*.

One gram of carbohydrate yields 4 calories, 1 gm. of fat yields 9 calories, and 1 gm. of protein yields 4 calories.

Joules

In the metric system of measure the unit of energy is the *joule*. It has been formally added to the national system of weights and measures and adopted by the United States. Nine tenths of the world already uses the metric system or is in the process of conversion.

The joule was named for James Prescott Joule (1818-1889). Joule was an English physicist who discovered the first law of thermodynamics and invented an electromagnetic engine. J. is the abbreviation used to indicate this measure. The conversion factor for changing calories (kilocalories) to joules (kilojoules) is 4.184. Thus one calorie equals 4.184 joules. For example, 55 calories would equal 230 joules. The fuel factors expressed in joules would be carbohydrates, 17 joules per gram; protein, 17 joules per gram; and fat, 38 joules per gram. The comparative fuel values of energy-producing foods as measured in calories and in joules are given in Table 4-1 for study purposes.

HUMAN ENERGY SYSTEM
Energy cycle and transformation

It is clear that energy is not created. When energy is spoken of as being produced, what is really meant is that it is being transformed. It is being changed in form and cycled

Table 4-1. Recommended daily calorie and joule allowances*

	AGE (YR.)	WEIGHT (LB.)	HEIGHT (IN.)	CALORIES	JOULES
Men	19 to 22	147 (67 kg.)	69 (172 cm.)	3,000	12,552
	23 to 50	154 (70 kg.)	69 (172 cm.)	2,700	11,297
	51+	154 (70 kg.)	69 (172 cm.)	2,400	10,042
Women	19 to 22	128 (58 kg.)	65 (162 cm.)	2,100	8,786
	23 to 50	128 (58 kg.)	65 (162 cm.)	2,000	8,368
	51+	128 (58 kg.)	65 (162 cm.)	1,800	7,531
	Pregnant			(+300)	(+1,255)
	Lactating			(+500)	(+2,092)
Infants	0 to ½	14 (6 kg.)	24 (60 cm.)	kg. × 117	kg. × 490
	½ to 1	20 (9 kg.)	28 (71 cm.)	kg. × 108	kg. × 452
Children	1 to 3	28 (13 kg.)	34 (86 cm.)	1,300	5,439
	4 to 6	44 (20 kg.)	44 (110 cm.)	1,800	7,531
	7 to 10	66 (30 kg.)	54 (135 cm.)	2,400	10,042
Boys	11 to 14	97 (44 kg.)	63 (158 cm.)	2,800	11,715
	15 to 18	134 (61 kg.)	69 (172 cm.)	3,000	12,552
Girls	11 to 14	97 (44 kg.)	62 (155 cm.)	2,400	10,042
	15 to 18	119 (54 kg.)	65 (162 cm.)	2,100	8,786

*From Food and Nutrition Board: Recommended dietary allowances, ed. 8, Washington, D. C., 1974, National Academy of Science, National Research Council.

throughout a system. In the human body the various metabolic processes convert chemical energy to other forms of energy for the body's work.

This chemical energy enters the system as stored potential energy in food. The ultimate source of power is the sun, with its vast reservoir of nuclear reactions. Then through the process of photosynthesis, using water and carbon dioxide as raw materials, plants transform the sun's energy into food storage forms. In the body these food sources are converted to the basic energy unit, glucose, which together with fatty acids is burned to release energy. Water and carbon dioxide are the end products of this process of oxidation.

After the food energy is taken into the body, it is converted in the process of metabolism to chemical energy in other products to do the body's work. This chemical energy is then changed to other forms of energy as this work is performed. For example, chemical energy is changed to *electrical energy* in brain and nerve activity. It is changed to *mechanical energy* in muscle contraction. It is changed to *thermal energy* in regulation of body temperature. It is changed to other types of *chemical energy* as in the synthesis of new compounds. In all these work activities of the body, heat is given off. This transformation of energy and its cycling through the body may be visualized in Fig. 4-1.

Energy control

In the human body the energy produced in its many chemical reactions, if "exploded" all at once, would be destructive. There must be some mechanism, therefore, by which energy is controlled in the human system so that it may support life and not destroy it. Several basic means of control are used by the body.

Chemical bonding. The main mechanism by which energy is controlled in the human system is *chemical bonding*. The chemical bonds that hold the elements of the compounds together consist of energy. As long as that compound remains constant, energy is being exerted to maintain it. It is in this sense that *potential energy* is stored in any chemical compound, such as in the sucrose or sugar consumed in food. When this com-

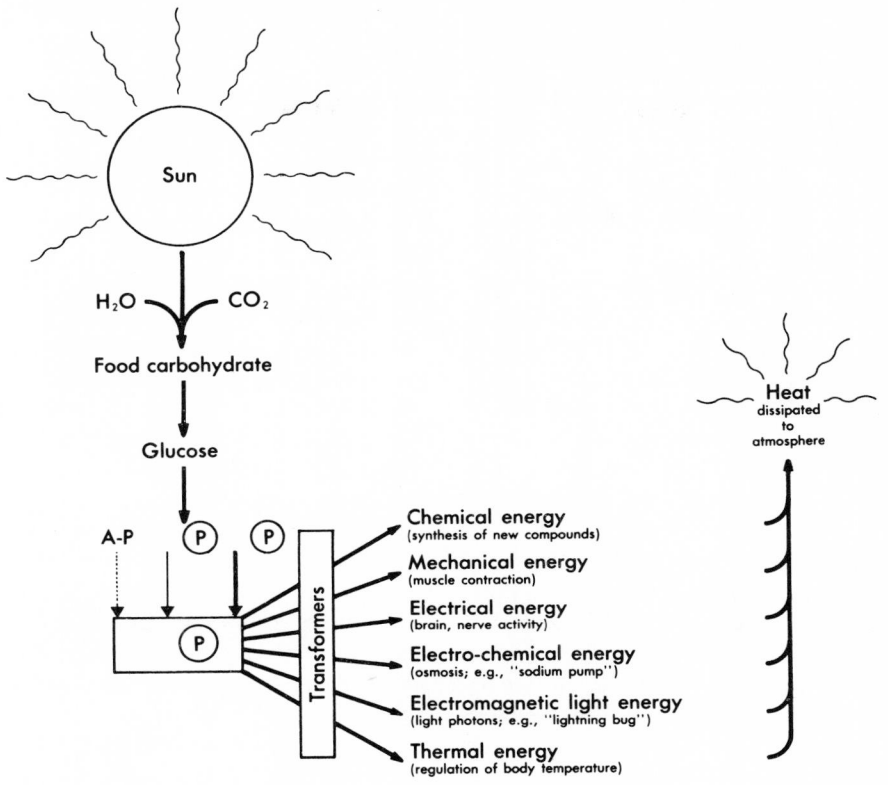

Fig. 4-1. Transformation of energy from its primary source (the sun) to various forms for biologic work by means of metabolic processes ("transformers").

pound is taken into the body and broken into its parts, energy is released and it becomes *free energy.*

There are three basic types of chemical bonds by which energy is transferred in the body. First are *covalent bonds* such as those that hold carbon atoms together in the core of an organic compound. Second are *hydrogen bonds*—weaker bonds that attach hydrogen to various compounds. But the very fact that they are less strong and can be broken easily makes them important in that they may be transferred or passed readily from one substance to another to help form still another substance. The third type of chemical bond is the strong *high-energy phosphate bond,* the main example of which is *adenosine triphosphate,* commonly called ATP. This is the

unique compound the human body uses to store energy for its cell work.

Controlled reaction rates. The many chemical reactions that make up the body's energy system must have controls. Some of the chemical reactions that break down proteins, for example, if left to themselves (as in sterile decomposition), would span several years. Therefore such reactions must be accelerated, or else it might take years to get the needed energy from a meal. At the same time they must be regulated so that too fast a reaction will not produce energy in a single explosion. The agents that control these reaction rates are enzymes, coenzymes, and hormones.

ENZYMES. There are many specific enzymes in every cell that control specific reactions in the cell. All enzymes that have been isolated thus far are protein substances. They are produced in the cells themselves, apparently under control of specific genes. One specific gene is believed to control the making of one specific enzyme, and there are thousands of enzymes in each cell. Each enzyme works on a particular substance, which is called its *substrate*. The enzyme and the substrate lock together to produce a new reaction product, and the original enzyme remains unchanged, ready to do its work over and over again. (See Fig. 4-2.)

COENZYMES. Many reactions require a partner to assist the enzyme in completing the reaction. These coenzymes in many instances involve several of the vitamins, especially the B vitamins, and some of the minerals.

HORMONES. The word "hormone" comes from a Greek word meaning "set in motion" or "to spur on." Hormones are secretions of the endocrine glands. They perform many regulatory functions in the body. In energy metabolism they act as chemical messengers to trigger or control enzymatic action. For example, the rate of oxidative reactions in the tissues (the body's basal metabolic rate) is controlled by thyroxine from the thyroid gland, which in turn is controlled by thyrotrophic hormone (TSH) from the anterior pituitary gland. Another familiar example is the controlling action of insulin from the pancreas on the rate of glucose use in the tissues.

Steroid hormones also have a capacity to regulate the cells' ability to synthesize enzymes.

Types of metabolic reaction. The two types of reaction constantly going on in energy metabolism are anabolism and catabolism. Each requires energy. *Anabolism* is the synthesis of a more complex substance. Energy is required to generate this synthesis. *Catabolism* is the breakdown of a more complex substance to simpler substances. This process releases free energy but also uses up some free energy for the breakdown. Therefore there is a constant energy deficit, which must be supplied by food. When food is not available, as in periods of fasting or starvation, the body draws for energy on its own stores.

1. *Glycogen.* Only a 12- to 48-hour reserve of glycogen exists in liver and muscle. This amount is quickly depleted.

2. *Protein.* Storage of energy as protein exists in limited amounts in the muscle mass but in greater volume than the glycogen stores.

3. *Fat.* The capacity for storage of energy in the adipose tissue is virtually unlimited. This stored fat provides needed energy, but the supply varies from person to person and from circumstance to circumstance.

ENERGY REQUIREMENTS

Individual energy needs are based on requirements to maintain the body's internal

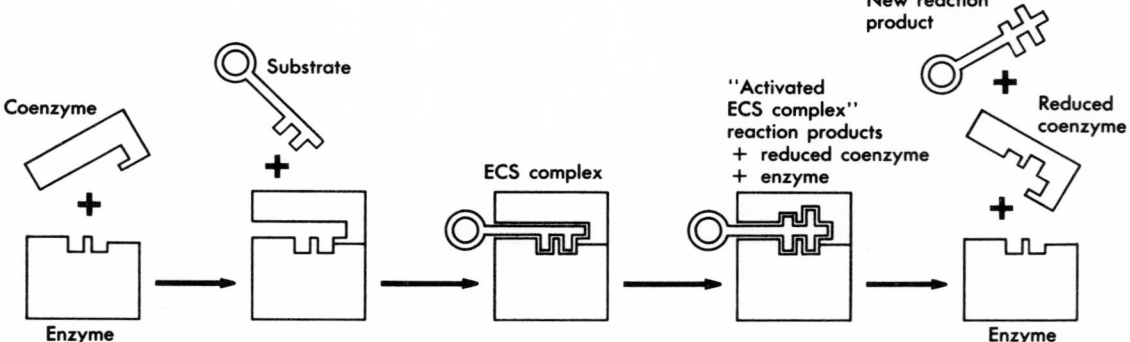

Fig. 4-2. Lock and key concept of the action of enzyme, coenzyme, and substrate to produce a new reaction product.

work. This is called a measure of *basal metabolism energy needs*. In addition to these needs, physical activities would be added to determine *total energy requirements*.

Basal energy metabolism requirements

Basal metabolism is a measure of the energy required to maintain the body in a state of rest. It measures the internal chemical activity of all the body work to maintain life. This involves all the involuntary activities of breathing, circulation, digestion, absorption, and other tissue activities.

Basal metabolic rate. The rate at which this energy is required is called the *basal metabolic rate*, or the BMR. It is interesting to compare the contribution of various body tissues to the rate of basal metabolism. Certain small but active tissues, such as the brain, liver, gastrointestinal tract, heart, and kidney, together make up less than 5% of the total body weight, yet they contribute about 60% of the total basal metabolic processes. Although resting muscle and adipose fat tissue are far larger in mass, they contribute much less to the body's BMR.

Methods of measuring BMR. Various methods are used for measuring the BMR. Formerly indirect measures were used that indicated the amount of oxygen consumed as a means of measuring the energy requirement. Today the new methods employ measurements of glandular activity such as that of the thyroid gland. The iodine uptake test is an example (p. 77). Whatever the form of the test, certain conditions are necessary for its accuracy. The patient must have had nothing to eat for the previous 12 hours, so that no digestive or absorptive activities are going on. He must be in a relaxed state in a quiet atmosphere, with at least 30 minutes of bed rest preceding the test. He should be lying down and fully awake, and the room temperature should be moderate.

Factors influencing BMR. Certain factors or states of health influence the BMR and should be considered when interpreting results of tests. The following situations usually increase the BMR:

1. During childhood the BMR slowly rises, levels off at about age 5, and then rises again just before puberty, after which it declines into old age.

2. Relative *sex* differences in body mass usually give a higher BMR to men than to women.

3. The BMR rises 20% to 25% during *pregnancy* because of the accelerated tissue growth process.

4. *Lactation* increases the BMR some 60%, or 1,000 calories.

5. *Fever* increases the BMR about 7% for each 1° F. rise in temperature.

6. *Colder climates* usually increase the BMR as more body heat has to be produced.

7. *Certain diseases* that involve increased cellular activity usually increase the BMR.

8. *Thyroid hormones* stimulate the BMR. Thus the principal use of BMR testing in clinical practice is in the diagnosis of thyroid disease.

Table 4-2. General approximations for daily adult basal and activity energy needs

		MAN (70 KG.) CALORIES	WOMAN (58 KG.) CALORIES
Basal energy needs (av. 1 cal./kg./hr.)		$70 \times 24 = 1,680$	$58 \times 24 = 1,392$
Activity energy needs			
Very sedentary	+20% basal	$1,680 + 336 = 2,016$	$1,392 + 278 = 1,670$
Sedentary	+30% basal	$1,680 + 504 = 2,184$	$1,392 + 418 = 1,810$
Moderately active	+40% basal	$1,680 + 672 = 2,352$	$1,392 + 557 = 1,949$
Very active	+50% basal	$1,680 + 840 = 2,520$	$1,392 + 696 = 2,088$

In *starvation* and *malnutrition* the BMR is usually lowered.

For a simple means of calculating the calories required for basal energy needs, compare the figures given in Table 4-2. This indicates that basal energy requirements average about one calorie per kilogram of body weight per hour. (One kilogram equals 2.2 pounds.)

Total energy metabolism requirements

In addition to basal energy requirements, the amount of physical activity would be added to determine one's total energy needs.

Muscular work. Exercise of any kind is the main additional factor that accounts for individual calorie requirements. Table 4-3 gives a comparison of the energy expenditure of a man and woman of average weight during some representative types of activities.

Mental effort. Mental effort such as studying demands few if any calories. Feelings of fatigue after periods of study are not the result of mental activity as such but various amounts of muscle tension involved.

Emotional state. Calories are used up during heightened emotional states because metabolic activity rises as muscle tension, restlessness, and agitated movements increase.

Table 4-3. Energy expenditure per hour during different activities for a man weighing 70 kg. and a woman weighing 60 kg.

ACTIVITY	CALORIES PER HOUR	
	MAN	WOMAN
Sleeping	65	56
Sitting at rest	100	85
Standing relaxed	105	90
Light exercise	170	143
Active exercise	290	244
Walking moderately fast	300	254
Walking upstairs	1,110	935

Diet. Food intake increases the expenditure of calories for digestion and absorption activities. Protein especially has a high specific dynamic action.

Thus the total daily energy requirement of an individual is the number of calories necessary to replace daily basal metabolic loss, plus loss from exercise and other activities. A person's weight is a general indicator of his state of energy balance between his energy requirement and the energy potential he takes in in the form of food.

CHAPTER **5** # PROTEINS: THE PROBLEM OF BUILDING TISSUE

As you have discovered thus far in your study of nutrition, the first major problem of the body, securing a fuel source and converting it into a system to supply energy, is solved by using carbohydrates and fats for this purpose. These nutrients provide the fuel, and the body provides a balanced system of chemical changes to get energy from them.

The second major problem the body must solve to survive and maintain health is that of *building tissue*. Any successful construction system requires four basic components:

1. Raw building materials
2. A means of changing the raw building materials to finished, ready-to-use building units
3. A means of carrying the finished building units to the construction site
4. A plan ("blueprint") and process for building and maintaining the specifically designed structures at the construction site

Body growth and maintenance requires constant building and rebuilding of body tissues. Healthy tissue is necessary for strength, vigor, and body functioning. The building material in food that enables us to accomplish this task is *protein*. The necessary components of a construction system listed above can be applied to the body's use of protein for this task.

GENERAL DEFINITIONS

The word "protein" comes from a Greek word meaning "primary" or "holding first place." A Dutch chemist first proposed the name in 1840 before much was known about this substance. However, he named it well. Proteins make up the basic structure of all living cells and are an essential life-forming and life-sustaining ingredient of the diet of all animal organisms. The amount of protein in the diets of different cultures varies. In countries with adequate nutrition it contributes from 10% to 15% of the total calories. In the average American diet, protein contributes approximately 14% of the total calories.

Proteins may be defined as organic substances that on digestion yield their constituent unit building blocks—*amino acids*. Proteins are found in animal foods such as meat, milk, cheese, and eggs. To a lesser extent proteins occur in plant foods such as grains and legumes. Entirely free protein, such as albumin in egg white, is rare in nature. Usually protein is found in connection with fats and carbohydrates. For example, in the animal food sources protein is usually associated with fat (meat, milk, cheese, egg yolk). In the plant food sources protein is usually associated with carbohydrate (grains, legumes).

Proteins may be further defined according

to their basic elements. Like carbohydrate and fat, protein contains carbon, hydrogen, and oxygen. But protein is unique in that it also contains *nitrogen* (16% of its total composition) and often other elements such as sulfur. The structure of protein is also different from that of either carbohydrate or fat. Proteins are much more complex compounds with high molecular weights. A given protein contains a specific number of specific amino acids linked in a sequence that is specific for that protein. It is this very *specificity* of protein structure in a definite amino acid sequence that gives various tissues their unique form, function, and character.

RAW BUILDING MATERIAL

Protein, therefore, is the body's vital building material; it is basic to life. Compare its use in the body to any basic building task. For any construction project the first requirement is an appropriate source of raw building material. If the structure were a house, for example, the raw source of the lumber to be used would be trees in the forest. These would have to be selected carefully for building quality, cut, trimmed, and sent to the lumber mill to be made into ready-to-use finished lumber.

Protein in the food we eat supplies the raw building material for our bodies. The individual building units in protein are called *amino acids*. The quality of a food protein as a building material may be classified either complete or incomplete, depending on which of these amino acid building units each protein food contains. Therefore, to determine the quality of protein, the quality of the constituent amino acids must first be determined.

AMINO ACIDS
Essential amino acids

The structural units of proteins, the amino acids, have been termed *essential* or *nonessential* on the basis of one major factor: whether the body can manufacture the particular amino acid. Consideration is also given

to how essential the amino acid is for normal growth and development.

On the basis of these distinctions in body dependence, eight amino acids have been demonstrated to be essential for adults. The eleven remaining amino acids are nonessential in the diet, although they are important in body activities. The body can manufacture them; therefore they are not as necessary for consideration in the diet. Following is a listing of the essential and nonessential amino acids:

Essential	*Nonessential*
Threonine	Glycine
Leucine	Alanine
Isoleucine	Aspartic acid
Valine	Glutamic acid
Lysine	Proline
Methionine	Hydroxyproline
Phenylalanine	Cystine
Tryptophan	Tyrosine
	Serine
	Arginine
	Histidine

Complete and incomplete proteins

According to the amount of essential amino acids that given protein foods possess, they have been broadly classified as complete or incomplete proteins. Complete protein foods are those that contain all the essential amino acids in sufficient quantity and ratio to supply the body's needs. These proteins are of animal origin: meat, milk, cheese, and eggs. Incomplete proteins are those deficient in one or more of the essential amino acids. They are of plant origin: grains, legumes, seeds, and nuts. In a mixed diet animal and plant proteins supplement one another. Even a mixture of plant proteins may provide an adequate balanced ratio of amino acids if planned carefully. The value of variety in the diet is therefore self-evident.

It is apparent that the protein requirement must be considered on the basis of quality, not merely quantity. It is obviously not only a matter of the total amount of protein needed but also of the specific amino acids needed. For example, gelatin alone is a rather worthless protein because it lacks three essential amino acids—tryptophan, valine, and isoleucine—and has only small amounts of leucine.

Various populations of the world may have few food sources of meat and dairy products and depend largely on plant sources to meet their protein requirement. Also, persons following vegetarian diets of various kinds need to plan food combinations to get sufficient protein. This may be accomplished by carefully planning a complementary combination of incomplete protein foods, so that the limited amino acid in one food will be supplied by another in the mixture. Thus, by combination of several incomplete protein foods, it is possible to obtain the essential amino acids. Securing sufficient protein is one of the significant world health problems today.

Basic structure of amino acids

As indicated by its name, an amino acid has a chemical structure that combines both acid and base (amino) factors. This important structure gives amino acids a unique buffering capacity.

This acid-base nature of amino acids also enables them to join one another to form the characteristic chain structure of protein. The amino (base) group of one amino acid joins the acid (carboxyl) group of another. This characteristic chain structure of amino acids is called a *peptide linkage*. Long chains of amino acids that are linked in this manner are called *polypeptides*. Proteins are formed, therefore, by long polypeptide chains that are coiled or folded back on themselves to form specific proteins.

FUNCTIONS OF PROTEIN
Tissue building

The primary function of dietary protein is the growth and maintenance of tissue. It does this by furnishing amino acids of appropriate numbers and types for efficient synthesis of specific cellular proteins. In addition, protein supplies amino acids for building other essential protein substances such as enzymes and hormones.

Energy

Protein also contributes to the body's overall energy metabolism. After removal of the nitrogenous portion of the amino acid (the amino group), the remaining part may be converted to fat or carbohydrate. If there is not sufficient carbohydrate or fat available in the diet for energy, then as much as 58% of the total dietary protein becomes available to be oxidized for energy. It is evident that sufficient nonprotein calories are needed in the diet to ensure that protein is used for its primary building purpose and not broken down unnecessarily to yield energy.

CHANGING RAW BUILDING MATERIAL TO FINISHED BUILDING UNITS

After the source of raw building materials—the food protein—is secured, it must be changed into the needed ready-to-use building units—the amino acids. This work is done by digestion.

Mouth. In the mouth only mechanical breaking up of the protein foods by chewing occurs. Here the food particles are mixed with saliva and passed as a semisolid mass into the stomach, where the main chemical digestion of protein begins.

Stomach. Because proteins are such complex structures, a series of enzymes is necessary to finally succeed in breaking them down to produce the amino acids. These chemical changes through a system of enzymes begin in the stomach. In fact, the stomach's chief digestive function in relation to all foods is the partial enzymatic breakdown of protein. Three agents in the gastric secretions help begin this task: pepsin, hydrochloric acid, and rennin.

PEPSIN. Pepsin is the main gastric enzyme specific for protein. It is first produced as an inactive substance, *pepsinogen,* by special cells in the mucosa of the stomach wall. Pepsinogen then requires hydrochloric acid for activation to the active enzyme pepsin. This active pepsin then begins breaking the peptide linkages of protein to produce smaller parts of the complex protein, called *proteoses* and *peptones*. However, these shorter chain polypeptides are still rather large protein derivatives. If the protein were held in the stomach longer, pepsin could continue this breakdown until individual amino acids resulted. However, with normal gastric emptying time, only the beginning stage is completed by the action of pepsin.

HYDROCHLORIC ACID. Hydrochloric acid is produced by special cells in the mucosa of the stomach wall. It is necessary to convert inactive pepsinogen to the active enzyme pepsin. Thus gastric hydrochloric acid is an important catalyst in gastric protein digestion. Clinical problems can be anticipated for patients who lack proper hydrochloric acid secretions.

RENNIN. Rennin is a gastric enzyme important in the infant's digestion of milk. Rennin and calcium act on the casein of milk to produce a curd; by coagulating milk, rennin prevents too rapid a passage from the stomach. In adults, however, rennin is apparently absent from the gastric secretion.

Small intestine. The difficult task of protein digestion begins in the stomach with enzymes activated by the acid medium of the stomach. It continues in the alkaline medium of the small intestine. A number of enzymes from both pancreas and intestinal cells continue the process of change to produce the final finished building units, the amino acids.

PANCREATIC SECRETIONS. Three enzymes are produced by the pancreas to continue the changes necessary to break down protein to simpler and simpler substances:

1. *Trypsin* is secreted first as an inactive substance, trypsinogen, and is activated by a hormone, enterokinase, which is produced by glands in the duodenal wall. This active enzyme, trypsin, then acts on protein and the large fragment proteoses and peptones carried over from the stomach to produce shorter chains of polypeptides and dipeptides.

2. *Chymotrypsin* is produced by special cells in the pancreas in its inactive precursor form, chymotrypsinogen. It is then activated by the trypsin already present. It continues the same protein-splitting action as trypsin.

3. *Carboxypeptidase*, as its name indicates, is a special enzyme that attacks the end of the peptide chain and splits off the acid (carboxyl)

Table 5-1. Summary of protein digestion

| | ENZYME | | | |
ORGAN	INACTIVE PRECURSOR	ACTIVATOR	ACTIVE ENZYME	DIGESTIVE ACTION
Mouth			None	Mechanical only
Stomach (acid)	Pepsinogen	Hydrochloric acid	Pepsin	Protein → proteoses and peptones
			Rennin (infants) (Ca necessary, for activity)	Casein → coagulated curd
Intestine (alkaline)				
Pancreatic juice	Trypsinogen	Enterokinase	Trypsin	Protein, proteoses, peptones → polypeptides, dipeptides
	Chymotrypsinogen	Active trypsin	Chymotrypsin	Proteoses, peptones → polypeptides, dipeptides Also coagulates milk
			Carboxypeptidase	Polypeptides → simpler peptides, dipeptides, amino acids
Intestinal juice			Aminopeptidase	Polypeptides → peptides, dipeptides, amino acids
			Dipeptidase	Dipeptides → amino acids

group. In doing so it produces still simpler peptides and some free amino acids.

INTESTINAL SECRETIONS. Glands in the intestinal wall produce two additional protein-splitting enzymes in the peptidase group:

1. *Aminopeptidase* attacks the amino (nitrogen-containing) end of the peptide chain. Through this action still shorter chain peptides and free amino acids are produced.

2. *Dipeptidase*, the final enzyme in this protein-splitting system, acts on the remaining dipeptides to produce free amino acids.

By this system of enzymes the pancreatic and intestinal secretions break down the large complex proteins into progressively smaller peptide chains and finally into amino acids that are split off from the ends of these chains. The end products of protein digestion, the amino acids, are now available as the finished, ready-to-use building units. They must now be carried by absorption into the intestinal mucosa and through the blood system to the cells for tissue synthesis.

A summary of protein digestion and the many changes and change agents required to break down so complex a substance is given in Table 5-1. The various enzyme names are not important. The whole system is presented here to illustrate that protein digestion is an involved, beautifully balanced process. This is because protein is a large, complex molecular structure, and a number of enzymes in sequence have to work on it to break it down for use as basic body-building material.

CARRYING FINISHED BUILDING UNITS TO CONSTRUCTION SITES

The construction sites in the body for building various kinds of necessary tissue protein are the *cells*. Each cell, depending on its particular nature and function, has a specific job to do and must be specifically structured to do that job.

Absorption of amino acids

After protein digestion the finished building units, the amino acids, are now ready to use in specific protein structures. These amino acids are water soluble. Therefore the task of carrying them to the cells is relatively simple compared with the more difficult task with fats, which are not water soluble. The larger task with proteins has already been accomplished in the many changes required to break down the food protein to the amino acids. The water-soluble amino acids are carried across the intestinal wall by a transport system using vitamin B_6 (pyridoxine) as a carrier. This is another example of the close relationships among the nutrients and their work in partnership. After crossing the intestinal wall they are carried by the blood to the cells for use in building specific tissue.

Absorption of peptides and whole proteins

A few larger fragments of short-chain peptides may remain after digestion and be absorbed as such. Even whole proteins are sometimes absorbed intact. These larger molecules apparently cannot be used in protein synthesis as can the free amino acids, but they may play a part in the development of immunity and sensitivity. For example, antibodies in the mother's colostrum (the pre-milk breast secretion) are passed on to her nursing infant.

BUILDING AND MAINTAINING SPECIFIC BODY STRUCTURES

All the various body structures, tissues, and organs are built of protein along with other materials as needed. Muscles, blood, bones, glands, nerves, skin, and other tissues are made up basically of protein. But each is unique, designed to carry out a particular task. Each kind of cell, depending on its specific task, has the specific "blueprint" in its nucleus for building the specific kind of proteins that it needs. It may build new tissues to bring about growth during childhood. It may rebuild and repair old tissue to maintain the body during adulthood.

All in all, the many metabolic processes and changes involved in protein metabolism form a fascinating array of complex and intricately interwoven chemical activities. Perhaps the metabolic activities of protein in building and rebuilding specific body structures can best be understood in broad terms under the basic concept of *balance*.

Concept of balance in protein metabolism

Throughout the body, many checks and balances exist. There is a constant ebb and flow of materials, a building up and breaking down of parts, and a depositing and mobilizing of constituents. Many body mechanisms maintain this internal stability or equilibrium. The body has built-in controls that operate as coordinated responses of its many parts to any situation that tends to disturb its normal condition or function. This resultant state of equilibrium is called *homeostasis.* The various mechanisms designed to preserve it are called *homeostatic mechanisms*. This balance between body parts and functions is life sustaining.

Increasingly, as more and more is being learned about human nutrition and physiology, older ideas of a rigid body structure are giving way to a concept of dynamic equilibrium—balance in the midst of constant change. All body constituents are in a constant state of flux, although some tissues are more actively engaged than others. This concept of dynamic equilibrium and balance has been described in carbohydrate and fat metabolism. However, it is especially striking in protein metabolism.

Protein turnover balance

The rate of protein turnover varies in different tissues. It is highest in the intestinal mucosa, liver, pancreas, kidney, and blood plasma. It is lowest in muscle, brain, and skin tissue. There is almost no protein turnover in collagen tissue.

Body protein exists in a balance between two compartments: the tissue protein and the plasma protein. These body stores are further balanced with dietary protein intake. Protein from one compartment may be drawn on to supply a need in the other. For example, dur-

ing fasting, reserves from the body protein stores may be used for tissue synthesis. But the interesting fact is that even when the intake of protein and other nutrients is adequate, the tissue proteins are still being constantly broken down and re-formed in a dynamic balance.

The adult body's state of stability, then, is the result of a balance between the rates of protein breakdown and protein resynthesis. In periods of growth the synthesis rate is higher so that new tissue can be formed and the child is in a state of positive protein balance. In conditions of starvation and wasting diseases and more gradually in the aging process, the rate of breakdown exceeds that of synthesis, the body deteriorates, and the person is in a state of negative protein balance.

Metabolic amino acid pool. Another part of this overall protein amino acid balance is the common metabolic pool of amino acids maintained in the liver. Amino acids derived from tissue breakdown and amino acids from dietary protein both enter this common reserve. Thus a balance of amino acids is constantly maintained to supply the body's total needs. Shifts and balances between tissue breakdown and dietary protein ensure the constant availability of a balanced mixture of amino acids. From this amino acid pool, specific amino acids are supplied as needed for specific tissue protein synthesis and to make up body losses. This overall protein–amino acid balance is summarized in Fig. 5-1.

Nitrogen balance. Another useful reference in indicating a person's state of protein balance is the concept of nitrogen balance. Total nitrogen balance involves all sources of nitrogen in the body, protein nitrogen as well as nonprotein nitrogen present in other compounds such as urea, uric acid, and ammonia and in other body tissues and fluids. The word "balance" refers to the balance between intake and output of a particular substance. Thus negative balance is a state in which the output of a substance exceeds its intake. Positive balance is a state in which the intake of a substance exceeds its output.

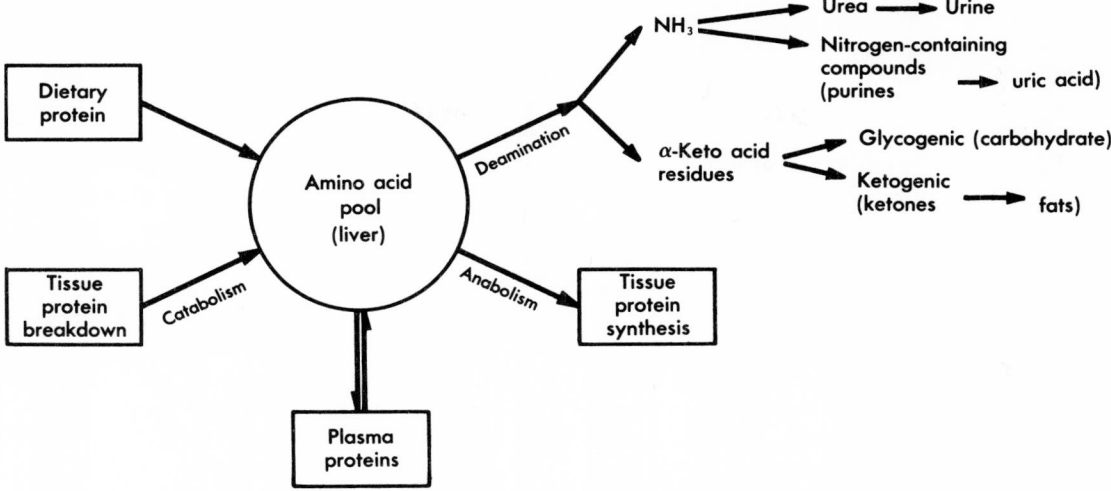

Fig. 5-1. Balance between protein compartments and amino acid pool.

Therefore total nitrogen balance is the net result of all nitrogen gains and losses in all the body protein. A person is in a state of negative nitrogen balance when his loss of body protein exceeds his input of food protein. Such a state exists in conditions such as starvation, a wasting disease, or long-term illness.

Anabolism-catabolism balance

Anabolism—tissue building. Anabolism is the building up of protein tissue through the synthesis of new protein. This building of protein tissue is a specific process governed by a specific pattern that requires specific amino acids to construct it. This specific characteristic has been called the "all-or-none" law. This means that all the necessary amino acids for a given protein must be present at the same time or the protein will not be formed. Specific selection and supply of amino acids are mandatory.

PROCESS OF TISSUE BUILDING. The overall process of building tissue may be summarized around four basic components:

1. *Blueprint.* The basic pattern for the specific protein is set by a substance in the nucleus called DNA (deoxyribonucleic acid). This specific pattern for the specific protein is then transferred to another chemical substance called RNA (ribonucleic acid).

2. *Building site.* After it receives the blueprint from the nucleus DNA, the messenger RNA goes out into the cell cytoplasm and attaches itself to the ribosomes for a building site on the endoplasmic reticulum. Thus a mold is set to guide the building of the specific protein.

3. *Building processes.* Three basic processes are involved in building the protein on the ribosomes:

   a. The specific amino acids required are activated by special enzymes and made ready for building.

   b. These amino acids are then placed in the building site mold in correct sequence by the partner fragments of transfer RNA. Thus they are guided into correct position ready to be joined.

   c. The amino acids are joined together in peptide linkages to form polypeptide chains for the new protein. The new protein is then released to serve its specific function.

CONTROL AGENTS. Several agents act as control factors for these intricate processes. These control agents include specific cell enzymes and coenzymes. Also, specific hormones control or stimulate the building of tissue. These include (1) the growth hormone, which stimulates extra tissue synthesis during the growth periods; (2) gonadotrophins, especially testosterone, which stimulate tissue building associated with puberty; and (3) thyroxine (in normal amounts), which regulates the rate of basal metabolism in the body.

Catabolism—tissue breakdown. Amino acids released as tissue protein is broken down or not used in tissue synthesis are further broken down and used for other purposes. Two main parts of the amino acid result: (1) the nitrogenous group, containing nitrogen (NH_2), and (2) the remaining nonnitrogen residue.

NITROGEN GROUP. The first step in the breakdown of amino acids is the splitting off of the nitrogen portion. This process, which takes place chiefly in the liver, is called *deamination.* The nitrogen is converted to ammonia and may be excreted in the urine as urea or used to form other nitrogen-containing compounds.

NONNITROGEN RESIDUE. The nonnitrogen residues are called *keto-acids.* These residues may be used to form either carbohydrates or fat substances. Certain amino acids tend to form carbohydrate substances, whereas other amino acids are used for fat substances. These residues may also be *reaminated* to form a new amino acid.

CONTROL AGENTS. As in the case of tissue building, cell enzymes and coenzymes are constantly at work controlling the various reactions involved. Hormones also influence catabolism. These include (1) large amounts of thyroxine, which stimulates excessive catabolism of muscle tissue, and (2) adrenal steroids, which stimulate the breakdown of amino acids and the conversion of the residue to glucose or glycogen.

PROTEIN REQUIREMENTS

Since protein is such an essential nutrient for tissue building and rebuilding, much study has been given to the question of how much protein the body actually requires. General requirements or recommendations for dietary protein intake have been developed on the basis of research pertaining to all age groups. These recommended amounts have been published as standards or guidelines by the Food and Nutrition Board of the National Academy of Sciences and National Research Council. These recommended amounts of protein are given in Table 5-2.

A study of these figures in Table 5-2 will indicate the increased need for protein per pound of body weight during the growth years of childhood. During adulthood the recommended amount levels off for maintenance purposes.

Factors influencing protein requirement

A number of factors influence the amount of protein a given individual requires. These include personal growth, diet, and conditions of stress in illness or disease.

Personal growth. Any period of growth increases the need for protein. These growth-related factors include age, body size, and general physical status. Special periods of rapid growth such as the growth of the fetus and maternal tissue during pregnancy require additional increases in protein. The expectant mother during pregnancy may require as much as 100 gm. of protein a day.

Diet. Other factors include the nature of the protein in the diet and its ratio, or pattern of amino acid structure. There must be sufficient nonprotein calories in the diet to have a protein-sparing effect, so that the total amount of protein will not be diminished for energy requirements. Also the digestibility and absorption of the protein is affected by the preparation and cooking of the food. The timing of the meals also plays a role; allowing time intervals between ingestion of protein foods apparently lowers the competition for absorption sites and enzymes.

Illness or disease. The presence of any illness or disease will usually increase the requirement for protein. Diseases accompanied by fever especially increase the requirement for protein because of the increase

Table 5-2. Required amounts of protein per day*

Men (154 lb.)†	56 gm.
Women (128 lb.)†	46 gm.
Pregnancy, last 4½ mo.	(+30 gm.)
Lactation	(+20 gm.)
Infants	
0 to 6 mo.	Kg. × 2.2 gm.
6 to 12 mo.	Kg. × 2.0 gm.
Children	
1 to 3 yr.	23 gm.
4 to 6 yr.	30 gm.
7 to 10 yr.	36 gm.
Boys	
11 to 14 yr.	44 gm.
15 to 18 yr.	54 gm.
Girls	
11 to 14 yr.	44 gm.
15 to 18 yr.	48 gm.

*From Food and Nutrition Board, National Academy of Sciences–National Research Council: Recommended dietary allowances, ed. 8, Washington, D. C., 1974, The Academy.
†0.422 gm. of protein per pound of ideal body weight.

Table 5-3. Foods high in protein

FOOD	APPROXIMATE AMOUNT	PROTEIN (GM.)
Beef, chuck roast	3 oz. cooked	23.4
Beef, hamburger	3 oz. cooked	20.5
Beef round	3 oz. cooked	24.7
Beef, club steak	4 oz. cooked	27.6
Lamb leg	3 oz. cooked	21.6
Liver (beef, calf, and pork)	3 oz. cooked	20.4
Pork loin	3 oz. cooked	20.7
Ham	3 oz. cooked	20.7
Veal, leg or shoulder	3 oz. cooked	25.2
Chicken	¼ broiler	22.4
Chicken, fryer	½ breast (4 oz. raw)	26.9
Chicken, hen, stewed	1 thigh or ½ breast	26.5
Duck, roasted	3 slices (3½ × 2¾ × ¼)	20.6
Goose, roasted	3 slices (3½ × 2¾ × ¼)	25.3
Turkey	3 slices (3½ × 2¼ × ¼)	27.8
Haddock	3 oz. cooked	20.2
Halibut	3 oz. cooked	21.0
Oysters	6 medium	15.1
Salmon	⅔ cup	20.5
Scallops	5 to 6 medium	23.8
Tuna	½ cup	15.9
Peanut butter	4 tbs.	15.9
Milk	1 cup	8.5
Cottage cheese	5 to 6 tbs.	19.5
American cheddar cheese	1 oz.	7.1

in basal metabolic rate and the general destruction of tissue. Traumatic injury requires extensive tissue rebuilding. Postsurgical states require extra protein for wound healing and to replenish losses. Extensive tissue destruction as in burns requires an extensive increase in protein intake for the healing process. Table 5-3 can serve as a guideline for a number of high-protein foods that may be used in such instances.

Measure of protein requirements

There is some confusion in the determination of requirements for protein. General terms such as minimum, average, adequate, and optimum have little meaning. Attempts to overcome this difficulty in establishing standards have brought into use the phrase, "recommended allowances" by the National Research Council. It is evident that both quantity and quality must be considered in establishing protein requirements.

Protein quantity. This measure would establish the total protein requirement. The United States' standard has generally been set for adults at 0.8 gm. per kilogram (2.2 pounds) of body weight. This amounts to about 56 gm. (about 1½ oz.) daily for a person weighing 70 kg. (154 pounds). Much more than this is needed during periods of physiologic stress caused by illness or normal stress of growth in pregnancy. The quantity standards as established by the National Research Council for protein throughout the life cycle have been listed in Table 5-2.

Protein quality. Since the value of a protein depends on its content of essential amino acids, in the final analysis the measure of protein requirements must be based on quality, that is, essential amino acid content.

Guidelines for such quality measure of protein have been established by the Food and Agriculture Organization, a division of the World Health Organization under the United Nations. This pattern is called a *provisional amino acid pattern* and is constructed according to the formula shown in Table 5-4. This pattern shows the relative requirements of the eight essential amino acids, beginning with the one required in least amount—tryptophan—and progressing toward those required in larger amounts, such as leucine and phenylalanine. According to this method of measuring protein quality, eggs and milk rank highest as reference proteins against which to measure other foods.

Table 5-4. Food and Agriculture Organization* amino acid proportionality pattern for the adult based on essential amino acid requirements

AMINO ACID	REQUIREMENT (MG.)	PROPORTIONALITY PATTERN	PATTERN SIMPLIFIED IN COMMON USE†
Tryptophan	250	1.0	1.0
Threonine	500	2.0	2.0
Isoleucine	700	2.8	3.0
Lysine	800	3.2	3.0
Valine	900	3.6	3.0
Total sulfur amino acid	950	3.8	3.0
(Methionine minimum)	(325)	(1.3)	
Leucine	1,050	4.2	3.4
Total aromatic amino acid	1,550	6.2	
(Phenylalanine minimum)	(325)	(1.3)	2.0

*Food and Agriculture Organization: Protein requirements, FAO Nutritional Studies, No. 16, Rome, 1957 (adapted).
†Leverton, R. M.: Amino acids. In Stefferud, A., editor: Food, the yearbook of agriculture, 1959, Washington, D. C., 1959, U. S. Department of Agriculture.

Vegetarian diets

Since protein quality based on amino acids present in foods used is a basis for measuring protein requirements, problems may arise for those persons consuming vegetarian types of diets in which less complete proteins from plant sources are used. Protein requirements in various vegetarian diets may be met by applying this same principle of combining complementary plant proteins to achieve the necessary balance of essential amino acids. Health workers working with persons on vegetarian diets should first explore the nature of their personal diet patterns, since there are at least four basic types of vegetarianism. Each would demand different approaches.

Lacto-ovovegetarian diet. This is an all vegetable diet supplemented with milk, cheese, and eggs. There would be no problem securing adequate protein with this combination; only meat is omitted.

Lactovegetarian diet. This is an all vegetable diet supplemented with only milk and cheese. Milk products add complete protein to this combination and enhance amino acids adequately. Only meat and egg are omitted.

Pure vegetarian, or "vegan," diets. A pure vegetarian diet is an all vegetable diet without any animal foods, dairy products, or eggs. Much more careful planning is required to achieve combinations providing the necessary amounts of the essential amino acids. A deficiency of B_{12} may become a problem.

Fruitarian diets. A fruitarian diet consists of raw or dried fruits, nuts, honey, and olive oil. Potential inadequacy is much greater here.

•　•　•

Combinations of complementary food proteins that achieve the necessary balance may include the following:

> Rice + black-eyed peas (a southern United States' dish called "Hopping John")
> Whole wheat or bulgur wheat + soybeans + sesame seeds (protein may be increased by the addition of yogurt)
> Cornmeal + kidney beans (a combination in many Mexican dishes; protein increased by the addition of cheese)
> Soybeans + peanuts + brown rice + bulgur wheat (an excellent sauce dish served over the rice and wheat)

Guidelines for such vegetable-protein combinations and interesting recipes for preparing these foods have been developed and tested.*

SUMMARY

This discussion of protein requirement is intended to help the student gain a sounder basis for teaching health practices to patients. So-called protein requirements are not as rigid as they may appear when listed in the National Research Council tables. The word "requirement" seems to have an inflexible meaning, which simply is not the case or the intention of the council.

The National Research Council's published standards for protein are intended to provide recommended guidelines. They are designed to cover a wide range of needs; to provide a margin of safety to cover stress situations, they are approximately double the minimum allowances. Therefore they are not absolute, rigid requirements but *flexible recommendations.* As such, they are intended to serve as guidelines and should be adapted as needed to the individual patient.

---

*Lappé, M.: Diet for a small planet, New York, 1971, Ballantine Books.

6 VITAMINS: THE PROBLEM OF REGULATION AND CONTROL

THE PROBLEM OF REGULATION AND CONTROL

You have seen how the body solves its two major problems of energy production and tissue building and rebuilding to maintain life and health. To do so requires thousands of interrelated physiologic activities, but to meet these two basic needs another major problem is created, that of regulation and control.

To maintain health and life, then, all the multiple body processes involved in energy production and tissue building must proceed in an organized, orderly fashion. Without such biologic balance, chaos, illness, and death would occur. Such order requires some kind of control agents. Some general types of control agents in the body such as hormones, enzymes, and coenzymes have been introduced. The remaining nutrients, the vitamins and minerals, mainly operate in the key role of *coenzymes*, or controllers of specific body functions. This chapter will discuss the role of the vitamins as control agents, and Chapter 7 will consider minerals in the same manner.

DISCOVERY OF VITAMINS

Over the past six decades the discoveries of the vitamins have formed a fascinating chapter in nutritional history. Numerous scientists have contributed to this unfolding story. The word *vitamin* was first used by Casimir Funk, a Polish chemist working at the Lister Institute in London in the early 1900s. He had little money to carry on his experimental work with pigeons, so he ordinarily fed them only the rice polishings that he could sweep up from the floor of a granary. Eventually, however, this source of food supply was closed to him, and he began to purchase some regular polished rice. After being fed the polished rice, the pigeons soon developed paralysis. Funk wondered whether the change of diet was related to the onset of the paralysis, so again he fed the birds the waste polishings: they recovered! Funk then tried to find some substance in the grain hulls that would account for the different response in the birds. In 1911 he discovered a nitrogen-containing material that he thought was an amine. (An amine is a nitrogenous substance produced from ammonia.) Because this substance was apparently vital to life, he called it *vitamine* (*vital-amine*). The final "e" was dropped later when other similarly vital substances turned out to be a variety of organic compounds. The name *vitamin* has been retained to designate compounds of this class of substances.

One by one, as the vitamins have been discovered, the list has grown. Two characteristics mark a compound for identification as a vitamin:

1. It must be a vital organic dietary substance that is not a carbohydrate, fat, protein, or mineral. It is necessary in only very *small* quantities to perform a particular metabolic function or to prevent an associated deficiency disease.

2. It cannot be manufactured by the body and therefore must be supplied in food.

Because of the intricacies of the human body, many such substances probably exist in addition to those already discovered. It may be that those vitamins that have been discovered were recognized first because they exist in relatively small quantities in food and so their deficiencies were more likely to occur to be observed and to be questioned.

Some of the vitamins were first discovered in the search for the causes of certain age-old diseases such as scurvy, beriberi, pellagra, and rickets. Others were discovered later as the result of studies of various body functions. In general, in cases of malnutrition, not just one but a number of vitamins may be lacking.

THE STUDY OF VITAMINS

Vitamins are usually classified according to their solubility in either fat or water. Although this distinction is sometimes an arbitrary one, it is still used for want of a better one. The fat-soluble group includes vitamins A, D, E, and K. The water-soluble group includes vitamin C and the B-complex vitamins.

To clarify the current concepts concerning each known vitamin, consider these questions as the basis for study:

1. What is the vitamin's nature—physical and chemical?
2. How does the body handle it?
3. What does it *do?* This is the most significant question.
4. How much is needed and where can it be obtained?

Some confusion exists concerning the naming of the vitamins. In the beginning, the vitamins were simply given letter names in the order of their discovery. However, as the discoveries increased rapidly, and some substances thought to be single elements turned out to be multiple, names were given to the vitamins to describe their chemical nature or function. Increasingly these names are being used, but some of the vitamins are still commonly referred to by their letter names. In the discussion that follows, an attempt is made to provide both names so that the student may differentiate one vitamin from another.

FAT-SOLUBLE VITAMINS
VITAMIN A (RETINOL)
General chemical and physical nature of vitamin A

Vitamin A was discovered in 1917 by E. V. McCollum and his co-workers at Johns Hopkins University in Baltimore. They demonstrated that an eye disease, xerophthalmia, was caused specifically by lack of a fat-soluble substance, which they called *vitamin A*.

Vitamin A is a primary alcohol of high molecular weight ($CO_{20}H_{29}OH$). It is a complex molecule. Because it has a specific function in the retina of the eye and because it is an alcohol, it has since been given the name *retinol*. However, it is still commonly called *vitamin A*.

Vitamin A is soluble in fat and ordinary fat solvents. Because it is insoluble in water, it is fairly stable in general cooking. However, it does oxidize readily on prolonged exposure to temperatures higher than those ordinarily used in cooking. In commercial preparations of vitamin A, antioxidants such as vitamin E have been used with it to preserve it.

Dietary forms of vitamin A

The two basic dietary forms of vitamin A are preformed vitamin A and provitamin A (carotene).

Preformed vitamin A. In its natural form, vitamin A is found only in animal sources, usually associated with fats, since it is fat soluble. Thus in this form it is found mainly in dairy products (the fat portion) and storage organs such as the liver.

Provitamin A (carotene). Since such a limited amount of vitamin A had been found in animal sources, investigators began to look for a precursor in plants that the animals consumed. They believed that the animals must convert such a precursor in their bodies to vitamin A: this indeed proved to be the case. The ultimate source of all vitamin A is plants. In plants the precursor of vitamin A—provitamin A—is a pigment substance called *carotene* ($C_{40}H_{56}$). It was first called carotene because it was identified in the yellow pigment of carrots. The body converts this carotene into vitamin A. Animals consume carotene in plants and make this conversion, so that our food sources of preformed vitamin A are from animal sources. Most of our vitamin A, about two thirds of that necessary in human nutrition, is supplied by carotene, which is found in deep yellow and green plants. Cooking these plants helps release the carotene crystals by weakening the cell walls, thus aiding their absorption in the intestine.

Absorption and storage of vitamin A

Vitamin A enters the body in two forms: as the preformed vitamin from animal sources and as carotene from plants. Since these are fat-related substances, the same materials that aid fat absorption also aid the absorption of vitamin A. These materials are bile salts, pancreatic lipase, and fat.

A warning must be given here about the nonfood fat, mineral oil. This oil is not digested by the body but goes through the gastrointestinal tract intact. If it is present in the intestine along with fat-soluble vitamins, such as vitamin A or carotene, it absorbs them and carries them out also. Therefore mineral oil should never be used with meals or be taken immediately before or after eating.

In the intestinal wall during absorption, some of the carotene is converted to vitamin A. Vitamin A and carotene then enter the lymphatic system following the same absorption route as fat and are carried through the thoracic duct into the portal vein and thence to the liver for storage and distribution. The liver is by far the most efficient storage organ: it contains about 90% of the total vitamin A in the body. Since liver has such a large storage capacity for vitamin A, there is a potential toxicity from large doses of this vitamin.

Certain intestinal diseases that change the absorptive surface tissue of the mucosa hinder absorption of vitamin A. Also conditions of the biliary tract affecting the flow of bile hinder vitamin A absorption. Age is also a factor: in the newborn and especially the premature infant, absorption is poor. With advancing age, the elderly person may experience increasing difficulty with absorption also.

Physiologic functions of vitamin A

Vitamin A has important functions in a number of human tissues. Its role in control of body functions is in vision and tissue growth:

1. *Vision.* The ability of the eye to adapt to changes in light is dependent on the presence of a light-sensitive pigment in the rods of the retina, a pigment commonly known as *visual purple.* A vitamin A compound is a vital part of this pigment. Hence, when the body is deficient in vitamin A, this adaption to light cannot be made as well, and the eye becomes increasingly sensitive to light changes. This may eventually cause night blindness or glare blindness. The condition is usually cured in about half an hour by an injection of vitamin A.

2. *Tissue growth.* Vitamin A has a vital role in the formation and maintenance of healthy functioning epithelial tissue, which forms the body's primary barrier to infection. The epithelium includes not only the skin but also the mucous membranes lining the ocular and oral cavities and the gastrointestinal, respiratory, and genitourinary tracts. Without vitamin A, these epithelial cells become dry and flat and gradually harden to form scales that slough off. This process is called *keratinization.* Keratin is protein that forms dry, scalelike tissue such as nails and hair. In the eye when the cornea dries and hardens in this way, the condition is called

xerophthalmia. This may progress to blindness in extreme deficiency of vitamin A. In general, in the absence of vitamin A, epithelial tissue is more prone to development of infections and tissue breakdown.

Vitamin A in its tissue growth function is also associated with normal growth and development. Therefore increased needs would be present in childhood and during pregnancy. Also, specific cells in the gums that develop the tooth buds (ameloblasts) by forming the enamel structure of the developing tooth depend on vitamin A for proper development and function.

Requirement of vitamin A

Since a number of variables modify an individual's vitamin A requirement, this need is difficult to establish precisely. These variables influencing requirement include the amount stored in the liver, the form in which it is taken (whether as carotene or as vitamin A), and the presence of illness or gastrointestinal defect. Thus to cover such variables the recommendations of the NRC allow a margin of safety above minimal needs. These recommendations may be compared throughout the life cycle in Table 6-1.

Vitamin A is commonly measured in international units (I.U.) or in retinol equivalents (RE). In general, carotene has one half or less the value of an equal quantity of vitamin A in the diet because of the differences in intestinal absorption and the necessity for conversion of carotene to vitamin A by the liver. One I.U. is equivalent to the biologic activity of 0.6 mcg. (0.006 mg.) of pure beta carotene or 0.3 mcg. of retinol. It can be seen from these figures how small the amount of vitamin required by the body is.

Hypervitaminosis A. In some instances large megadoses of vitamin A have been advocated. It is clearly possible to take toxic amounts of this vitamin, since its storage capacity is high. Vitamins are substances that are vital in *small* amounts, but too much of some vitamins can be dangerous. Hypervitaminosis A is manifested by joint pains, thickening of long bones, loss of hair, and jaundice. Such a case has been reported in an infant whose mother mistakenly gave vitamin A concentrate (recommended dosage in

Table 6-1. National Research Council recommended daily vitamin A allowances (revised 1973)

	AGE (YR.)	VITAMIN A ACTIVITY	
		(RE)*	(I.U.)
Men	All	1,000	5,000
Women	All	800	4,000
Pregnancy		1,000	5,000
Lactation		1,200	6,000
Infants	0.0 to 0.5	420†	1,400
	0.5 to 1.0	400	2,000
Children	1 to 3	400	2,000
	4 to 6	500	2,500
	7 to 10	700	3,300
Boys	11 to 14	1,000	5,000
	15 to 18	1,000	5,000
Girls	11 to 14	800	4,000
	15 to 18	800	4,000

*Retinol equivalents.
†Assumed to be all as retinol in milk during the first 6 months of life. All subsequent intakes are assumed to be one half as beta carotene when calculated from international units. As retinol equivalents, three fourths are as retinol and one fourth is as beta carotene.

drops) in amounts required for liver oil (recommended dosage in *teaspoons*).

Food sources of vitamin A

The few animal sources of preformed vitamin A include liver, kidney, cream, butter, and egg yolk. The major contributors are the yellow and green vegetables and fruits, which are sources of carotene. These include carrots, sweet potatoes, squash, apricots, spinach, collards, broccoli, and cabbage. A number of commercial products may be fortified with vitamin A. Margarine, for example, is fortified with 15,000 I.U. of vitamin A per pound.

In summary, therefore, vitamin A deficiency may occur for three basic reasons:
1. Inadequate diet intake
2. Poor absorption because of lack of bile or defective absorbing surface in the intestine
3. Inadequate conversion of carotene because of liver or intestinal disease

VITAMIN D (CALCIFEROL)
General chemical and physical nature of vitamin D

Vitamin D was discovered in 1922, also by Dr. McCollum's group at Johns Hopkins University. He discovered it during his studies of vitamin A because it is similar in chemical nature. Vitamin D has since been identified not as one but as a group of sterols varying in potency. All forms are soluble in fat but not in water. They are heat stable and not easily oxidized. Of the two D vitamins most important in nutrition, one is produced from body cholesterol by exposure to sunlight. Thus vitamin D is unique among the vitamins in two respects: (1) it occurs naturally in only a few common foods (mainly in fish oils), and (2) it can be formed in the body by exposure of the skin to ultraviolet rays, either from the sun or from a sunlamp. The general name *calciferol* has been given to vitamin D, indicating its function in relation to calcium metabolism and its chemical nature as a sterol.

Absorption and storage of vitamin D

Since vitamin D is fat soluble, its absorption also requires the presence of bile salts. Vitamin D, like vitamin A, is also absorbed by mineral oil, so, if mineral oil is taken, it should be ingested separately from food. Diseases of the intestine affecting the absorbing surface also hinder the absorption of vitamin D.

After being absorbed, vitamin D is carried to the liver and other organs for use; it is stored in the liver, as is vitamin A. Thus the potential for toxic quantities of vitamin D in the body is also present.

Physiologic functions of vitamin D

Vitamin D in the body is predominately associated with calcium and phosphorus. It helps to regulate and control the metabolism of these two minerals in two ways:

1. *Absorption of calcium and phosphorus.* Vitamin D is to aid the absorption of calcium from the small intestine. Since it makes the cell membrane more permeable to calcium, phosphorus also follows.

2. *Bone formation.* After the absorption of calcium and phosphorus through the intestinal wall, vitamin D continues to work in partnership with these minerals in their deposition in the bones to form bone tissue. Vitamin D directly increases the rate at which these minerals form bone and maintain it.

This basic function of vitamin D in the proper calcification of bone tissue is therefore associated with the disease *rickets*, a condition that results from a deficiency of vitamin D. The bones in the absence of vitamin D do not properly form from the softer collagenous tissue. Hence, as the child grows and begins to bear weight, the bone structures become deformed. (Note the children in Fig. 6-1.)

Requirement of vitamin D

Similar difficulties exist in setting requirements for vitamin D as for vitamin A. Variables arise from a lack of knowledge of precise body needs and the limited number of food

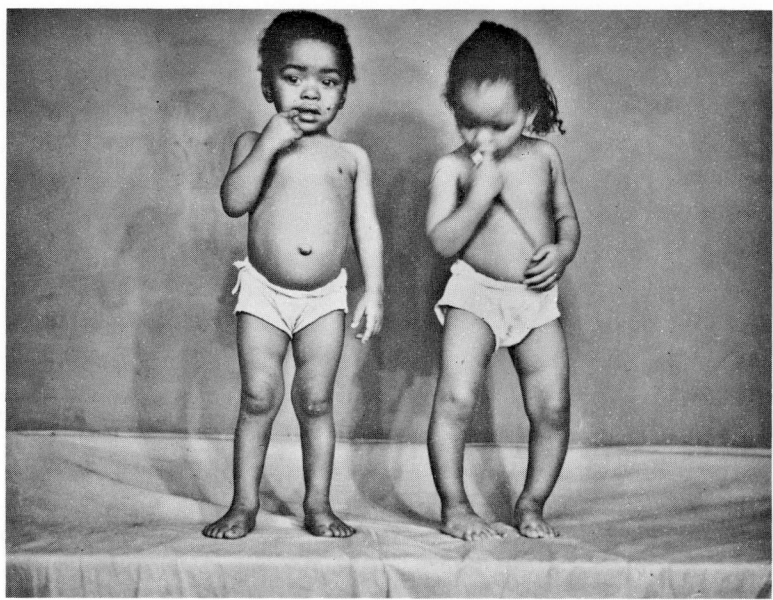

Fig. 6-1. Rachitic children. Note the knock-knees on the child on the left and the bowlegs on the child on the right. (From Therapeutic notes, Parke, Davis & Co., Detroit; courtesy Dr. Tom Spies and Dr. Orson D. Bird.)

sources available. Also the degree to which the body is able to produce vitamin D in response to irradiation by sunlight is not precisely known. A person's way of living determines the degree of exposure to sunlight and therefore would influence the individual needs for additional vitamin D. For example, a city person living in a high-rise apartment or a tenement and working indoors may need more than a farmer who works outside all day. Elderly persons or invalids who do not go outside may also need supplementary vitamin D. Growth demands in childhood and in pregnancy and lactation necessitate increased intake.

The NRC recommends 400 I.U. daily for children and for women during pregnancy and lactation. No statement is made concerning adult needs, which indicates that, in most instances, general exposure to sunlight is sufficient. One I.U. of vitamin D is equivalent to the biologic activity of 0.025 mcg. of pure crystalline vitamin D_3.

Hypervitaminosis D. As with vitamin A, it is possible to take in excess quantities of vitamin D and so to produce toxicity—a special danger in infant feeding practices in which fortified milk, fortified cereal, and variable vitamin supplements are used. The small infant needs only 400 I.U. daily. The amount in all the preceding items could easily total 4,000 I.U. or more. Since vitamin D is now commonly added to many infant foods, the need for supplementation with vitamin D preparations should be reconsidered.

Symptoms of vitamin D toxicity are calcification of soft tissues, such as lungs and kidney, and bone fragility. Renal tissue is particularly prone to harden, or calcify, thus reducing glomerular filtration and overall function of the kidney.

Food sources of vitamin D

Few natural food sources of vitamin D exist. The two basic vitamins, D_2 and D_3, occur only in yeast and fish liver oils. Thus the main food sources are those to which crystalline vitamin D has been added or in which vitamin D has been produced by irradiation. Milk, because it is so commonly used, has proved to be the most practical carrier. Now it is a widespread commercial practice to standardize the added vitamin D content to milk at 400 I.U. per quart. Milk is also a good companion for the vitamin because it provides calcium and phosphorus as well. Butter substitutes such as margarine are also fortified with vitamin D.

VITAMIN E (TOCOPHEROL)
General chemical and physical nature of vitamin E

Vitamin E was discovered in 1922 in connection with studies concerning the reproductive responses of rats and was identified as an alcohol. Because of this early function in rats and its chemical nature, it was named *tocopherol* from a Greek word meaning *childbirth* or *to bring forth* and from its chemical nature as an alcohol. Since then, tocopherol has come to be known as the antisterility vitamin, but this effect has been demonstrated only in the rat and not in man, despite all advertising claims for its contribution to potency or virility and the like.

Vitamin E also has been found to be not a single vitamin but a group of related vitamins. It is stable to heat and also to acids but not to alkalies; it is insoluble in water. One of its most important chemical characteristics is resistance to oxidation. This gives it an important role as an *antioxidant*.

Absorption and storage of vitamin E

Vitamin E is believed to be absorbed like the other fat-soluble vitamins through the aid of bile salts and fats. Storage takes place in different body tissues, but especially in adipose fat tissue.

Physiologic functions of vitamin E

Although exact mechanisms are unclear, recent studies indicate several significant functions of vitamin E in relation to human metabolism:

1. It is an effective antioxidant and as such is being used in commercial products to retard spoilage. It is added to therapeutic forms of vitamin A to protect the vitamin from oxidizing before it is absorbed.

2. It seems to preserve the integrity of red blood cells by protecting them from breakdown of the cell walls. Vitamin E therapy has effectively controlled certain anemias in infants.

3. It may also protect the structure and function of muscle tissues. Various stages and forms of muscle degeneration and lesions have been found in patients with low plasma vitamin E levels, for example, patients with cystic fibrosis or kwashiorkor.

4. It protects unsaturated essential fatty acids, such as linoleic acid, from oxidative breakdown. The amount of vitamin E required by a person has been directly linked with the amount of polyunsaturated fatty acids in the diet.

Requirement of vitamin E

Vitamin E is clearly an essential nutrient. The NRC recommendation is for a daily allowance of 15 I.U. for men and 12 I.U. for women, increased to 15 I.U. during pregnancy and lactation. A summary of the various age group requirements is given in Table 6-2.

Food sources of vitamin E

The richest sources of vitamin E are the vegetable oils. Curiously enough, these are also the richest sources of polyunsaturated fatty acids, which vitamin E protects from oxidation. Other food sources include wheat germ, milk, eggs, muscle meats, fish, cereals, and leafy vegetables.

VITAMIN K (MENADIONE)
General chemical and physical nature of vitamin K

In 1929 the work of a Swedish chemist working with a hemorrhagic disease in chicks led to the discovery of vitamin K. He deter-

Table 6-2. Vitamin E recommended dietary allowances, National Research Council (revised 1973)

	AGE (YR.)	VITAMIN E ACTIVITY* (I.U.)
Infants	0.0 to 0.5	4
	0.5 to 1.0	5
Children	1 to 3	7
	4 to 6	9
	7 to 10	10
Boys	11 to 14	12
	15 to 18	15
Girls	11 to 14	10
	15 to 18	11
Men	All	15
Women	All	12
Pregnancy		15
Lactation		15

*Total vitamin E activity, estimated to be 80% α-tocopherol and 20% other tocopherols.

mined that the basic factor was a blood-clotting vitamin, which he called *vitamin K,* from the Swedish word for its function—*koagulationsvitamin.*

As with most of the vitamins, further study showed that vitamin K was not one but a group of substances of similar biologic activity. The first vitamin K was isolated from alfalfa. A second one was isolated from putrified sardine meal. A third vitamin K has been made synthetically and has wide clinical use: it is *menadione,* one of several vitamins that are synthetic products with similar structures and properties. A water-soluble form of menadione is available for clinical use in patients in whom a fat-soluble form would be less readily absorbed and metabolized.

Vitamin K is synthesized by the normal intestinal bacteria, so an adequate supply is generally present. However, since the intestine of a newborn infant is sterile at birth, the supply of vitamin K is inadequate until normal bacterial flora of the intestine develop about the third or fourth day of life. Thus a prophylactic dose of vitamin K is usually given to all newborns. Vitamin K is fairly stable, although it is sensitive to light and irradiation. Thus clinical preparations of vitamin K should be kept in dark bottles.

Absorption and storage of vitamin K

The natural fat-soluble vitamins require bile salts for absorption, since they are fat soluble. They are absorbed with other fat-related products by way of the lymphatic system and then into portal blood and transported to the liver. Vitamin K is apparently stored in the liver in small amounts.

Physiologic function of vitamin K— blood clotting

The major function of vitamin K is to control the synthesis of prothrombin by the liver. Prothrombin is the material necessary to initiate the blood-clotting mechanism. Hence without vitamin K this whole vital process of blood clotting cannot go forward. Vitamin K acts either as an enzyme or coenzyme to control this important reaction. If liver damage, however, has led to hemorrhage, vitamin K would not be an effective therapeutic agent, since, in the absence of functioning liver tissue, vitamin K cannot act.

Clinical applications. A number of clinical situations, therefore, have important relationships with vitamin K:

1. *Obstetrics.* Since the intestinal tract of the newborn is sterile, the infant has no vitamin K during the first few days of life until normal bacterial flora develop. During this immediate postnatal period, therefore, hemorrhage may occur. This condition is called *hemorrhagic disease of the newborn.* Hence a preventive dose of vitamin K is usually given to the infant soon after delivery.

2. *Biliary disease and surgery.* Any condition of the biliary tract affecting the flow of bile will prevent the proper absorption of vitamin K. Therefore bleeding tendencies would be present in any obstruction of the gallbladder ducts or after surgical removal of the gallbladder.

3. *Intestinal disease.* Vitamin K deficiency is common in diseases such as celiac disease and sprue, which affect the absorbing surface

of the small intestine or in other diarrhea-type diseases such as ulcerative colitis that cause rapid loss of intestinal content. In such cases intravenous administration of vitamin K may be indicated.

4. *Antibiotic therapy.* Prolonged use of antibiotics may kill the normal bacterial flora of the intestine. A vitamin K deficiency may occur because this bacterial flora is one of the major sources of vitamin K.

5. *Anticoagulant therapy.* Use of heparin or bishydroxycoumarin (Dicumarol) in anti-coagulant therapy for coronary thrombosis or blood-clotting disease processes may counter-act the action of vitamin K. Dicumarol is almost like vitamin K in structure, so that it can act as an *antimetabolite,* or antagonist, to vitamin K because it gets in the way of the vitamin in the important liver reaction that forms prothrombin. Thus it prevents the normal reaction of vitamin K and prothrombin, which accounts for its anticoagulant action. In case of an overdose of the anti-coagulant, vitamin K may be used as an antidote.

Requirement of vitamin K

No requirement for vitamin K is stated, since a deficiency is unlikely except in the clinical situations indicated. An adequate amount is usually ensured for two reasons: (1) the intestinal bacteria constantly synthe-size a supply, and (2) the amount the body needs is apparently extremely small. The liver, however, must produce prothrombin, if vitamin K is to be effective.

Food sources of vitamin K

The items from which the natural vitamins were originally extracted—alfalfa and putri-fied sardine meal—are hardly human foods. However, small amounts of vitamin K may be found in green leafy vegetables, such as cab-bage, spinach, kale, and cauliflower. Lesser

Table 6-3. Summary of fat-soluble vitamins

VITAMIN	FUNCTION	RESULTS OF DEFICIENCY	FOOD SOURCES
A (retinol)	Vision cycle—adaptation to light and dark	Night blindness Xerophthalmia	Retinol (animal food): liver, egg yolk, cream, butter or fortified margerine, and whole milk
Provitamin A (carotene)	Tissue growth, especially skin and mucous mem-branes Toxic in large amounts	Susceptability to epithelial infection; changes in skin and membranes and in tooth formation	Carotene (plant foods): green and yellow vege-tables and fruits
D (calciferol)	Absorption of calcium and phosphorus Calcification of bones Toxic in large amounts	Rickets Faulty bone growth; poor tooth development	Fortified or irradiated milk Sunshine Fish oils
E (tocopherol)	Antioxidant—protection of materials that oxidize easily Normal growth Reproduction (in animals)	Protection of Vitamin A and unsaturated fatty acids Breakdown of red blood cells, anemia Sterility (in rats)	Vegetable oils Vegetable greens
K (menadione)	Normal blood clotting Toxic in large amounts	Bleeding tendencies, hemorrhagic disease	Green leafy vegetables Cheese Egg yolk Liver Intestinal bacteria synthesis—main source

amounts are found in tomatoes, cheese, egg yolk, and liver. However, the main source remains bacterial synthesis.

A summary for review of the fat-soluble vitamins is presented in Table 6-3.

WATER-SOLUBLE VITAMINS
VITAMIN C (ASCORBIC ACID)
Discovery

The history and recognition of vitamin C is associated with the search for a cause of the ancient hemorrhagic disease, *scurvy*. Documents describing this disease are as ancient as an Egyptian papyrus that dates from about 1500 B.C. The Greek father of medicine, Hippocrates, was concerned about scurvy. Crusaders of the thirteenth century observed the toll of the disease in their ranks. Jacques Cartier, exploring America in 1536, provided a clue to the cause of the disease when he wrote in his log that he cured his dying men "almost overnight simply by giving them a brew made from pine needles and bark." Officers of sailing vessels contributed further bits of information. In 1600 Captain Lancaster of the East India Company stated that he kept his crew hearty merely by "the addition of a mandatory three spoonfuls of lemon juice every morning." In 1753 the English naval surgeon, James Lind, concluded that the key must lie in a food factor in citrus fruit. The result was the official order for one ounce of lemon or lime juice daily in every British sailor's food ration. The name that stuck with the sailors was "limies."

Thus the ground was laid for the research of Norwegian scientists who in 1907 reproduced the disease in animals by feeding them a diet deficient in foods containing ascorbic acid. In 1928 an American scientist, while working on cell oxidation in adrenal tissue, isolated a substance from the adrenal glands and later from cabbage and from orange juice, which he believed to be a hexuronic acid derivative. He did not test it at that time for antiscorbutic effect. Finally, in 1932 Charles Glen King and W. A. Waugh, at the University of Pittsburgh, isolated and identified a hexuronic acid in lemon juice and demonstrated that it prevented or cured scurvy. The name *ascorbic acid* was given to the substance because of its antiscorbutic, or "antiscurvy," properties. At last the centuries-old scourge of scurvy had been defeated.

General chemical and physical nature of vitamin C

Vitamin C is soluble in water but not in fat. It is an unstable, easily oxidized acid. It can be destroyed by oxygen, alkalies, and high temperatures.

Interestingly, the chemical structure of vitamin C is almost identical with that for glucose. Glucose is the natural precursor of vitamin C in almost all of the animal and plant world. Plants make the conversion from glucose to produce the vitamin. Almost every animal species can also make ascorbic acid from glucose and hence does not require the vitamin in the diet. In the main, the only exceptions include man, monkeys, and guinea pigs, so these three species require vitamin C in the diet to prevent scurvy and bleeding tendencies.

Since vitamin C is easily destroyed by heat and exposure to air or to alkalies, vitamin C foods should be cooked in as little water as possible for a brief period of time and kept covered. Also soda should never be added as a coloring agent to foods during cooking. Vegetables should not be cut into small pieces until the time of cooking, since the more surface is exposed to air, the greater is the destruction of vitamin C. Also juices should not be left uncovered.

Absorption and storage of vitamin C

Vitamin C is easily absorbed from the small intestine. However, absorption is hindered by a lack of hydrochloric acid or by bleeding from the gastrointestinal tract.

Vitamin C is not stored in single tissue depots in the body as, for example, is vitamin A in the liver but is more generally distributed throughout the body tissues. Since it is not stored, it is important to get the daily requirement of vitamin C every day.

Sufficient vitamin C for needs in early infancy is present in breast milk. Cow's milk does not contain an adequate supply for the requirements of the human infant, so formulas must be supplemented with ascorbic acid.

Physiologic functions of vitamin C

Intercellular cement substance. The well-established basic role of vitamin C in human nutrition concerns the provision of an intercellular cementing substance that is necessary to build supportive tissue. Vitamin C is required to build and maintain bone matrix, cartilage, dentine, collagen, and connective and general body tissues. *Collagen* is a protein substance that exists in many tissues of the body, such as the white fibers of connective tissue. The term is derived from two Greek words that mean glue and to produce. Evidently, therefore, vitamin C must help provide the glue.

Blood vessel tissue particularly is weakened without the cementing substance of vitamin C to provide firm capillary walls. Therefore vitamin C deficiency is characterized by fragile, easily ruptured capillaries with resultant diffuse tissue bleeding. Clinical conditions include easy bruising, pinpoint hemorrhages of

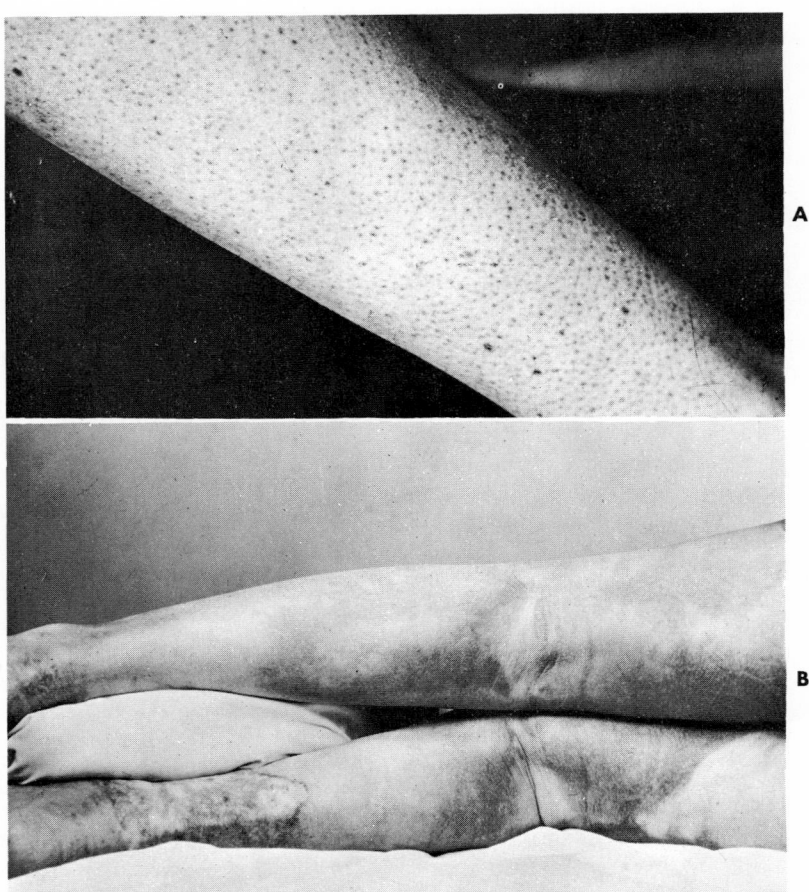

Fig. 6-2. A, Perifollicular hemorrhages of early scurvy. **B,** Ecchymosis of scurvy. (From Merck report, Rahway, N. J., May, 1956, Merck & Co., Inc.)

the skin, bone and joint hemorrages, easy bone fracture, poor wound healing, and soft, bleeding gums with loosened teeth (gingivitis). Some effects of vitamin C deficiency can be seen in Fig. 6-2.

General body metabolism. Broad activities in general metabolism include vitamin C. For example, more vitamin C is found in metabolically active tissues, such as those of the adrenal glands, brain, kidney, liver, and pancreas. Vitamin C is closely related to protein in tissue growth, building, and rebuilding and in cell metabolic processes. Vitamin C is especially required in periods of stress when adrenal hormones are produced in greater quantities.

Vitamin C also helps in the formation of hemoglobin and the development of red blood cells in two ways: (1) it aids in the absorption of iron, and (2) it influences the removal of iron from its transport complex so that it is available to tissues producing the hemoglobin.

Wound healing. For the extensive tissue rebuilding following surgery or injury, more vitamin C is needed. Especially where extensive tissue is involved, such as in severe burns, a great deal of vitamin C may be necessary.

Fevers and infections. Infections deplete tissue stores of vitamin C and necessitate additional intake. Optimum tissue stores of vitamin C help maintain resistance to infection. Just how large a therapeutic dose may be required to maintain this prevention of infection is not known. Much controversy continues concerning the effectiveness of massive doses of vitamin C in the prevention of the common cold. As yet there is not sufficient evidence to substantiate claims for such megadoses. The result is that vitamin C beyond the level at which tissue saturation is maintained is excreted in the urine. Hence one may only be producing expensive urine, rather than maintaining great therapeutic value. Fevers also deplete tissue stores of vitamin C, since they accompany infection and produce a catabolic effect on tissue.

Stress. Any body stress—injury, fracture,

Table 6-4. National Research Council daily allowances for vitamin C (revised 1973)

	AGE (YR.)	VITAMIN C (MG.)
Men		45
Women		45
Pregnancy		60
Lactation		60
Infants	0 to 1	35
Children	1 to 10	40
Boys	11 to 18	45
Girls	11 to 18	45

general illness, shock, or emotional stress—calls on tissue stores of vitamin C. This seems indicated by the large concentration of vitamin C in adrenal tissue.

Growth. Additional vitamin C is needed during growth periods, such as infancy and childhood, and during pregnancy to supply the demand for fetal growth and maternal tissues.

Requirement of vitamin C

The need for vitamin C varies with the state of the individual. However, for a person in health, the NRC's recommendation is 45 mg. daily for an adult. This allows some margin to cover variances of tissue demand. Table 6-4 gives the various allowances for different age groups.

Food sources of vitamin C

Because of the ease with which vitamin C can be oxidized, the handling, preparation, cooking, and processing of any food source should be considered in evaluating its contribution of the vitamin. Well-known sources include citrus fruit and tomatoes. Good additional sources include cabbage, sweet potatoes, white potatoes, and green and yellow vegetables. Other sources are seasonal, local, or regional foods such as strawberries, melons, chili peppers, green peppers, guavas, pineapples, chard, kale, turnip greens, broccoli, and asparagus.

Table 6-5. Summary of vitamin C (ascorbic acid)

FUNCTIONS	CLINICAL APPLICATIONS	FOOD SOURCES
Intercellular cement substance; firm capillary walls and collagen formation Helps prepare iron for absorption and release to tissues for red blood cell formation	Scurvy (deficiency disease) Sore gums Hemorrhages, especially around bones Tendency to bruise easily Stress reactions Growth periods Fevers and infections Wound healing; tissue formation Anemia	Citrus fruits, tomatoes, cabbage, potatoes, strawberries, melons, chili peppers, broccoli, chard, turnip greens, green peppers, asparagus

A summary of vitamin C and its role in the body is given in Table 6-5.

B-COMPLEX VITAMINS
Discovery

The story of the B vitamins is a compelling one because it is a history of many people dying of a puzzling age-old disease, which other people observed and sought to cure. Eventually a common everyday food was found to hold the answer. The paralyzing disease was beriberi. It had plagued the Orient for centuries and caused many persons in many lands to search for a solution. As early as 1882, a Japanese naval medical officer, Takaki, reported that he had cured beriberi in sailors of the Japanese navy by giving them less rice and more vegetables, barley, meat, and canned milk. Later, in 1897, a Dutch doctor working in a prison in the Netherlands East Indies reported that he could cure the disease simply by changing the diet from polished rice to cheap natural unmilled rice. His first theory was that the disease resulted from a poison in the polished rice that was neutralized by an antidote in the hulls. Although his theory was wrong, his observation was an important clue. One of his associates offered another clue in 1901 with the suggestion that the disease was caused by something vital that was present in the hulls but absent in the polished rice. Then, in 1911, Casimir Funk isolated the vital nitrogen compound in the hulls that he called a *vitamine* (p. 40).

The international search gained momentum in the field and the laboratory as the years continued. A dedicated American, R. R. Williams, in the foreign service as chief chemist of the Philippine Bureau of Science from 1909 to 1916, applied these new findings. He made tremendous strides in control and eradication of beriberi in infants by using extracts of rice polishings to feed them. In 1916 another American scientist, E. V. McCollum, then at the University of Wisconsin, named the food factor *water-soluble B* because he thought that it was a single vitamin. The widening search, however, proved that vitamin B was not a single substance but about a dozen vitamins and vitamin-related factors. The B-complex family of vitamins is now recognized.

The B vitamins, originally believed to be important only in preventing the deficiency diseases that led to their discovery, have now been identified with many important metabolic functions. They serve as vital control agents in many reactions as coenzymes in energy metabolism and tissue building and rebuilding.

In this discussion seven of these B vitamins will be considered:

GROUP I: CLASSIC DISEASE FACTORS
      Thiamine

Riboflavin
Niacin
GROUP II: MORE RECENTLY DISCOVERED
    COENZYME FACTORS
Pyridoxine
Pantothenic acid
GROUP III: BLOOD-FORMING FACTORS
Folic acid
Vitamin B_{12}

Classic disease factors

Thiamine (B_1)

DISCOVERY. The search of many persons for the cause of beriberi led eventually to a successful conclusion. In 1924 Dutch workers isolated and identified thiamine hydrochloride from rice polishings as the beriberi preventive material. Subsequently, in 1935, the American workers, Williams and his associates, finally synthesized thiamine. The answer to the puzzle of beriberi was found. The basic metabolic functions of thiamine were essentially clarified during the 1930s.

GENERAL CHEMICAL AND PHYSICAL NATURE OF THIAMINE. Thiamine is a water-soluble, fairly stable vitamin. However, it is destroyed by alkalies. Thiamine gets its name from its ringlike chemical structure.

ABSORPTION AND STORAGE OF THIAMINE. Thiamine is absorbed more readily in the acid medium of the first section of the intestine, the duodenum. In the lower duodenum the acidity of the food mass is counteracted by alkaline intestinal secretions. Thiamine is not stored in large quantities in the tissue. The tissue content is highly relative to increased metabolic demand, as in fever, increased muscular activity, pregnancy, and lactation. The tissue stores also depend on the adequacy of the diet and on its general composition. For example, carbohydrate increases the need for thiamine, whereas fat and protein spare thiamine.

PHYSIOLOGIC FUNCTIONS OF THIAMINE. The main function of thiamine as a control agent in metabolism is related to energy metabolism. It serves as a coenzyme in key reactions that produce energy from glucose or that convert glucose to fat for tissue storage. Thus the manifestations of beriberi (muscle weakness, gastrointestinal disturbances, and neuritis) can be traced to problems related to these basic functions of thiamine.

CLINICAL EFFECTS OF THIAMINE DEFICIENCY. If thiamine is not present in sufficient amounts to provide the key energizing control agent in the cells, clinical effects will be reflected in the gastrointestinal, nervous and cardiovascular systems.

1. *Gastrointestinal system.* Symptoms of deficiency include loss of appetite, indigestion, severe constipation, loss of muscle tone, and deficient hydrochloric acid secretion. The cells of the smooth muscles and the secretory glands are not able to receive sufficient energy from glucose. Hence they cannot do their proper work in digestion to provide still more glucose. Thus a vicious cycle ensues as deficiency continues.

2. *Nervous system.* The central nervous system is extremely dependent on glucose for energy to do its work. Without sufficient thiamine to help provide this need, nerve activity is diminished, and general apathy and fatigue result. If thiamine deficiency continues, damage or degeneration of myelin sheaths, the covering of nerve fibers composed of fatty material, causes increased nerve irritation, which produces pain and prickling or deadening sensations. Paralysis may gradually result if the process continues unchecked.

3. *Cardiovascular system.* If the thiamine deficiency persists, the heart muscle weakens and cardiac failure may result. Also smooth muscle of the vascular system may be involved, causing the blood vessels to dilate. As a result of this cardiac failure, edema (fluid accumulation in the tissues) may be observed in the lower legs (Fig. 6-3).

REQUIREMENT OF THIAMINE. The requirement for thiamine in human nutrition is usually stated in terms of carbohydrate and energy metabolism needs, as expressed in caloric intake. The average adult requires from 0.23 to 0.5 mg. per 1,000 calories. The NRC recommends, therefore, 0.5 mg. per 1,000 calories, with a minimum of 1 mg. for

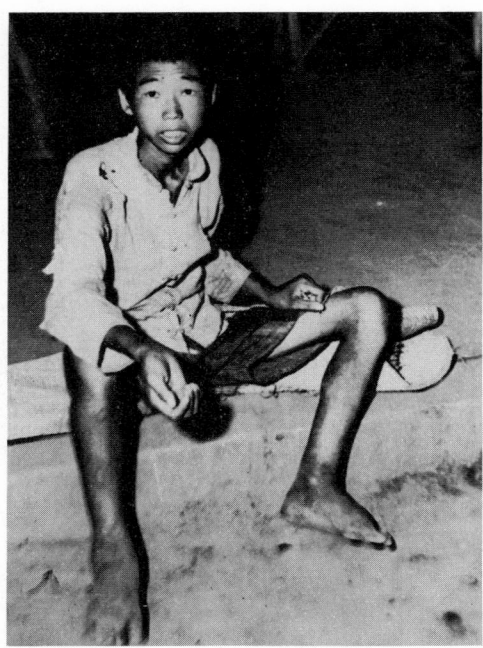

Fig. 6-3. Chinese refugee boy suffering from multiple nutritional deficiencies. Note the edema in feet and legs, characteristic of wet beriberi. (UNRRA photograph released by FAO.)

any intake between 1,000 and 2,000 calories. The correlations of thiamine with calories are shown in Table 6-6.

CLINICAL APPLICATIONS. Several important factors influence thiamine requirements and should be recognized in the care of patients. Increased thiamine is required in the following situations:

1. During growth periods of infancy, childhood, and especially adolescence
2. During pregnancy and lactation because of growth demands, increased metabolic rate, and energy requirements
3. Larger body size and tissue volume, with its greater cellular energy requirements
4. Fevers and infections because of increased cellular energy requirements
5. During old age or chronic illness at any age to avoid deficiencies

FOOD SOURCES OF THIAMINE. Good sources are lean pork, beef, liver, whole or enriched grains, and legumes. Eggs, fish, and a few vegetables are fair sources. Thiamine is less widely distributed in food than some of the other vitamins such as A and C, and the

Table 6-6. National Research Council allowances for thiamine in relation to calories (revised 1973)

	AGE (YR.)	CALORIES	THIAMINE (MG.)
Men	19 to 22	3,000	1.5
	23 to 50	2,700	1.4
	51+	2,400	1.2
Women	19 to 22	2,100	1.1
	23 to 50	2,000	1.0
	51+	1,800	1.0
Pregnancy		(+300)	(+0.3)
Lactation		(+500)	(+0.3)
Infants	0.0 to 0.5	Kg. × 117	0.3
	0.5 to 1.0	Kg. × 108	0.5
Children	1 to 3	1,300	0.7
	4 to 6	1,800	0.9
	7 to 10	2,400	1.2
Boys	11 to 14	2,800	1.4
	15 to 18	3,000	1.5
Girls	11 to 14	2,400	1.2
	15 to 18	2,100	1.1

quantities of thiamine in these foods are less than the naturally available quantities of vitamins A and C. Therefore a deficiency of thiamine is a distinct possibility in the average diet. This is especially true when calories are markedly curtailed as in some "crash" weight reduction programs and in some highly inadequate special therapeutic diets.

Riboflavin (B₂)

DISCOVERY. Although as early as 1897 a London chemist named Blythe had observed in milk whey a water-soluble pigment with peculiar yellow-green fluorescence, it was not until 1932 that riboflavin was actually discovered by workers in Germany. It was given the chemical group name *flavins* from the Latin word for *yellow*. Later, because the vitamin was found also to contain a sugar named *ribose*, the term *riboflavin* was officially adopted.

GENERAL CHEMICAL AND PHYSICAL NATURE OF RIBOFLAVIN. Riboflavin is a yellow-green fluorescent pigment that forms yellowish brown, needlelike crystals. It is water soluble and relatively stable to heat but is easily destroyed by light and irradiation. It is stable in acid media and is not easily oxidized. However, it is sensitive to strong alkalies.

ABSORPTION AND STORAGE OF RIBOFLAVIN. Absorption seems to occur readily in the upper section of the small intestine and is helped by combining with phosphorus in the intestinal mucosa. Storage is relatively limited, although some amounts are found in liver and kidney. Day-to-day tissue turnover needs must be supplied in the diet.

PHYSIOLOGIC FUNCTIONS OF RIBOFLAVIN

Coenzyme in protein metabolism. Just as thiamine is a partner in carbohydrate metabolism, riboflavin is a vital factor in protein metabolism. It acts as an important control agent, for example, in removing the nitrogen group (NH₂) from certain amino acids (p. 35). This process is called *deamination*. It also helps in other reactions involving amino acids in tissue-building functions.

Coenzyme in carbohydrate metabolism. Riboflavin is also a part of key enzyme systems in the production of energy in the cell. It acts as a control agent at several vital points. Thus riboflavin acts as a control agent in both energy production and tissue building and rebuilding.

CLINICAL EFFECTS OF RIBOFLAVIN DEFICIENCY. Manifestations of riboflavin deficiency center around tissue inflammation and breakdown.

1. *Wound aggravation.* Even minor tissue injuries easily become aggravated and do not heal easily.

2. *Mouth.* The lips become swollen and crack easily, and characteristic cracks develop at the corners of the mouth (cheilosis).

3. *Nose.* Cracks and irritations develop at the nasal angles.

4. *Tongue.* The tongue becomes swollen and reddened (glossitis).

5. *Eyes.* Extra blood vessels develop in the cornea (corneal vascularization), and the eyes burn, itch, and tear.

6. *Skin.* A scaly, greasy eruption may develop, especially in skin folds (seborrheic dermatitis).

Since nutritional deficiencies are usually multiple rather than single, riboflavin deficiencies seldom occur alone: they are likely to occur in conjunction with deficiencies of other B vitamins and of protein, with which they work.

REQUIREMENT OF RIBOFLAVIN. The body's requirement for riboflavin is related not so much to total caloric intake as it is to body size and metabolic and growth rate. All these are related to protein intake. Tissue stores of riboflavin are not maintained when the dietary intake is less than 1 mg. daily. About 1.3 mg. or more daily is necessary to maintain tissue reserves. For practical purposes the recommendations for riboflavin of the NRC are stated in terms of metabolic body size. The relation of riboflavin to protein intake is shown in Table 6-7.

CLINICAL APPLICATIONS. Attention should be given to certain risk groups or clinical situations in which riboflavin requirements

Table 6-7. National Research Council allowances for riboflavin in relation to protein (revised 1973)

	AGE (YR.)	PROTEIN (GM.)	RIBOFLAVIN (MG.)
Men	19 to 22	52	1.8
	23 to 50	56	1.6
	51+	56	1.5
Women	19 to 22	46	1.4
	23 to 50	46	1.2
	51+	46	1.1
Pregnancy		(+30)	(+0.3)
Lactation		(+20)	(+0.5)
Infants	0.0 to 0.5	Kg. × 2.2	0.4
	0.5 to 1.0	Kg. × 2.0	0.6
Children	1 to 3	23	0.8
	4 to 6	30	1.1
	7 to 10	36	1.2
Boys	11 to 14	44	1.5
	15 to 18	54	1.8
Girls	11 to 14	44	1.3
	15 to 18	48	1.4

may be increased and deficiencies more likely to occur:

1. Cheap, high-starch diets, which are limited in protein foods.

2. Gastrointestinal disorders or chronic illness. In these cases food intake is affected by such disorders as lack of appetite, poor food tolerance, or prolonged use of too limited a special diet.

3. Wound healing, as in surgical procedures, trauma, and burns, increases the need for riboflavin because of the increased need for protein for tissue building.

4. Periods of normal body stress such as growth periods, pregnancy, and lactation increase the need for riboflavin.

FOOD SOURCES OF RIBOFLAVIN. The most important food source is milk. One of the pigments in milk, *lactoflavin,* is the milk form of riboflavin. Each quart of milk contains 2 mg. of riboflavin, which is more than the daily requirement. Other good sources are the active organ meats, such as liver, kidney, and heart, and some vegetables. Cereals are poor sources unless they are enriched by commercial processing. This is now common practice, however.

Since riboflavin is water soluble and destroyed by light, the worth of food sources may depend on the manner of preparation. Considerable loss can occur in open, excess-water cooking. Therefore covered containers and limited water are indicated.

Niacin (nicotinic acid)

DISCOVERY. The discovery of niacin was also the result of man's age-old struggle with disease. In this case, the disease is pellegra, which is characterized by a typical dermatitis and often has fatal effects on the nervous system. The unraveling of the mystery of pellagra forms a classic example of the interworking of talents and techniques from medicine, public health, epidemiology, nutrition, and nursing.

Pellagra was first observed in eighteenth century Spain and Italy, where it was endemic in populations subsisting largely on corn. In the early 1900s Joseph Goldberger, a United States public health physician studying the problem of pellagra, worked in an orphanage in the rural southern United States. He noticed that, although the majority of the children in the orphanage had pellagra to some degree, a few of them did not. Finally, he discovered that the few who did not have pellagra were sneaking into the pantries at night and eating from the orphanage's limited supply of milk and meat. His investigations established the relationship of the disease to a certain food factor, which he called the P-P (pellagra preventive factor), or vitamin G. It was not until 1937, however, that Conrad Elvehjem, a scientist at the University of Wisconsin, definitely associated the vitamin with pellagra, by using it to cure a related disease, black tongue in dogs.

GENERAL CHEMICAL AND PHYSICAL NATURE OF NIACIN

Relation of niacin to tryptophan. As further study of the vitamin and pellagra continued, a new mystery developed concerning the relation of niacin to the essential amino acid, tryptophan. Again curious observations were made. Why was pellagra rare in some population groups whose diets were actually low in niacin, whereas it was common in other groups whose diets were higher in niacin? And why did milk that was low in niacin have the ability to cure or prevent pellagra? Why was pellagra so common in groups subsisting on diets high in corn?

At the University of Wisconsin in 1945, Willard Krehl and his associates finally made the key discovery: tryptophan can be used by the body to make niacin; it is a precursor of niacin. Here again was a vital link of a B vitamin with protein. Milk prevents pellagra because it is high in tryptophan. Almost exclusive use of corn contributes to pellagra because corn is low in tryptophan. Some populations subsisting on diets low in niacin may never have pellagra because they happen also to be consuming adequate amounts of tryptophan.

This tryptophan-niacin relationship led to the development of a unit of measure called *niacin equivalent.* In persons with average physiologic needs, approximately 60 mg. of tryptophan are calculated to produce 1 mg of niacin. Thus the amount of tryptophan was designated as a niacin equivalent. Dietary requirements are now usually given in terms of total milligrams of niacin and its equivalents.

Chemical nature of niacin. Two forms of niacin exist. Niacin (nicotinic acid) is easily converted to its amide form, *nicotinamide,* which is water soluble and stable to acid and heat.

PHYSIOLOGIC FUNCTION OF NIACIN—COENZYME IN TISSUE OXIDATION. Niacin is a partner with riboflavin as a control agent in the cell coenzyme system that converts protein to glucose and oxidizes glucose to release controlled energy.

CLINICAL EFFECTS OF NIACIN DEFICIENCY. Since niacin and riboflavin have close interrelationships as control agents in cell metabolism, clinical evidences of their deficiency closely parallel. When one is deficient, the other is usually deficient as well. General niacin deficiency is manifest as weakness, lassitude, loss of appetite, indigestion, and various skin eruptions. More specific symptoms include the skin and nervous system. Skin areas exposed to sunlight are especially affected, developing a dark, scaly dermatitis. If deficiency continues, the central nervous system becomes involved, and confusion, apathy, disorientation, and neuritis develop.

REQUIREMENT OF NIACIN. The minimum amount of niacin necessary for tissue stores is about 9 mg./1,000 calories. Many factors affect this requirement, including age and growth periods, pregnancy and lactation, illness, tissue trauma, or injury, body size, and physical activity. The NRC recommends 6.5 mg./1,000 calories and not less than 12 niacin equivalents at intakes of less than 2,000 calories. These recommendations are about 50% higher than the minimum requirements to provide a margin of safety to cover variances in individual needs. These recommendations also allow for the contribution of tryptophan in terms of niacin equivalents from the dietary protein sources. Table 6-8 indicates these niacin requirements throughout the life cycle.

FOOD SOURCES OF NIACIN. Meat is a major source of niacin. Peanuts, beans, and peas

Table 6-8. National Research Council allowances for niacin equivalents in relation to calories and protein (revised 1973)

	AGE (YR.)	CALORIES	PROTEIN (GM.)	NIACIN (MG. EQUIVALENT)
Men	19 to 22	3,000	52	20
	23 to 50	2,700	56	18
	51+	2,400	56	16
Women	19 to 22	2,100	46	14
	23 to 50	2,000	46	13
	51+	1,800	46	12
Pregnancy		(+300)	(+30)	(+2)
Lactation		(+500)	(+20)	(+4)
Infants	0.0 to 0.5	Kg. × 117	Kg. × 2.2	5
	0.5 to 1.0	Kg. × 108	Kg. × 2.0	8
Children	1 to 3	1,300	23	9
	4 to 6	1,800	30	12
	7 to 10	2,400	36	16
Boys	11 to 14	2,800	44	18
	15 to 18	3,000	48	20
Girls	11 to 14	2,400	44	16
	15 to 18	2,100	48	14

are also good sources. Enrichment makes good sources of all the grains. Otherwise corn and rice are poor because they are low in tryptophan; oats are also low in niacin; vegetables and fruits generally are poor sources.

More recently discovered coenzyme factors

Pyridoxine (B₆)

DISCOVERY. Continuing his work with B vitamins, Joseph Goldberger suggested in 1926 that the group of vitamins contained a factor that cured a particular dermatitis in rats. Because of this property, the factor was at first called *adermine*, or the rat anti-dermatitis factor. In 1939 the vitamin factor was synthesized and its chemical structure distinguished by having a pyridine ring so it was named *pyridoxine*. In 1944 the substance was isolated in animal tissue, and two companion products were synthesized. Later, in 1945, the companion phosphate forms were identified. Thus the activity of another B vitamin in metabolic enzyme reactions throughout the body was clearly and systematically brought into view.

GENERAL CHEMICAL AND PHYSICAL NATURE OF PYRIDOXINE. As with a number of the vitamins, pyridoxine is not a single vitamin, but a group of them. Three basic forms in the body undergo conversion to the phosphate form (B_6-PO_4), which is by far the most potent and active one. The term *pyridoxine*, or simply B_6, is usually used to indicate the entire group as well as one of its components. Pyridoxine is water soluble and heat stable. It is sensitive, however, to light and alkalies.

ABSORPTION AND STORAGE OF PYRIDOXINE. Pyridoxine is absorbed in the upper portion of the small intestine and is usually found throughout the body tissues, which is evidence of its many essential metabolic activities.

PHYSIOLOGIC FUNCTIONS OF PYRIDOXINE *Coenzyme in protein metabolism.* In its active phosphate forms (B_6-PO_4), pyridoxine is an active coenzyme control agent in many types of reactions governing the use of amino acids in the body:

1. Deamination and transamination are reactions that move nitrogen from one compound to another. Through these key re-

actions controlled by pyridoxine, new amino acids are formed, and carbon residues for energy are made available.

2. Pyridoxine helps in reactions producing *serotonin,* a potent blood vessel constrictor, which stimulates cerebral activity and brain metabolism.

3. Sulfur transfer reactions are controlled by pyridoxine. These reactions help produce new sulfur-containing amino acids from other precursor sulfur-containing amino acids.

4. Pyridoxine controls the formation of niacin from tryptophan.

5. Pyridoxine controls reactions that help incorporate two amino acids into *heme,* part of the essential protein core of hemoglobin.

6. Pyridoxine acts as an essential carrier for amino acids in absorption and entry into cells.

Coenzyme in carbohydrate and fat metabolism. To a lesser extent, pyridoxine also plays a part in carbohydrate metabolism, in helping to control reactions to produce energy. It also participates in the conversion of the essential fatty acid, linoleic acid, to another fatty acid. Thus pyridoxine plays a large controlling role in energy metabolism and in tissue building and rebuilding.

CLINICAL EFFECTS OF PYRIDOXINE DEFICIENCY. It is evident from such an impressive list of metabolic activities that pyridoxine may hold a key to a number of clinical problems.

Anemia. A hypochromic type of anemia has been observed in several patients even in the presence of a high serum iron level. The anemia was subsequently cured by supplying pyridoxine. This is related to its role in the formation of heme.

Central nervous system disturbances. Since pyridoxine is an important control agent in the formation of regulatory compounds in brain activity, it helps to control related neurologic conditions. In infants deprived of the vitamin there is an increasing hyperirritability that progresses to convulsive seizures. For example, a classic object lesson occurred in the early 1950s when infants fed a com-

mercial milk formula in which most of the pyridoxine content had been carelessly destroyed by high-temperature autoclaving subsequently had convulsions. The seizures ceased soon after a pyridoxine-supplemented formula was administered.

Physiologic demands of pregnancy. Pyridoxine deficiencies during pregnancy have been demonstrated. Fetal growth, in addition to creating greater maternal metabolic demands, also increases the pyridoxine requirement.

REQUIREMENT OF PYRIDOXINE. Although pyridoxine is a vital material, the amount required is small, so that a deficiency is unlikely. Since it is involved in amino acid metabolism, the need for pyridoxine varies with dietary protein intake. The NRC has set a recommended allowance of 2 mg. per day for adults to assure a safe margin for variances in individual needs.

FOOD SOURCES OF PYRIDOXINE. Pyridoxine is fairly widespread in foods, but many sources provide only small amounts. Good sources include yeast, wheat and corn, and liver, kidney and other meats. Milk, eggs, and vegetables have limited amounts.

Pantothenic acid

DISCOVERY. The presence of pantothenic acid in all forms of living things and the amount of it throughout body tissues accounts for the name given it by its discoverer. Pantothenic comes from a Greek word that means in every corner or from all sides: thus it is widespread in nature. It was isolated and synthesized by Roger J. Williams of the University of Texas between 1938 and 1940.

Intestinal bacteria synthesize considerable amounts of pantothenic acid. This, together with its widespread natural occurrence, makes deficiencies unlikely.

PHYSIOLOGIC FUNCTIONS OF PANTOTHENIC ACID—COENZYME ROLE IN METABOLISM. The basic coenzyme role of pantothenic acid in overall body metabolism relates to its structure. It is an essential constituent in its active form of a key enzyme (CoA). This activating agent is a control for a large number of key chemical reactions in the body. Some of these include the following:

1. Enzyme CoA forms the key compound active acetate, the important common molecule in the process of energy production in the cell (p. 15).

2. Active acetate is a precursor of cholesterol and, as such, of steroid hormones and vitamin D.

3. Active acetate prepares two key amino acids for the production of heme in hemoglobin synthesis.

4. Active acetate activates amino acids so that they may combine in key synthesis reactions.

REQUIREMENT OF PANTOTHENIC ACID. Studies indicate that adults show a daily excretion rate from 2.5 to 9.5 mg. Since pantothenic acid is so widespread in nature, a deficiency is not likely. Thus no recommendation has been made for it. The daily intake of pantothenic acid in an average American diet of from 2,500 to 3,000 calories is about 10 to 20 mg. Only under extreme metabolic stress is any deficiency likely.

FOOD SOURCES OF PANTOTHENIC ACID. Food sources of pantothenic acid are widespread. Yeast and metabolically active tissues such as liver and kidney are rich sources. Egg, especially the yolk, and skimmed milk contribute more. Fair additional sources include lean beef, cheese, legumes, broccoli, kale, sweet potatoes, and yellow corn.

Blood-forming factors

Folic acid (B₉)

DISCOVERY. The isolation and identification of folic acid are associated with laboratory studies of anemias and growth factors in animals. In 1945 folic acid was obtained from liver and finally synthesized. The vitamin was given the name *folic acid* from the Latin word *folium,* meaning leaf, because a major source of its extraction was dark green, leafy vegetables such as spinach. A reduced form of folic acid has since been discovered—*folinic acid.*

GENERAL CHEMICAL AND PHYSICAL NA-TURE OF FOLIC ACID. Folic acid is a substance made up of three acids, one of which is an amino acid. It is water soluble and forms yellow crystals. As with many of the B vitamins, folic acid is a group of related compounds that have similar actions in the body and is absorbed throughout the small intestine. Apparently some small amount may be synthesized by intestinal bacteria.

PHYSIOLOGIC FUNCTIONS OF FOLIC ACID. The basic metabolic role of folic acid is to act as a necessary coenzyme control agent in a number of key reactions that attach carbon to compounds. Some of these actions contribute to the following synthesis of key materials:

1. *The formation of purines.* Purines are part of a group of materials called *nucleoproteins* and are essential constituents of all living cells, especially nuclear material. As such they are involved in cell division and the transmission of inherited traits.

2. *The formation of thymine.* Thymine is also an essential nucleoprotein that forms a key part of DNA—the important material from the cell nucleus that transmits genetic characteristics.

3. *The formation of hemoglobin.* Folic acid helps form heme, the iron-containing part of the core protein in hemoglobin.

CLINICAL APPLICATIONS

Anemias. A deficiency of folic acid produces a nutritional megaloblastic anemia. Immature large red blood cells are formed, which are unable to carry oxygen properly. This condition has occurred in pregnancy and in infancy. Apparently fetal development increases the demand for folic acid. For this reason folic acid supplementation is usually recommended during pregnancy.

Sprue. Folic acid is effective in the treatment of sprue, a gastrointestinal disease characterized by intestinal lesions, malabsorption defects, diarrhea, anemia, and general malnutrition. Response to folic acid has been excellent. Both the blood-forming and the gastrointestinal defects have been corrected.

REQUIREMENT OF FOLIC ACID. Folic acid

requirements have been set by the NRC at 0.4 mg. daily for adults. During pregnancy twice this amount, 0.8 mg. daily, is recommended. For lactation, 0.6 mg. is needed. Stress such as disease and growth increases the requirement.

FOOD SOURCES OF FOLIC ACID. Liver, kidney, fresh green leafy vegetables, and asparagus are rich sources of folic acid. Fruit, milk, poultry, and eggs are relatively poor sources.

Cobalamin (B_{12})

DISCOVERY. The discovery of vitamin B_{12} is associated with the search for the specific agent in the control of pernicious anemia. At first the disease was thought to be associated with a deficiency of folic acid. However, although folic acid helped in initial red blood cell regeneration in patients with pernicious anemia, it was not permanently effective and did not control the nerve problems associated with the disease. When folic acid was found to be lacking in full effectiveness, the search continued for the remaining piece in the disease puzzle.

In 1948 two groups of workers, one in America and one in England, crystallized a red compound from liver, which they numbered vitamin B_{12}. In the same year, it was clearly shown that this new vitamin could control both the blood-forming defect and the neurologic involvement in pernicious anemia. Soon afterward, a method was discovered for producing the vitamin through a process of fermentation with microorganisms: this remains the main source of commercial supply today. The vitamin was named *cobalamin* because at the core of its structure is a single red atom of cobalt.

GENERAL CHEMICAL AND PHYSICAL NATURE OF VITAMIN B_{12}. Thus continued study of the vitamin's chemistry revealed this unique nature, with cobalt at the center. It is a complex red crystalline compound of high molecular weight. It occurs in a protein complex in foods, so that its food sources are almost entirely of animal origin. The ultimate source, however, might be designated as microorganisms in the gastrointestinal tract of herbivorous animals. Such microorganisms are found in large amounts in the rumen (first stomach, containing cud) of cows. Apparently some synthesis occurs in the intestinal bacteria of man also, although the amount supplied from this source is not known.

ABSORPTION OF VITAMIN B_{12}. Two gastric secretions are necessary to prepare vitamin B_{12} for absorption. It is the only human nutrient known to require exposure to stomach secretions before it can be absorbed. Hydrochloric acid in the stomach prepares the vitamin, and in this free form it is then able to combine with an *intrinsic factor*, which is also a component of the gastric secretions: it is a mucoprotein enzyme, which is secreted by glands in the stomach. This combined material of B_{12} and intrinsic factor then allows B_{12} to be absorbed. Thus the defect in pernicious anemia turns out to be an absorption defect because of the lack of the vital carrier intrinsic factor to absorb B_{12}.

STORAGE OF VITAMIN B_{12}. Vitamin B_{12} is stored in active body tissues. Organs holding the greatest amounts are the liver, kidney, heart, muscle, pancreas, testes, brain, blood, spleen, and bone marrow. This widespread storage indicates significant metabolic functions of the vitamin in the body. Even these amounts stored are very minute, but because they are so vital the body apparently holds tenaciously to its small supply, and the stores are very slowly depleted. For example, a characteristic type of anemia caused by loss of gastric secretions necessary for absorption of vitamin B_{12} develops after surgical removal of the stomach: this is called a postgastrectomy anemia. Because of the extensive storage of vitamin B_{12}, this anemia does not become apparent until three to five years after the surgery.

PHYSIOLOGIC FUNCTIONS OF VITAMIN B_{12}

Coenzyme in protein metabolism. Vitamin B_{12} is closely related to protein metabolism, and its requirement increases as protein intake increases. It acts as an important coenzyme control agent in the synthesis of nucleic acid and other vital proteins in the cell.

Table 6-9. Summary of selected B-complex vitamins*

VITAMIN	FUNCTION	RESULTS OF DEFICIENCY	FOOD SOURCES
Thiamine (B_1)	Normal growth Coenzyme in carbohydrate metabolism; normal function of heart, nerves, and muscle	Beriberi GI: Loss of appetite, gastric distress, indigestion, deficient hydrochloric acid CNS: Fatigue, neuritis, paralysis CV: Heart failure, edema of legs especially	Pork, beef, liver, whole or enriched grains, legumes
Riboflavin (B_2)	Normal growth and vigor Coenzyme in protein and energy metabolism	Ariboflavinosis Wound aggravation, cracks at corners of mouth, glossitis (smoothness of tongue), eye irritation and sensitivity to light, skin eruptions	Milk, liver, enriched cereals
Niacin (nicotinic acid)— precursor: tryptophan	Coenzyme in energy production Normal growth, health of skin, normal activity of stomach, intestines, and nervous system	Pellagra Weakness, lack of energy, and loss of appetite Skin: scaly dermatitis CNS: neuritis, confusion	Meat, peanuts, enriched grains
Pyridoxine (B_6)	Coenzyme in amino acid metabolism: protein synthesis, heme formation, brain activity Carrier for amino acid absorption	Anemia CNS: hyperirritability, convulsions, neuritis Pregnancy: anemia	Wheat, corn, meat, liver
Pantothenic acid	Coenzyme in formation of active acetate: fat, cholesterol, and heme formation and amino acid activation	Unlikely due to widespread occurrence and intestinal bacteria synthesis	Liver, eggs, milk, beef, cheese, legumes, broccoli, kale, sweet potatoes, yellow corn Intestinal bacteria synthesis
Folic acid	Growth and development of red blood cells	Certain types of anemia; megaloblastic (large immature red blood cells)	Liver, green leafy vegetables, asparagus, eggs
Cobalamin (B_{12})	Normal red blood cell formation, nerve function, and growth	Pernicious anemia (B_{12} is necessary extrinsic factor, which combines with intrinsic factor of gastric secretions for absorption)	Liver, meats, milk, eggs, cheese

*Key: GI, gastrointestinal; CNS, central nervous system; CV, cardiovascular.

Formation of red blood cells. The well-established role of vitamin B_{12} in formation of red blood cells and, therefore, in the control of pernicious anemia has two relationships: (1) the absorption defect related to the necessity for intrinsic factor to ensure getting B_{12} into the system and (2) an indirect effect on red blood cell formation through activation of folic acid coenzymes. Within the developing red blood cell, building activities that are dependent on folic acid for control are indirectly controlled by vitamin B_{12}. Perhaps this link with folic acid explains why folic acid may control pernicious anemia only temporarily and why folic acid must be supplemented by B_{12} if the pernicious anemia is to be corrected over a long period.

CLINICAL APPLICATIONS

Pernicious anemia. The discovery of B_{12} as a specific controlling factor in pernicious anemia was a great clinical breakthrough. Now a patient with this defect can be given from 15 to 30 mcg. of B_{12} daily in intramuscular injections during a relapse and can then be maintained afterward by an injection of about 30 mcg. every 30 days.

Sprue. Like folic acid, vitamin B_{12} has been effective in the treatment of the intestinal disease sprue. However, it seems most effective when used in conjunction with folic acid.

Therefore its role may again be indirect, in that it facilitates the action of folic acid.

REQUIREMENT OF VITAMIN B_{12}. The amount of B_{12} needed for normal human metabolism appears to be very small. Daily minimum requirements have been from 0.6 to 1.2 mcg., with a range upward to approximately 2.8 mcg. The ordinary diet easily provides this much and more. For example, one cup of milk, one egg, and four ounces of meat provide 2.4 mcg. of vitamin B_{12}. The NRC recommends a daily intake of 3 mcg. for adults. This amount allows a margin of safety to cover a variety of individual needs, absorption, and body stores.

FOOD SOURCES OF VITAMIN B_{12}. Vitamin B_{12} is supplied almost entirely by animal foods. The richest sources are liver, kidney, and lean meat. Milk, eggs, and cheese supply additional amounts. A natural dietary deficiency is rare. The only reported deficiencies (general nervous symptoms, sore mouth and tongue, and amenorrhea) have come from a group of true vegetarians called *Vegans*, who live in Great Britain, and from other vegetarian groups in India and America.

A summary of these selected B-complex vitamins is given in Table 6-9 for study and review.

7 MINERALS: THE PROBLEM OF REGULATION AND CONTROL

One remaining group of nutrients is essential to man—the minerals. They also act in the body as control agents and contribute to energy production and body building and maintenance.

Minerals are inorganic elements widely distributed in nature, many of which have vital roles in metabolism. Their metabolic roles are as varied as are the minerals themselves. These substances, which appear so inert in comparison with the complex organic vitamin compounds, fulfill an impressive variety of metabolic functions: building, activating, regulating, transmitting, and controlling. For example, ionized sodium and potassium exercise all-important control over shifts in body water. Dynamic calcium and phosphorus provide structure for the framework of the body. Oxygen-hungry iron gives a core to heme in hemoglobin. Brilliant red cobalt is the atom at the core of vitamin B_{12}. Iodine is the necessary constituent of thyroid hormone, which in turn controls the overall rate of body metabolism. Thus, far from being static, inert body materials, the minerals are active participants, helping to control many of the overall metabolic processes of the body.

Minerals differ from the vitamins also in that varying amounts are required in the body to perform their many functions, whereas vitamins occur in extremely small amounts in the body, as has been shown. For example, calcium forms a relatively large amount of the body weight—about 2%. Most of this calcium is in the skeletal tissue. An adult weighing 150 pounds has about 3 pounds of calcium in the body. On the other hand, iron is present in small amounts. This same adult has only about 3 gm. (about 1/10 ounce) of iron in the body.

Thus the body minerals are usually classified into two main groups according to the amount used in the body for various necessary control and building functions. The *major minerals* are those present in larger amounts. The *trace minerals* are those present in smaller amounts. Other minerals present in the body in small amounts have functions that are not entirely clear. These three groups of minerals include the following:

GROUP I: MAJOR MINERALS
Calcium (Ca)
Magnesium (Mg)
Sodium (Na)
Potassium (K)
Phosphorus (P)
Sulfur (S)
Chlorine (Cl)

GROUP II: TRACE MINERALS
Iron (Fe)
Copper (Cu)
Iodine (I)

Manganese (Mn)
Cobalt (Co)
Zinc (Zn)
Molybdenum (Mo)
GROUP III: FUNCTION UNKNOWN
Fluorine (F)
Aluminum (Al)
Boron (B)
Selenium (Se)
Cadmium (Cd)
Chromium (Cr)
Vanadium (V)

Seven of the minerals most commonly encountered in general nutritional care of patients are discussed here and summarized in Table 7-1, p. 79.

Consider these basic questions in the study of mineral control agents:

1. Where is the mineral located in the body?

2. What does it do? Where and how does it act?

3. What is the clinical significance of the mineral? What are some of its relationships to health and disease?

4. How much is required in food, and what are these sources?

MAJOR MINERALS
Calcium

Of all the minerals in the human body, calcium is present in by far the largest amount. The total amount of body calcium is in constant balance with food sources of calcium from the outside as well as with tissue calcium within the body among its various parts. A number of balanced mechanisms are constantly at work to maintain these levels within normal ranges. The balance concept can be applied, therefore, at three basic levels to understand better the vital role of calcium in body metabolism: (1) the intake-absorption-output balance, (2) the bone-blood balance, and (3) the calcium-phosphorus blood serum balance.

Intake-absorption-output balance. The first level at which body calcium is controlled is the balance between the amount of dietary calcium taken in daily, the amount that is absorbed, and the amount that leaves the body.

CALCIUM INTAKE. The average adult American diet contains about 700 to 1,200 mg. of calcium. Most of this comes from dairy products and some from green leafy vegetables and grains. For example, each of the following food items contributes about 300 mg. of calcium:

1 cup milk
1 ounce cheese
1 cup dark greens (except spinach, chard, beet greens)
1 serving oysters
1 serving salmon (with bones)
2 servings ice cream

About 300 mg. of calcium are contained in the remainder of the diet. Each quart of milk contains about 1 gm. of calcium.

ABSORPTION OF CALCIUM. Not all this diet calcium gets absorbed, however, because absorption is affected by a number of factors. Generally speaking, only about 10% to 30% of the total calcium taken in is absorbed. The remaining 70% to 90% is unabsorbed and carried out with the feces. Compare the following factors that increase or decrease the amount of calcium absorbed. Obviously the state of the body and its general need for calcium will play a large role.

Factors increasing absorption

1. *Vitamin D.* An optimum amount of this control agent is necessary for absorption of calcium.

2. *Body need.* During periods of growth and when body stores are depleted, more calcium is absorbed.

3. *Calcium level in the body fluids.* When these levels are low, more calcium will be absorbed.

4. *Acidity.* Generally, a lower pH (higher acidity) favors solubility of calcium and, consequently, its absorption. For this reason a dietary protein increase helps absorb calcium by providing amino acids to contribute the intestinal acidity. Lactose (milk sugar) also aids absorption of calcium by providing lactic acid. It is interesting that the only source of

lactose in our diet is milk, which also contributes the major amount of calcium—a fortunate combination.

Factors decreasing absorption

1. *Vitamin D.* A deficiency hinders absorption.

2. *Binders.* Certain substances combine with calcium and prevent its absorption. Fatty acids, from excess fat in the diet or from poor absorption of fats, combine with the free calcium to form insoluble calcium soaps—a process called *saponification.* Other binding agents include oxalic acid, as in spinach, and phytic acid, which is found in the outer hulls of many cereal grains, especially wheat. These materials produce calcium oxalate and calcium phytate, both insoluble compounds, and thus prevent the absorption of calcium.

3. *Alkalinity.* Calcium is insoluble in an alkaline medium and therefore is poorly absorbed.

CALCIUM OUTPUT. The overall body calcium balance is maintained first, therefore, at the point of absorption. A large unabsorbed amount, varying according to body need, is excreted in the feces. A small amount of calcium may be excreted in the urine, about 200 mg. daily. This urine excretion depends on the levels of calcium in the body fluid.

Bone-blood balance. The second major level of calcium balance in the body is between the calcium in the bones and the calcium in blood.

CALCIUM IN THE BONES. In health the body maintains a constant turnover of the calcium in the bone tissue, which is the major site of calcium storage. However, this is not a static storage. Like a checking account at the bank in which the client must maintain a constant minimum balance, regular deposits and withdrawals of money occur; despite this continual movement of money, a definite balance is always maintained in the account. In the same manner calcium is constantly being deposited in bone tissue and withdrawn for various uses, causing constant turnover. All the while a dynamic equilibrium is maintained. In certain conditions or diseases, the withdrawals may exceed the deposits,

and a state of calcium imbalance occurs. Conditions such as immobility because of a body cast or diseases such as osteoporosis would cause such excess withdrawals. By far the largest amount of body calcium is in the bone tissue with some in the teeth: this calcium in bone is about 99% of that in the body.

CALCIUM IN THE BLOOD. The remaining small amount of calcium, about 1% of the total, is circulating in the blood and body fluids. Although this is a relatively small amount, it plays a vital role in controlling body functions. This calcium in the blood is in two main forms:

1. *Bound calcium.* About half the calcium in the blood is bound in the plasma proteins and hence is not free or diffusable—able to move about or to enter into other activities. A small amount of the bound calcium is a part of other complexes, such as citrate.

2. *Free ionized calcium.* These are free particles of calcium, carrying electric charges and hence in an active form, freely moving about and diffusing through membranes to control a number of body functions, including blood clotting, transmission of nerve impulses, muscle contraction and relaxation, membrane permeability, and activation of enzymes. This is a good illustration of a small amount of a nutrient doing a great deal of metabolic work because it is activated.

Calcium-phosphorus serum balance. A third level of calcium balance is that which calcium maintains with phosphorus in the blood serum. The amounts of these minerals in the blood serum are normally maintained in a definite relationship because of their relative solubility. This relationship is called the *serum calcium to phosphorus ratio.* This ratio is the product (solubility product) of calcium × phosphorus, expressed in milligrams of each mineral per 100 ml. of serum.*

---

*Since the serum level of calcium is normally 10 mg./100 ml. and that of phosphorus is normally 4 mg./100 ml. in adults (5 mg./100 ml. in children), the normal calcium to phosphorus ratios are $10 \times 4 = 40$ for adults and $10 \times 5 = 50$ for children. Briefly expressed, then, the ratios are Ca:P = 40 for the adult and Ca:P = 50 for the child.

This is an important ratio between these two minerals in the blood. Thus any situation that causes an increase in the phosphorus level would cause a resulting decrease in the calcium level. Such a condition of decreased calcium brings on tetany-like responses. Tetany is a condition marked by spastic contractions of the muscles and by muscular pain. It is caused by a decrease in serum calcium because calcium is necessary for normal muscular contraction.

Control agents for calcium balance. These three vital levels of calcium balance in the body are carefully controlled by two basic control agents working together: *parathyroid hormone (PH)* and *vitamin D*. The cooperative action of these two factors is a good example of *synergistic* behavior of metabolic controls. Synergism is an important biologic concept. It is the cooperative action of two or more factors that in acting together produce a total effect greater than the sum of their separate effects. Many biologic and physiologic interactions provide examples of synergism. Consider the interdependent relationship of these two control agents.

PARATHYROID HORMONE. The parathyroid gland is particularly sensitive to changes in the circulating plasma level of free ionized calcium. When this level drops, the parathyroid gland releases its hormone, which acts in three ways to restore the normal calcium level:

1. It stimulates the intestinal mucosa to increase the absorption of calcium.

2. It withdraws more calcium rapidly from the bone compartment.

3. It causes the kidney to excrete more phosphate.

These combined activities then restore calcium and phosphorus to their correctly balanced ratio in the blood.

VITAMIN D. Vitamin D mainly controls the absorption of calcium. However, it also affects the deposit of calcium and phosphorus in bone tissue. Thus these two agents balance

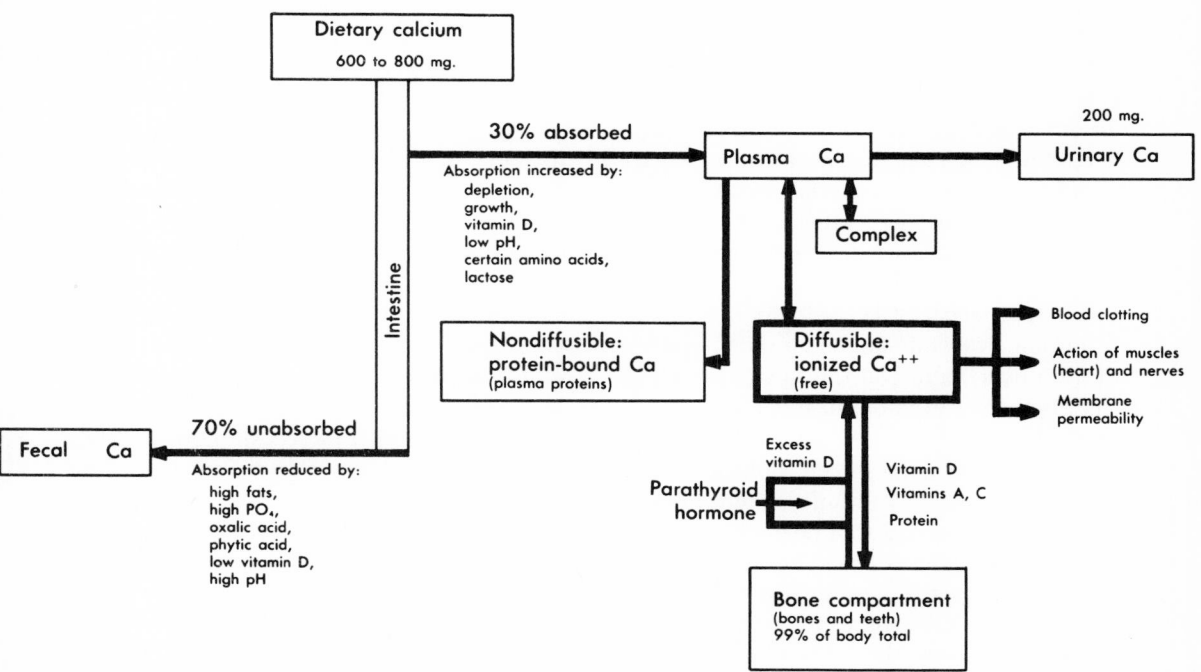

Fig. 7-1. Calcium metabolism. Note the relative distribution of calcium in the body.

each other, with vitamin D acting more to control calcium absorption and bone deposit, and parathyroid hormone acting more to control calcium withdrawal from bone and kidney excretion of the partner phosphorus.

The overall relationship of the various factors involved in these vital calcium balances in the body may be visualized in Fig. 7-1.

Physiologic functions of calcium

BONE AND TEETH FORMATION. The physiologic function of 99% of the calcium in the body is to build and maintain the skeletal tissue. This is done by a constant balance between depositing the calcium in bone and withdrawing it. Calcium phosphate deposits are also important to *tooth formation*. As the teeth develop, special cells in the gum form the tooth. The mineral exchange continues as in the bone but mainly in the dentine and cementum. Little occurs in the enamel, once the tooth is formed.

BLOOD CLOTTING. The remaining 1% of the body's calcium contributes to vital physiologic functions such as blood clotting. Calcium ions help to bond and stabilize the fibrin threads needed for development of the clotting process.

MUSCLE CONTRACTION AND RELAXATION. Ionized serum calcium helps to initiate muscle contraction. Then, as the calcium particles are rebound to the muscle fibers, they bring about contraction. This vital function of calcium in the contraction-relaxation cycle of the heart muscle is significant.

NERVE TRANSMISSION. Calcium is required for normal transmission of nerve impulses. Calcium ions operate at the tips of the many nerve branches and help to excite the muscle fiber.

CELL WALL PERMEABILITY. Ionized calcium controls the passage of fluid through the cell walls by affecting cell wall permeability.

ENZYME ACTIVATION. Calcium ions are important activators of specific enzymes, especially the one that releases energy for muscle contraction. They play a similar role with other enzymes, including lipase, which digests fat, and with some members of the protein-splitting enzyme system.

Clinical application

TETANY. As noted, any decrease in the level of ionized serum calcium causes muscular spasms and pain. This condition is called *tetany* from a Greek word that means to stretch. Sometimes a newborn infant fed undiluted cow's milk may develop such tetany-like muscle spasms because of the intake of excess phosphorus in relation to calcium in the cow's milk. The ratio of phosphorus to calcium in cow's milk is greater than in human milk, and the kidneys of these infants cannot clear this phosphate load. Phosphorus, therefore, accumulates in the blood. This rise in blood phosphorus causes a decrease in the serum calcium, which in turn, causes the typical muscle spasms of tetany. This is one of the reasons that milk fed to a newborn is diluted in formula preparation.

RICKETS. A deficiency of vitamin D causes rickets. When inadequate calcium and phosphorus are absorbed, proper bone formation cannot take place.

RENAL CALCULI. By far the majority of kidney stones are composed of calcium. A predisposing factor for the formation of kidney stones may be an increase in the amount of calcium that must be excreted in the urine as calcium is mobilized, or withdrawn from the bone. Thus conditions that cause excess withdrawal and excretion of calcium may lead to the formation of calcium stones. Such a condition is prolonged immobilization of the body because normal muscle tension on the bones is necessary for calcium balance. Such a state would be caused by a full body cast, for example, which would immobilize the body for a long period. In such situations dietary calcium should be adequate but should not exceed the usual daily allowances. If kidney stones have already occurred, the amount of calcium in the diet should be somewhat reduced.

Requirement of calcium. The NRC's recommended allowances for calcium are 800 mg. daily for men and women, increased to

1.2 gm. during pregnancy and lactation. Infants younger than 1 year should have 360 to 540 mg., and children should have from 800 to 1,200 mg. daily.

Food sources of calcium. Dairy products supply the bulk of dietary calcium: milk and cheese give large amounts. Secondary sources contribute much smaller quantities: these include egg yolk, green leafy vegetables, legumes, nuts, and whole grains.

Phosphorus

The human body contains about half as much phosphorus as it does calcium. An adult weighing 150 pounds would have about 1.5 pounds of phosphorus in the body to 3 pounds of calcium.

Phosphorus has often been called the *metabolic twin* of calcium. It is involved with calcium in many body functions in human nutrition, and its balance in the body is controlled by the same agents.

Intake-absorption-output balance. The first level at which body phosphorus is controlled, as with its companion mineral, calcium, is the balance between the amount eaten in the diet, the amount of this absorbed, and the amount that leaves the body.

PHOSPHORUS INTAKE. The ideal diet ratio of phosphorus to calcium is about 1:1, especially during pregnancy, lactation, and childhood. Adults may require a little more phosphorus to calcium for general maintenance. The average adult diet contains about 1 gm. of phosphorus, from 900 to 1,200 mg.

ABSORPTION OF PHOSPHORUS. The same factors that control calcium absorption also determine the amount of phosphorus absorbed. These factors include vitamin D, the diet ratio with calcium, and the amount of body need. For example, during growth or periods of illness or body depletion, more phosphorus is absorbed. Phosphorus differs from calcium, however, in that much more of the phosphorus taken in is absorbed. About 70% of the dietary phosphorus is absorbed, usually much more than with calcium, perhaps because of the greater meta-bolic demand for phosphorus in general cell work.

PHOSPHORUS OUTPUT. The remaining 30% of the dietary phosphorus is unabsorbed and passes out of the body in the feces. Unlike calcium control, however, the main control agent of the body balance of phosphorus is the kidney. The urine output of phosphorus is higher than with calcium. In health on an average diet an adult usually excretes about 600 to 1,000 mg. of phosphorus daily compared with about 200 mg. of calcium. It can reabsorb more or less phosphorus according to blood phosphorous level needs. When the diet is deficient in phosphorus, for example, the kidney will reabsorb more and return it to the blood. If the blood level rises, it will excrete more. This variable excretion of phosphorus according to need is under the control of the parathyroid hormone.

Bone-blood-cell balance. The second main level of phosphorus balance is inside the body with a constant interchange between the amount combined with calcium in the bones and teeth, the amount circulating in the blood in ratio with calcium, and the amount in the cells helping to produce energy.

PHOSPHORUS IN THE BONES. About 80% of the body's phosphorus is located in the bones and teeth combined with calcium as calcium phosphate. This bone phosphorus is in a constant turnover balance with the rest of the body tissue.

PHOSPHORUS IN THE BLOOD. The remaining 20% of body phosphorus is in the circulating body fluids—the blood and cell fluids. This serum phosphorus exists in the blood in direct relationship to calcium (p. 66), under the same close control of the parathyroid hormone (PH). In the blood phosphorus helps in many key metabolic functions, some of which will be described.

PHOSPHORUS IN THE CELLS. Phosphorus is a vital material in cell metabolism, especially in energy production.

Control agents for phosphorus balance. Since calcium and phosphorus work so closely together, as has been seen, this inner balance

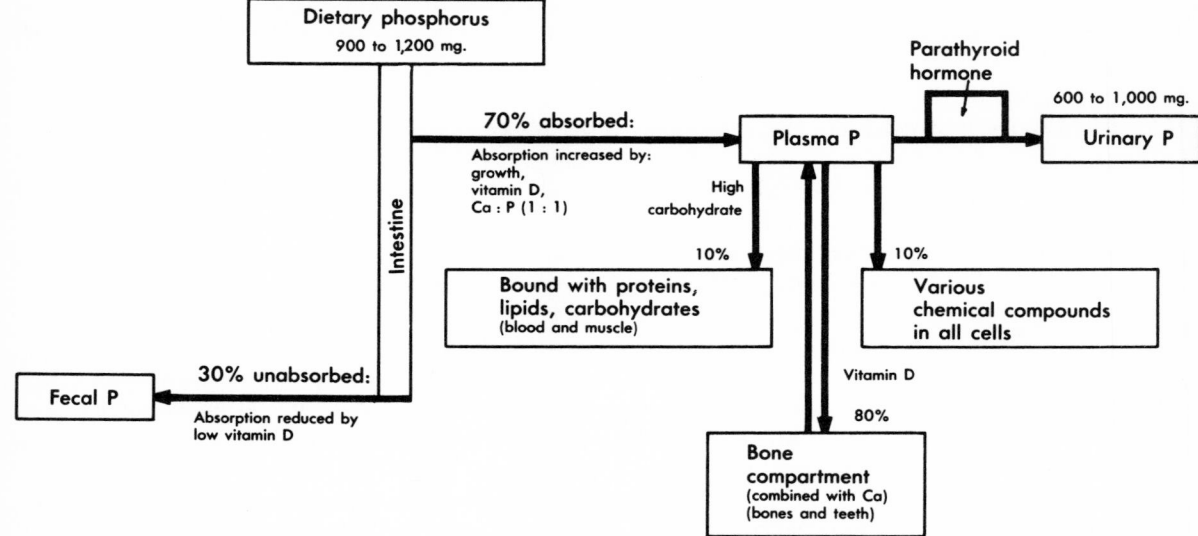

Fig. 7-2. Relative distribution and interchange of phosphorus in the body.

of phosphorus is under the direct control of the same two agents controlling calcium balance—vitamin D and parathyroid hormone.

These various balance relationships of phosphorus may be visualized in Fig. 7-2.

Physiologic functions of phosphorus. Eighty percent of the body phosphorus contributes to mineralization of bones and teeth. As a component of calcium phosphate, it is constantly being deposited and reabsorbed in the dynamic process of bone formation.

The remaining 20% of body phosphorus is intimately involved in overall human metabolism, playing several vital roles.

ABSORPTION OF GLUCOSE AND GLYCEROL. By combining with phosphorus, glucose and glycerol are absorbed more easily from the intestine.

TRANSPORT OF FAT. Fats combine with phosphorus as phospholipids to help provide a transport form for fat in the blood.

ENERGY METABOLISM. Phosphorus is an essential part of key cell compounds, especially for glucose oxidation and finally energy production. A key power compound containing high-energy phosphate bonds is ATP, adenosine triphosphate (p. 16). This is the unique chemical compound in the cell that controls energy production and release.

BUFFER SYSTEM. The phosphate buffer system helps to control acid-base balance in the blood.

• • •

It is evident that such extensive metabolic functions would have much application in periods of growth and high metabolic body demands.

Requirement of phosphorus. During growth, pregnancy, and lactation, the ideal diet ratio of phosphorus to calcium is 1:1. In ordinary adult life the intake of phosphorus to calcium should be a bit more, from 1 to 1.5 times that of calcium. In general, since these two minerals are found in the same food sources, if calcium needs are met, adequate phosphorus will be assured.

The new 1973 NRC dietary allowances list a specific quantitative recommendation for phosphorus. It indicates that an allowance equal to that of calcium will meet the needs of most ages, except infancy. For the infant the proportion of phosphorus should be somewhat lower than that of calcium.

Food sources of phosphorus. Milk and milk products are the most significant sources of phosphorus, as they are for calcium. However, because the role of phosphorus in cell metabolism is great, an additional food source of phosphorus is lean meat.

Sodium

Sodium is crucially important to many metabolic activities. Thus it is one of the more plentiful major minerals in the body. A person weighing 154 pounds would have about 4 ounces or so in his body. About one third of this body sodium is in the skeleton as inorganic bound material. The remaining two thirds is free ionized sodium. It is a major electrolyte in the body fluids outside the cells. The body's sodium balance may also be viewed in its intake-absorption-output balance mechanisms.

Intake-absorption-output balance

SODIUM INTAKE. A wide variance occurs in the amount of sodium ingested in the diet. It may range from about 4 gm. of sodium in the average 10 gm. of table salt consumed daily to an amount much higher in a high salt user. In the diet of persons who have a "heavy hand with the salt shaker," the amount may be twice the average intake or more. In any case, the average use of sodium in the adult diet is about ten times the amount the body actually requires for metabolic balance. Salt is an acquired taste, however, and in high salt users the intake can be large.

ABSORPTION OF SODIUM. Most of the sodium taken into the body is absorbed—about 95% of it. Thus the body must maintain its body balance of sodium elsewhere. It does this through kidney excretion. In abnormal states such as diarrhea much larger amounts of sodium go through the body and are lost in the multiple stools.

SODIUM OUTPUT. The main route of body sodium output is under control of the kidneys, which regulate about 95% of the body's sodium excretion. The remaining 5% of sodium excreted in the daily diet would, therefore, be excreted normally in the feces. The output of sodium by the kidneys is under the control of a major hormone, *aldosterone*, a sodium-conserving hormone from the adrenal gland. In response to loss of sodium or water, the body responds by secreting more aldosterone to reabsorb more sodium and hence more water.

Physiologic functions of sodium. The major body sodium is in the form of free ionized particles circulating in the body fluids. As such it controls a number of basic body functions:

1. *Water balance.* Ionized sodium is the major cation (a particle—ion—carrying a positive electrical charge) of the fluid outside the cell. As such it has a major role in controlling the internal shifts of water throughout the body. (See p. 80.) In this capacity, sodium would have a large effect on the cardiovascular system and water circulation. For example, in disease states such as congestive heart failure when normal blood pressures and circulation begin to fail, fluid accumulates in the tissues. This condition is called *edema*. Sodium concentration in these fluids contributes to the edema. Normally these shifts of water from one part of the body to another are the means whereby substances in solution in the body water can circulate between the cells and the fluid that surrounds them. Such shifts also protect the body against large fluid losses.

2. *Acid-base balance.* Through its association with chloride and bicarbonate ions, ionized sodium is an important factor in the regulation of the acid-base balance of the body. It contributes a major component of the base partner of the body's main buffer system: the carbonic acid–sodium bicarbonate buffer system.

3. *Cell permeability.* Sodium helps to control and operate what has been called a sodium *pump* in cell walls. This pump helps to exchange sodium and potassium across the cell wall. It also helps to make the cell wall more permeable to other materials. A major material that the sodium pump helps carry across the cell wall is glucose.

4. *Muscle action.* Sodium ions play a large part in transmitting electrochemical impulses along nerve muscle membranes. In this way sodium helps to maintain normal muscle action. Potassium and sodium ions balance the response of nerves to stimulation, the travel of nerve impulses to muscles, and the resulting contraction of the muscle fibers.

Requirement of sodium. As indicated, the body apparently can function on a rather wide range of dietary sodium. Thus no specific dietary requirement for sodium is stated. The average American diet contains about 4 to 6 gm. of sodium in the average 10 to 12 gm. of table salt consumed daily.

Food sources of sodium. Common salt as used in cooking and for seasoning and preserving is the main dietary source of sodium. Other natural food sources include milk, meat, egg, and certain vegetables such as carrots, beets, spinach and other leafy greens, celery, artichokes, and asparagus.

Potassium

Like sodium, potassium is a vital mineral element associated with water balance. It acts in balance with sodium as a major control for water distribution in the body. Potassium is about twice as plentiful as sodium in the body. An average man, weighing 154 pounds would have about 9 ounces of potassium in the body. By far the largest amount of this potassium is in free ionized form, located inside the body cells. As such it has a large role in cell metabolism.

Intake-absorption-output
potassium balance
POTASSIUM INTAKE. The average American diet contains 2 to 4 gm. of potassium, which is distributed widely in foods.

ABSORPTION OF POTASSIUM. The potassium in the diet is easily absorbed from the small intestine. Thus almost all the potassium consumed is absorbed. Potassium also constantly circulates in the gastrointestinal secretions, being reabsorbed as an aid in the digestive process. However, diseases such as prolonged diarrhea have a danger of excess potassium loss.

POTASSIUM OUTPUT. Little potassium, therefore, is lost in the feces under normal conditions. Urinary excretion is the principal route of output. However, the kidney guards the body supply of potassium carefully. The ability of the kidney to filter, reabsorb, secrete, and excrete potassium is remarkable. Though these mechanisms it can maintain normal serum potassium levels even in the face of large variances in potassium intake. The hormone of the adrenal gland, aldosterone, which controls sodium absorption and excretion, also influences potassium excretion. As a part of the aldosterone process that conserves sodium, ionized potassium is excreted in exchange for ionized sodium.

Physiologic functions of potassium. In its major role as a circulating electrolyte in body fluids, potassium helps to control a number of important body functions:

1. *Water and acid-base balance.* As the major cation of the fluid inside the cells, ionized potassium functions in balance with the ionized sodium outside the cells to maintain the normal osmotic pressures and water balance that maintain the integrity of the cellular fluids (p. 80).

2. *Muscle action.* Ionized potassium also plays a significant role in the activity of skeletal and cardiac muscle. It works with sodium and calcium to regulate neuromuscular stimulation, transmission of electrochemical impulses, and contraction of muscle fibers. This effect of ionized potassium on muscle action is particularly significant in the action of heart muscle. Even small variations in serum potassium concentrations are reflected in electrocardiographic changes. Variances in serum level of low serum potassium may cause muscle irritability and paralysis: the heart may even develop a gallop rhythm and finally cardiac arrest.

3. *Carbohydrate metabolism.* When blood glucose is converted to glycogen for storage in the liver or muscle, potassium is stored with the glycogen. For this reason, diabetics who are under treatment for diabetic acidosis usually are given replacement of serum potassium along with the glucose and insulin.

4. *Protein synthesis.* Potassium is also required for the storage of nitrogen as muscle protein. When muscle tissue is broken down, potassium is lost together with the nitrogen in muscle protein. Thus replacement therapy also includes potassium as well as amino acids to ensure nitrogen retention. About one third of the cell's supply of potassium is bound with the cell protein. Any situation involving extensive breakdown of tissue such as burns, for example, also involves the release of more potassium and hence an elevating effect on the blood potassium.

Requirement of potassium. No dietary requirement is specified for potassium. The usual diet contains an ample amount, about 2 to 4 gm. daily. Thus no deficiency is likely, except in clinical situations. Such a situation may occur with the continuous use of certain diuretic drugs, such as chlorothiazide (Diuril) or acetazolamide (Diamox). For this reason such drugs are given in interrupted doses, and the patient receives potassium replacement or extra food sources of potassium.

Food sources of potassium. Potassium is widely distributed in natural foods. Legumes, whole grains, leafy vegetables, meats, and certain fruits such as oranges, bananas, and dried prunes supply considerable amounts. Many other foods are supplementary sources.

OTHER MAJOR MINERALS

Three additional minerals are assigned to the major mineral group because of the extent of their occurrence in the body. These are magnesium, chloride, and sulfur.

Magnesium

The body of an average adult man contains about 25 gm. of magnesium, or a little less than an ounce. About 70% of this magnesium is combined with the calcium and phosphorus in bone. The remaining 30% is distributed in various soft tissues and body fluids. It is an active ion in body fluids and is important as a control agent in cell metabolism. It acts as an enzyme activator for energy production and tissue protein synthesis. It also aids in normal muscle action.

Chloride

Chloride accounts for about 3% of the body's total mineral content. It is mainly a part of the body fluids outside the cells. In these fluids ionized chlorine is the major anion (a particle—ion—carrying a negative electrical charge) balancing with sodium. As such it helps to control water balance and acid-base balance.

Sulfur

Sulfur occurs in some form throughout the body. It is present in all cells, usually as an essential constituent of cell protein; it contributes structural bonds to proteins and also acts as an important component in energy metabolism.

TRACE MINERALS

Seven essential minerals have been grouped as trace elements because they occur in the body in such small amounts. These include iron and its "twin," copper, which help to build red blood cells. Iodine is related to basal metabolism control. Cobalt is an essential part of vitamin B_{12}. Manganese, zinc, and molybdenum all contribute to essential enzyme systems in the cell.

Of these seven elements, two of the most significant in human nutrition are discussed here—iron and iodine.

Iron

Trace minerals are so called because a very small amount of them occurs in the body and is required for their specific function: iron is such a mineral. For example, a 150-pound man has only about 3 gm. (1/10 ounce) of iron in his body. Even though iron occurs in such small amounts in the body, it plays a vital role in blood building and energy production.

Iron balance in the body is controlled at two main levels: (1) the dietary amounts, both that which is absorbed and that which is excreted and (2) the amounts in the blood and tissues, especially the liver and that constantly being used in hemoglobin.

Intake-absorption-output balance

IRON INTAKE. Iron enters the body in foods

in a form that cannot be used as such by the body. First it must be acted on by the hydrochloric acid of the stomach and prepared for absorption. The average diet contains about 10 to 20 mg. of iron distributed in a number of foods. Because no large food sources of iron exist, sometimes the diet may be deficient in this mineral. In times of increased need for iron, such as during pregnancy, iron supplements may have to be used.

ABSORPTION OF IRON. The main point of control of the body's iron balance is at the point of absorption in the intestine. A special protein compound in the intestinal mucosal cells receives the iron and transports it in the body. The amount of this protein in the cells of the intestinal wall, as well as the degree to which it is already saturated with iron, determines the amount of iron from food that will be absorbed and enter the body. This mechanism has been called the *ferritin mechanism* because the name of the iron compound formed is *ferritin*. Thus it acts as a sort of "ironstat" to control the amount of iron in the body. Through the operation of this mechanism, only about 10% to 30% of the dietary iron is absorbed, and the remaining 70% to 90% is eliminated in the feces. A variety of factors influence the absorption of iron.

Factors increasing the absorption of iron

1. *Body need.* In deficiency states or in periods of extra demand, as in growth or pregnancy, the amount of ferritin in the intestinal mucosa is lower, and more iron is absorbed. When the tissue reserves are ample or saturated, iron is rejected or excreted.

2. *Ascorbic acid (vitamin C).* As an acid, vitamin C aids in absorption of iron by helping to change dietary iron to the form in which it can be absorbed.

3. *Hydrochloric acid.* This normal constituent of stomach secretions provides the optimum acid medium for the preparation of iron for absorption and use. Thus any condition that reduces the amount of hydrochloric acid secreted by the stomach affects iron absorption.

4. *Binding agents.* An adequate amount of calcium helps to bind and remove agents such as phosphate and phytate, which if not removed would combine with the iron and hinder its absorption.

Factors decreasing iron absorption

1. *Binding agents.* Certain binding agents, such as phosphate, phytate, and oxalate, remove iron from the body. Therefore a diet high in these materials leads to a decrease in iron absorption.

2. *Reduced hydrochloric acid.* Surgical removal of stomach tissue (gastrectomy) reduces the number of cells that secrete hydrochloric acid. The necessary acid medium for iron preparation is therefore not provided.

3. *Infection.* Severe infection hinders iron absorption.

4. *Malabsorption syndromes.* Any disturbance that causes diarrhea or malabsorption will hinder iron absorption.

IRON OUTPUT. Since the absorption mechanism controls the iron intake in the body, the output of iron from the body, about 70% to 90% of that taken in, is largely in the feces. Thus an exceedingly small amount of iron is excreted in the urine (only about 0.1 mg.) daily. During the reproductive years in women, some iron (about 20 mg.) is lost in the monthly menstrual flow. The iron cost of a pregnancy is high—about 400 to 900 mg., including some fetal deposit of iron during the growth of the child.

Blood-tissue-hemoglobin balance. Once the iron has been absorbed, it is maintained in an interdependent balance among that in the blood, the tissues, and the hemoglobin of red blood cells.

IRON IN THE BLOOD. Iron in the blood, other than that in red blood cells, is carried in a transport compound called *transferrin.* This is a protein-iron complex designed to carry the iron to the tissues for use by the body.

IRON IN THE TISSUES. The iron is delivered to the tissues, especially those involved in building red blood cells—mainly the liver, spleen, and bone marrow. Here the iron is

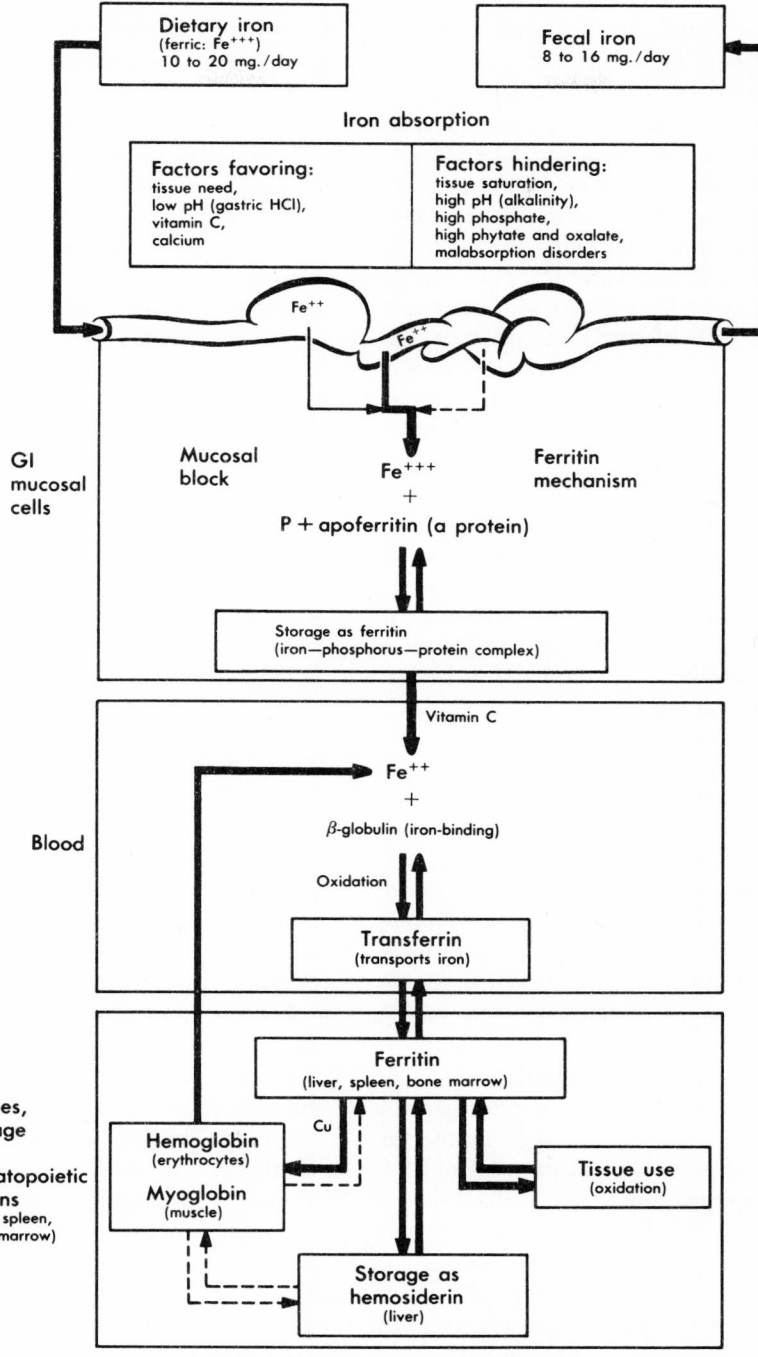

Fig. 7-3. Summary of iron metabolism, showing its absorption, transport, main use in hemoglobin formation, and storage forms (ferritin and hemosiderin).

reconverted to the storage form, ferritin, and drawn on as needed for formation of red blood cells. It is also drawn from this storage for general tissue metabolism. It may also be stored as another compound in the liver called *hemosiderin*. Hemosiderin may be thought of as a reserve storage account, much like a back-up savings account in the bank.

IRON IN HEMOGLOBIN. From these storage compounds iron is constantly being withdrawn for hemoglobin synthesis as needed. In the average adult from 20 to 25 mg. of iron is involved daily in hemoglobin synthesis. The body carefully conserves the iron that it uses in this synthesis. Red blood cells are destroyed after an average life-span of about 120 days. About 90% of the iron that is released when the cells are broken down is conserved and used over and over again. This is another example of the intricate interbalances that maintain life in the body.

The factors involved in iron intake-absorption-output balance and in the blood-tissue-hemoglobin balance are summarized in Fig. 7-3 for reference and review.

Physiologic functions of iron. Thus iron serves two main functions in the body, both of which support energy production and tissue building:

1. *Hemoglobin formation.* Iron is the core of the heme molecule, the central part of the fundamental protein of hemoglobin. Hemoglobin in the red blood cell is the oxygen transport unit of the blood that carries oxygen to the cells for energy metabolism and general cell work.

2. *Cellular oxidation.* Although in smaller amounts, iron also functions in the cells as a vital component of enzyme systems for the oxidation of glucose to produce energy.

Clinical applications. These functions of iron in the body have widespread applications in patient conditions.

NORMAL LIFE CYCLE. During periods of rapid growth, the demand for iron is greater. Thus during pregnancy, to supply deposits in the growing fetus and to supply the increasing maternal blood volume, more iron is re-

quired. After birth the infant draws on fetal storage in the liver. However, this iron storage is enough to last only 3 to 6 months. After that time iron must be supplied by the diet. Since milk, the first food of the infant, has little or no iron in it, solid food additions must be supplied to provide this needed iron. During continued growth in childhood and especially in adolescence more iron is needed. The need of women for iron during childbearing years makes their adult requirement for iron greater than that of men.

ANEMIAS. Because of its role in producing red blood cells, a deficiency of iron in the diet results in inadequate production of red blood cells—a condition called *anemia*. Various kinds of anemias may be listed according to cause:

1. *Nutritional anemia.* An inadequate supply of iron in the diet throughout the life cycle

2. *Hemorrhagic anemia.* Excessive blood loss, such as in wounds or injury

3. *Pernicious anemia.* The inability to form hemoglobin in the absence of other necessary factors such as vitamin B_{12}

4. *Postgastrectomy anemia.* Lack of gastric hydrochloric acid necessary to liberate iron for absorption after removal of the stomach

5. *Malabsorption anemia.* The presence of iron-binding agents or infections or inflammations on the absorbing surface that decrease or hinder the absorption of iron

6. *"Milk anemia."* Feeding older infants only milk, which is lacking in iron

Requirement of iron. The recommended allowances of the NRC list a general daily adult dietary intake of 10 mg. of iron for men and 18 mg. for women during the childbearing years. The ordinary diet probably cannot supply this larger quantity of iron to meet pregnancy demands, and fortification with iron supplements is desirable. Growth requirements gradually increase during the growing period and level off at the larger requirement for girls. Iron needs vary with age and situation, and these allowances are designed to provide margins for safety.

Food sources of iron. Organ meats, especially liver, are by far the best sources of iron. Other food sources include meats, egg yolks, whole wheat, seafood, green leafy vegetables, nuts, dried fruit, and legumes.

Iodine

Intake-absorption-output balance. Iodine is a trace element associated mainly with the thyroid gland. Little of its major balance in the body is controlled at the first level of intake-absorption-output.

IODINE INTAKE. About 100 to 200 mg. of iodine are needed daily in the diet to supply the basal requirement (about 25 mcg.) that is absorbed—an *exceedingly* small amount required to fulfill basic body needs. This iodine is eaten mainly in the form of iodized table salt.

ABSORPTION OF IODINE. The iodine ingested in the diet is absorbed in the small intestine and carried throughout the body with the aid of protein. About one third of the iodine absorbed into the body system is taken up by the thyroid gland. The remainder is excreted in the urine.

IODINE OUTPUT. About two thirds of the iodine absorbed by the body is excreted in the urine usually within two or three days after being eaten.

Blood-thyroid-TSH balance. Since the one function of iodine is to produce *thyroxine*, the hormone synthesized by the thyroid gland, the main balance is controlled between the blood and the thyroid gland.

IODINE IN THE BLOOD. Some free iodide (I^-) is in the blood from intestinal absorption; however, it does not remain long. According to need, this blood supply of iodine is constantly being taken up by the thyroid gland to produce its hormone, thyroxine. Thus the main blood iodine is bound in thyroxine for transport to the cells. This transport form of iodine in the blood is called *protein-bound iodine (PBI)*.

IODINE IN THE THYROID GLAND. The cell membranes of the thyroid gland have a tremendous specific capacity to take up, or trap, iodine. They accomplish this through an active transport mechanism called the *iodine pump*. Once inside the gland, the cells of the thyroid gland can concentrate iodine twenty-five times or more. This concentrated and activated iodine is then used by the thyroid gland to produce thyroxine through successive stages of production (T_1, T_2, T_3, and T_4). The iodine is attached to a protein base, the amino acid tyrosine, to produce the hormone. The thyroid hormone is then released to the blood supply to regulate the rate of basal metabolism.

TSH-THYROXINE BALANCE. The balance maintained between these two hormones, TSH (thyroid-stimulating hormone) and thyroxine, is an excellent example of hormonal control of body function by the master gland, the *pituitary*. In this case, the pituitary hormone TSH controls the blood level and hence the cells' supply of thyroxine.

The body cells require a constant supply of thyroxine to control the rate of cell metabolism. After the thyroxine is used by the body, the blood level of this thyroid hormone drops. This decrease in thyroxine level in the blood triggers the pituitary gland to put out its special thyroid-stimulating hormone (TSH), which in turn makes the thyroid gland take up more iodine and produce more needed thyroxine.

When the final product, thyroxine, is released by the thyroid gland into the bloodstream, the increased blood level then signals the pituitary to cut off its secretion of TSH. This type of finely balanced cycle is called a *negative feedback mechanism*, which controls hormonal balance in the body. A summary of these balances that control the use of iodine in the body are illustrated in Fig. 7-4.

Two tests are commonly used to measure the amount of iodine action in the body. One is the PBI test, which measures the amount of iodine that is bound to thyroxine and in transit in the plasma. The second is the radioactive ^{131}I test, which uses radioactive iodine to measure the uptake and use of iodine by the thyroid gland.

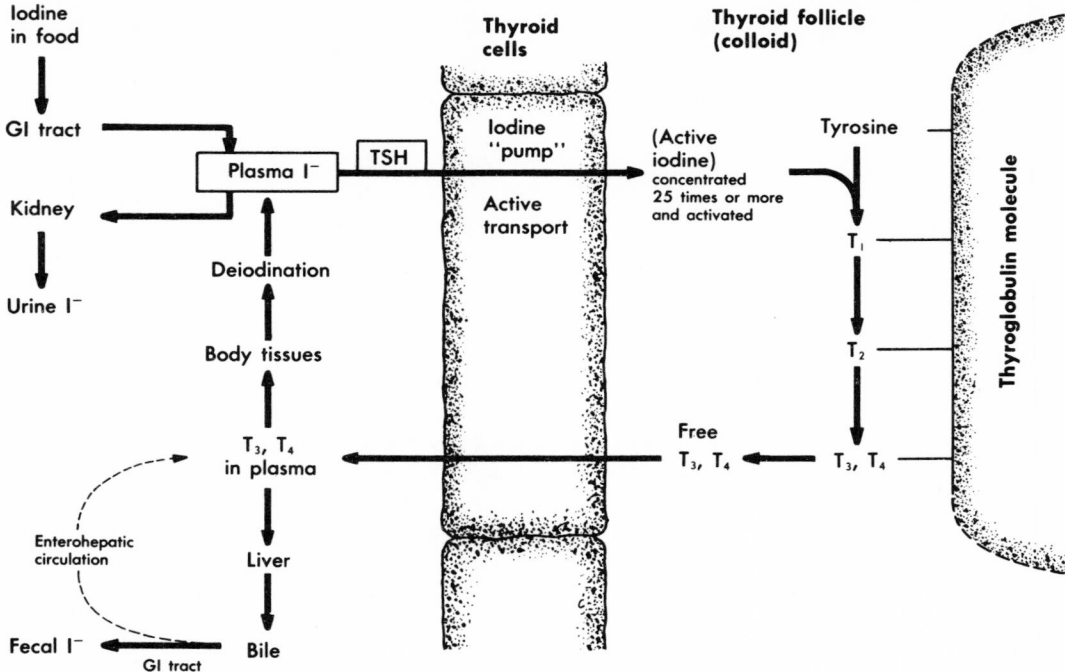

Fig. 7-4. Summary of iodine metabolism, showing active iodine pump in the thyroid cells and the synthesis of thyroxine in the colloid tissue of the thyroid follicles. (TSH = thyroid-stimulating hormone; T_1 = monoiodotyrosine; T_2 = diiodotyrosine; T_3 = triiodothyronine; T_4 = tetraiodothyronine.)

Physiologic function of iodine. The only known function of iodine in human metabolism is its role in the synthesis of the thyroid hormone, which in turn stimulates cell oxidation, apparently by increasing oxygen uptake and work of the enzyme system in handling glucose. Therefore iodine exerts tremendous controlling influence on overall body metabolism.

Clinical applications. This main function of iodine has two main areas of application: (1) the normal growth cycle and (2) goiter.

GROWTH. Clearly, during growth, when basal metabolic rates are increased, the demand also increases for iodine to produce the necessary thyroid hormone. Such periods occur during pregnancy, childhood, and especially adolescence.

GOITER. Goiter is a classic disease, characterized by great enlargement of the thyroid

gland, which enlarges because it is starved for iodine. When iodine is insufficient in the diet, the gland cannot produce a normal quantity of thyroxine, and the blood level remains low. In response, the pituitary continues to put out TSH. These large quantities of TSH constantly stimulate the thyroid gland to produce the needed thyroxine, but without iodine it cannot. The only response that the iodine-starved gland can make is to increase the amount of colloidal tissue of which it is composed; thus the gland becomes increasingly engorged. It may attain a tremendous size, weighing 500 to 700 gm. (1 to 1½ pounds) or more.

Requirement for iodine. The NRC has recommended daily adult allowances of 140 mcg. for young men because of their generally larger body size and 100 mcg. for young women. These needs normally decrease with age, of course, as the body's metabolic activity gradually lessens. The demand is increased during periods of accelerated growth.

Food sources of iodine. Seafood provides a considerable amount of iodine. However, the quantity in other natural food sources varies widely, depending on the iodine content of the soil in which the food is grown. The average diet falls somewhat below the requirement. The commercial iodizing of table salt (1 mg. to every 10 gm. of salt) provides the main dietary source of iodine; thus labels should be checked to ensure that the salt purchased is iodized.

Fluorine

One additional trace mineral, the function of which is not clearly defined, is fluorine. The only relationship thus far established for this mineral in human metabolism is its

Table 7-1. Summary of some essential minerals

MINERAL	FUNCTION	RESULTS OF DEFICIENCY	FOOD SOURCES
Calcium (Ca)	Bone formation	Rickets Porous bones	Milk, cheese, green leafy vegetables,
	Tooth formation	Poor tooth formation	whole grains, egg
	Blood clotting	Slow-clotting blood	yolk, legumes, nuts
	Muscle contraction and relaxation	Tetany, decrease in free serum calcium	
	Heart action		
	Nerve transmission		
Phosphorus (P)	Bone formation	Rickets	Milk, cheese, meat,
	Overall metabolism of carbohy- drates and fat	Poor growth	egg yolk, whole grains, legumes, nuts
Sodium (Na)	Water balance, osmotic pressure	Imbalances in water shifts and control	Table salt (NaCl) Milk, meat, eggs,
	Acid-base balance	Imbalances in buffer system	baking soda, baking powder, carrots,
	Glucose absorption, muscle action	Losses in gastro- intestinal disorders	beets, spinach, celery
Potassium (K)	Water balance in cells	Water imbalance	Whole grains, meat,
	Acid-base balance	Heart action (irregular beat, cardiac arrest)	legumes, fruits, vegetables
	Muscle and nerve action	Tissue breakdown—	
	Protein synthesis	potassium loss	
Iron (Fe)	Hemoglobin formation, carrying oxygen to cells for oxidation of nutrients to produce energy	Anemia Poor growth Inability to meet demands of pregnancy	Liver, meats, egg yolk, whole grains, enriched bread and cereal, dark green vegetables, legumes, nuts
Iodine (I)	Synthesis of thyroid hormone, which regulates basal metabolic rate, cell oxidation	Goiter Impaired metabolic rate	Iodized salt Seafood
Fluorine (F)	Dental health, prevention of dental caries by application to formed teeth	Small amount prevents dental caries Excess causes dental fluorosis (mottled teeth	Fluoridated water (1 ppm F)

association with dental health. *Dental caries* has been demonstrated to be largely preventable by the addition of small amounts of the mineral to fluorine-poor drinking water or by the topical application of fluoride solution to young developing teeth. Public health authorities advocate the fluoridation of public drinking water low in fluoride content in the amount of 1 ppm. The exact mechanism by which fluorine helps to prevent dental caries is unknown.

A summary for some of these essential minerals is provided in Table 7-1 for study and review.

WATER BALANCE

In patient care water balance in the body frequently has to be closely watched. Intake and output of water may have to be measured carefully to monitor some disease condition. Water is an essential nutrient basic to life but is often overlooked in a general discussion of the basic nutrients. The earth is a water planet, and life on it is maintained by a constant supply of adequate and safe water.

The principles governing water balance may be summarized under several headings. Since some of the minerals discussed previously are part of this balance, a review of some basic principles is included here. These main aspects of water balance involve three interdependent factors: (1) the water itself, (2) the particles in solution in the water, and (3) the separating membranes throughout the body that control flow.

Overall water balance

The adult body is about 65% water, which performs three functions that are essential to life: (1) it helps give structure and form to the body, (2) it furnishes the aqueous environment that is necessary for cell metabolism, and (3) it provides the means for maintaining a stable body temperature.

Body water and its distribution. The total body water is divided into two major categories in the body according to its placement: the total water outside the cells (the extracellular fluid—ECF) and the total water inside the cells (the intracellular fluid—ICF).

The total collective water inside the body cells amounts to about twice that outside the cells. This is not surprising, since the cells carry on the major body work. A small amount of the water outside the cells is circulating in the blood. The remaining amount is in interstitial and transit water, bathing the cells and moving from place to place.

The infant is much more vulnerable to water loss and hence the danger of dehydration than is an adult. This is for two reasons: (1) infants have much more water in their bodies than adults—about 75% of total body weight is water—and (2) more of this total body water is located outside the cells and hence is more readily lost.

Overall water balance: intake and output. Water enters the body in three main forms: (1) as preformed water in liquids that are drunk, (2) as preformed water in foods that are eaten, and (3) as a product of cell oxidation. Water leaves the body through the kidneys, the skin, the lungs, or the feces. These routes of water intake and output must be in constant balance. This overall body water balance is illustrated in Fig. 7-5.

Solutes

Solutes in the body water are a variety of particles in solution with varying concentrations. Two main types of particles control water balance in the body: electrolytes and plasma protein.

Electrolytes. As was seen in the preceding discussion of minerals, several minerals provide the major electrolytes for the body. Electrolytes are small inorganic substances that dissociate in solution and carry an electric charge. Hence in any solution they are constantly in balance between those carrying a positive charge (cations) and those carrying a negative charge (anion). The sodium ion is the major cation of the water outside the cell. The potassium ion is the major cation of the water inside the cell. The constant balance between these two electrolytes, sodium outside and

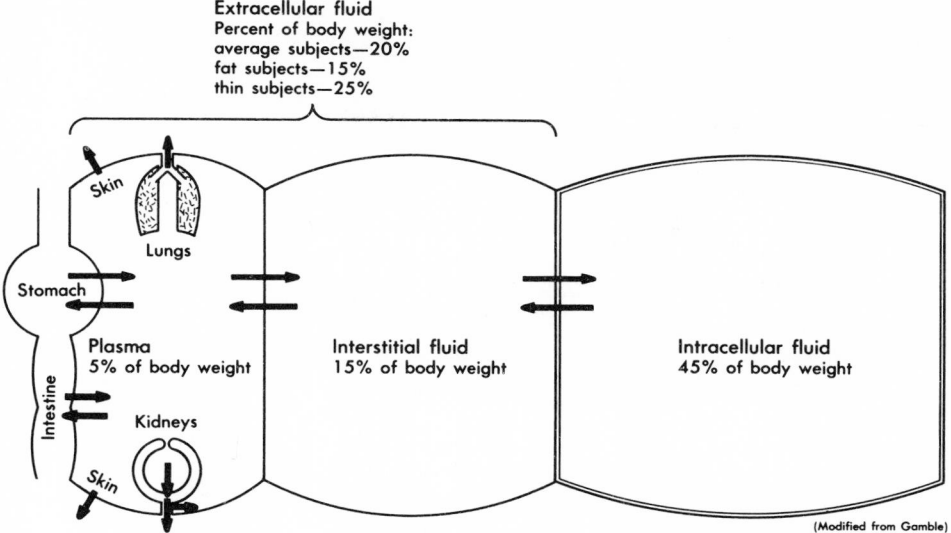

Fig. 7-5. Body fluid compartments. Note the relative total quantities of water in the intracellular compartment and in the extracellular compartment.

potassium inside the cell, maintains water balance between these two compartments. Other electrolytes include calcium, magnesium, chloride, sulfate, and phosphate. These electrolytes because of their small size can diffuse freely across most membranes of the body.

Plasma protein. Plasma protein, mainly in the form of albumin, is an organic compound of large molecular size. As such, it does not diffuse as freely across membranes as the electrolytes and is retained in the blood vessels. Thus it is a major substance in the body water that controls water shifts in the body and preserves blood volume. Cell protein helps to preserve cell water.

Organic compounds of small molecular size. Other organic compounds of small size are in solution in the body water but ordinarily do not influence shifts of water unless they occur in abnormally large concentrations. Glucose, for example, is one of these solutes. Only when it is in abnormal concentrations, as in uncontrolled diabetes, does it influence water loss from the body.

Separating membranes

Capillary wall. The capillary wall is a fairly free membrane because it is thin and porous. Thus water and small enough particles can move freely across this membrane. However, larger particles such as protein cannot. These plasma protein molecules remain in the capillary vessel to exert a pressure control that keeps the water in circulation.

Cell wall. The cell wall is a thicker membrane, to protect the cell contents. It is constructed in sandwich fashion with outer layers of protein and an inner structure of fat material. Special transport mechanisms are necessary to carry substances across the cell wall.

Forces moving water and solutes across membranes

As a result of the presence of these separating membranes, certain forces are created that control the movement of water and particles in solution in it.

Osmosis. Through the pressure created by osmosis, water molecules are moved from a

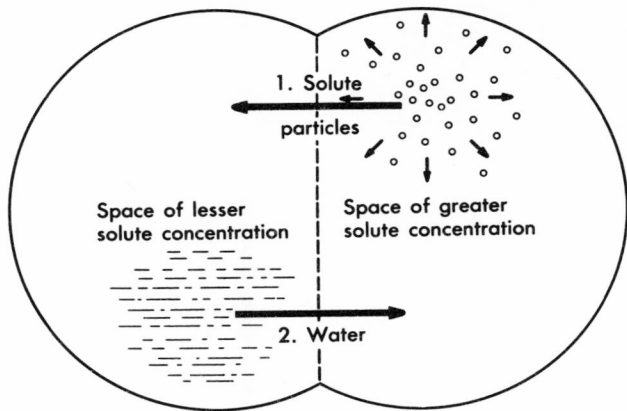

Fig. 7-6. Movement of molecules, water, and solutes by osmosis and diffusion.

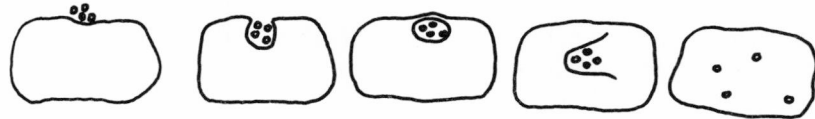

Fig. 7-7. Pinocytosis—engulfing of large molecules by the cell.

space of greater concentration of water molecules to a space of lesser concentration of water molecules. The effect of this movement is to distribute water molecules more evenly throughout the body and thus provide a solvent base for materials the water must carry.

Diffusion. Diffusion is a force similar to osmosis but applying to the particles in solution in the water. It is the force by which these particles move outward in all directions from a space of greater concentration to a space of lesser concentration of particles. The relative movements of water molecules and solute particles by osmosis and diffusion are compared in Fig. 7-6.

Filtration. Water is forced or filtered through membranes when there is a difference in pressures on the two sides of the membrane. This difference in pressure would be the result of differences in concentration of the particles in solution.

Active transport. Particles in solution vital to body processes must move throughout the body across membranes even when the pressures are against their flow. Thus some means of energy-driven active transport is necessary to carry these particles across the separating membranes. Usually these active transport mechanisms require some kind of a carrier partner to help them across.

Pinocytosis. Sometimes larger particles such as proteins and fats enter cells by the interesting process of pinocytosis (Fig. 7-7). The word means cell drinking. In this process these larger molecules are engulfed by the cell and carried into its center and across. For example, this is one of the mechanisms by which fat is absorbed from the small intestine.

Control mechanisms

Capillary fluid shift mechanism. Water is constantly circulated through the body by the blood vessels. It must, however, get out of the blood vessels to service the tissues and then be drawn back into circulation to maintain the normal flow. The body's means of maintaining this constant flow of water and the materials it is carrying to and from the cell is maintained by a balance of pressures. It is a filtration process operating by the differences in osmotic pressure on either side of the capillary wall.

When blood first enters the capillary system, the blood pressure forces water and small solutes (glucose, for example) out into the tissues to bathe and nourish the cells. The plasma protein particles (mainly albumin), however, are too large to go through the pores of capillary walls. Hence the protein remains in the vessel to exert the necessary pressure to draw the fluid back into circulation after it has bathed the cells.

ADH mechanism. ADH is a hormone produced by the pituitary gland. Its major function is to cause reabsorption of water by the kidney; hence it is a water-conserving mechanism. In any stress situation with threatened or real loss of body water, this hormone is triggered to conserve precious body water.

Aldosterone mechanism. A second important hormonal process that governs the renal control of water and electrolyte balance is the aldosterone mechanism. As indicated in the discussion of sodium, this mechanism is primarily a sodium-conserving device, but it also exerts a secondary control over water. This mechanism is sometimes called the *renin-angiotensin mechanism* because these are intermediate substances used to trigger the adrenal glands to produce the aldosterone hormone. Both ADH and aldosterone may be activated by stress situations such as body injury or surgery. They also operate to compound problems of water balance in such disease conditions as congestive heart failure, when the failing heart muscle cannot maintain the normal amount of blood output.

8 DIGESTION-ABSORPTION-METABOLISM PROCESS

Up to this point, for purposes of study the many dynamic processes that the body uses to solve its primary survival problems of energy production and tissue building and rebuilding have been examined in separate sections as these changes applied to each of the nutrients in turn. Foods must be transformed into simpler substances in a successive interrelated system of balanced change into other still simpler chemical substances that the cells can use to sustain life.

Thus the basic concepts used in this study to see how the body solves these problems have been those of *change* and *balance*. All these many changes whereby food is prepared for use by the body comprise the overall digestion-absorption-metabolism process.

However, of necessity, to understand this overall process, these food and nutrient changes have been examined first in separate sections; yet the parts do not exist alone but make up one continuous *whole*. This is the other aspect of the balance concept—that of *wholeness*, or body *integrity;* so an understanding of the science of nutrition requires that, at this point, the parts be put together and the overall process be viewed as one continuous, interdependent whole— a *dynamic unit.*

This, then, is the purpose of this final chapter in Part I—to help summarize this initial study by putting the parts back together, to see it all as one process. To achieve this picture of the digestion-absorption-metabolism process as a whole, the general principles related to each phase should be noted. Then the fate of food components may be followed as they travel *together* through the successive parts of the gastrointestinal tract and into the body cells. For study reference, the respective components of the gastrointestinal tract and their relative position in the overall system should be carefully reviewed (Fig. 8-1).

Why is this intricate complex of biochemical and physiologic activities so necessary? Two reasons are apparent. First, food as it naturally occurs and as it is eaten is not a single component but a mixture of substances. If these are to release their energy for use, they must be separated into their respective components so that each one may be handled by the body as a separate unit. Second, because in most instances the still simpler chemical units that make up these nutrient components are still unavailable to the body, some additional means of changing their form must follow. The intermediate units must be broken down, simplified, re-

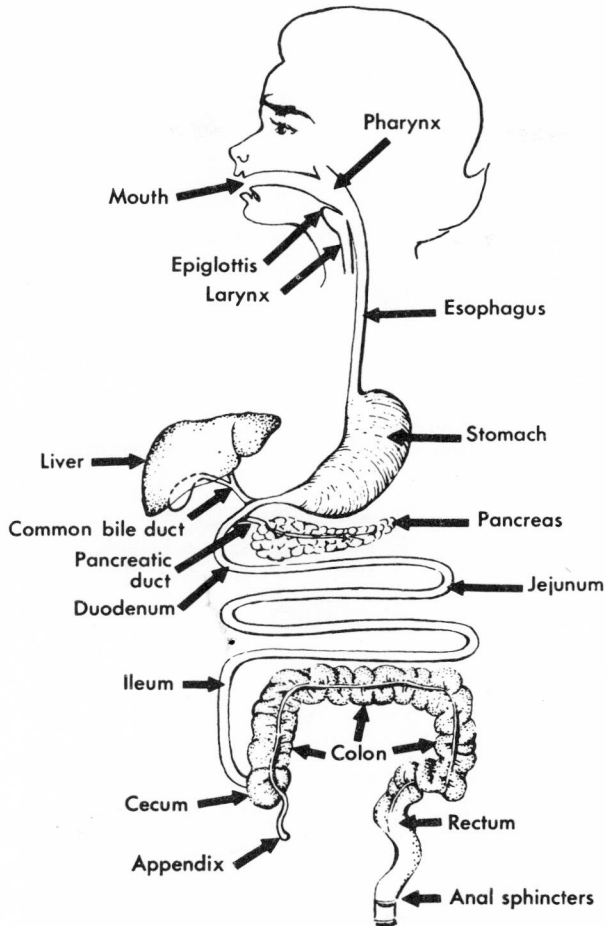

Fig. 8-1. The gastrointestinal system. Note the relative position of the successive parts. (From Stacy, R. W., and Santolucito, J. A.: Modern college physiology, St. Louis, 1966, The C. V. Mosby Co.)

grouped, and rerouted. This exceedingly complex chemical work must take place because man, whose life is developed and sustained in a fantastic internal chemical environment, is the most highly organized and intricately balanced of all organisms. This view of the human body as an integrated physiochemical organism is basic to an understanding of human nutrition.

DIGESTION
Basic principles of digestion

Digestion achieves the initial preparation of food for use by the body. Two basic types of action are involved: mechanical activities and chemical reactions.

Gastrointestinal motility. Mechanical digestion takes place through a number of neuromuscular self-regulatory processes. These actions work together to move the food components along the alimentary tract at the best rate for digestion and absorption of the nutrients.

TYPES OF MUSCLES. Four types of muscle in the stomach and intestine contribute to this motility: (1) a layer of circular contractile rings that break up, mix, and churn the food particles; (2) longitudinal muscles that help to propel the food mass along; (3) sphincter muscles that act as valves (the pyloric, ileocecal, and anal valves) and control passage of material to the next segment in the intestine; and (4) a thin mucosal layer of smooth muscle that can raise intestinal folds to increase the absorbing surface.

TYPES OF MUSCLE ACTION. The interaction of these four types of muscles in the gastrointestinal tract produce two general types of muscular action: (1) a general muscle tone, or tonic contraction, which ensures continuous passage and valve control and (2) periodic rhythmic contractions that mix and propel the food mass along. These alternating muscular contractions and relaxations that force the contents forward are known by the term *peristalsis*. The layers of smooth muscle that make up the wall of the gastrointestinal tract are shown in Fig. 8-2.

NERVE CONTROL OF MUSCLE ACTION. Specific nerves regulate these muscular actions: a complex, interrelated network of nerves within the gastrointestinal wall extends all the length from the esophagus to the anus. This network of nerves controls muscle tone of the gastrointestinal wall, regulates the rate and intensity of periodic muscle contractions, and coordinates the various movements.

Gastrointestinal secretions. Food is di-

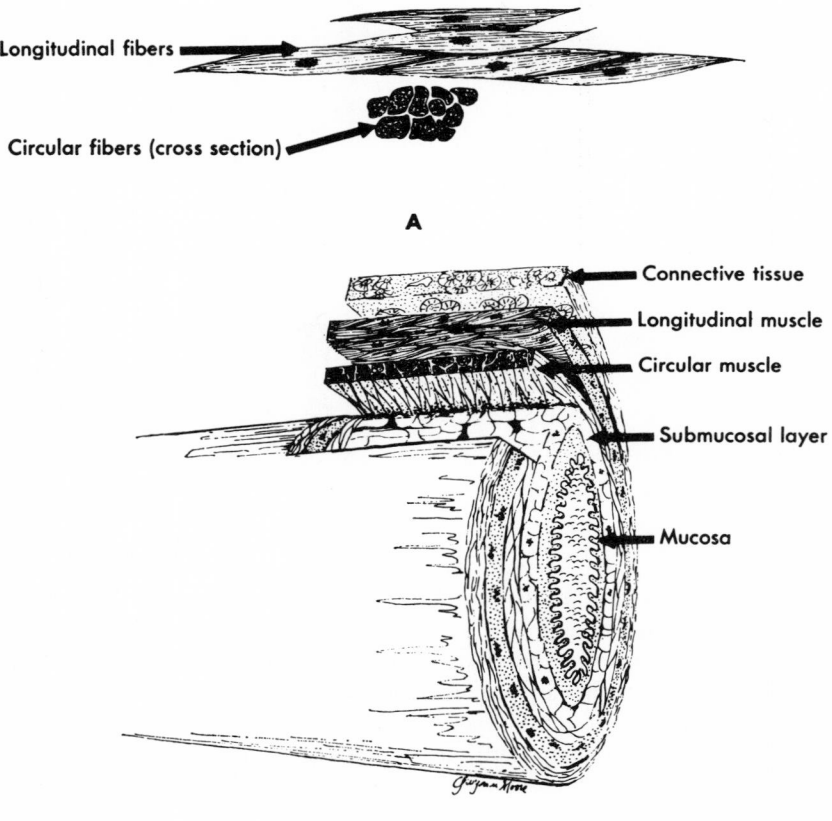

Fig. 8-2. Layers of smooth muscle in the intestinal wall. **A,** Microscopic appearance of muscle tissue. **B,** Arrangement of layers of muscle. (From Stacy, R. W., and Santolucito, J. A.: Modern college physiology, St. Louis, 1966, The C. V. Mosby Co.)

gested chemically by the action of a number of secretions; generally, these secretions are of four types:

1. *Enzymes.* Enzyme action is specific: each enzyme works on a particular nutrient. These enzymes are always specific in type and quantity for the breaking down of a given nutrient.

2. *Hydrochloric acid and buffer ions.* These materials produce the degree of acidity or alkalinity necessary for the activity of these enzymes.

3. *Mucus.* Mucous material lubricates and protects the gastrointestinal tract.

4. *Water and electrolytes.* Water, the basic transport material, must be present in quantities sufficient to carry, or circulate, the substances being produced.

All these secretions are produced by special cells in the mucosal tissue of the gastrointestinal tract or in accessory organs adjacent to it. The secretory action of these special cells or glands may be stimulated locally by the presence of food, by the sensory nerve network stimuli, or by hormones specific for certain foods.

Digestion in the mouth and esophagus

Mechanical digestion

MASTICATION. Initial biting and chewing begins the breaking up of food into smaller particles. The teeth and other oral structures are particularly suited for this function: incisors cut and molars grind. Tremendous force is supplied by the jaw muscles: 55 pounds of muscular pressure is applied through incisors, and 200 pounds is applied through the molars. This chewing of food makes it possible for an enlarged surface area of the food to be exposed constantly to enzyme action. Also the fineness of the food particles eases the continued passage of material through the gastrointestinal tract.

SWALLOWING. The process of swallowing this mixed mass of food particles and its passage down the esophagus are accomplished by peristaltic waves controlled by nerve reflexes. Muscles at the base of the tongue are responsible for the process of swallowing. In the usual upright eating position, gravity aids this movement of food down the esophagus. However, it is more difficult for a bed patient in a flat position. Swallowing and food movement through the intestinal tract, especially through the area of the stomach, is usually accomplished more easily if the patient lies on the left side.

ENTRY INTO THE STOMACH. At the point of entry into the stomach, the gastroesophageal constrictor muscle relaxes to allow food to enter; then it constricts again to prevent regurgitation of stomach contents up into the esophagus. When regurgitation does occur, through failure of this mechanism, the patient feels it as "heartburn." Clinical conditions such as *cardiospasm,* caused by failure of the constrictor muscle to relax properly, hinder normal food passage at this point. *Hiatus hernia* may also create a problem. Hiatus hernia is a protrusion of the stomach into the thorax through an abnormal opening in the diaphragm. This outpouching of the stomach wall allows food to be held in this area.

Chemical or secretory digestion. Three pairs of salivary glands—parotid, submaxillary, and sublingual—secrete a digestive material containing *ptyalin,* an enzyme specific for starches. A mucous material that lubricates and binds the food particles is also secreted. Stimuli such as sight, smell, taste, and touch—and even the thought of likes or dislikes in foods—influence secretions.

Because food remains in the mouth only a short time, however, starch digestion by ptyalin is largely unimportant and is terminated by the acid medium of the stomach. The secretions of mucous glands that line the esophagus aid in swallowing and movement of the food mass toward the stomach.

Digestion in the stomach

Mechanical digestion. The major parts of the stomach are shown in Fig. 8-3. The three main areas of the stomach are the first section, or fundus; the body, or middle portion; and the antrum, or pylorus, the small end.

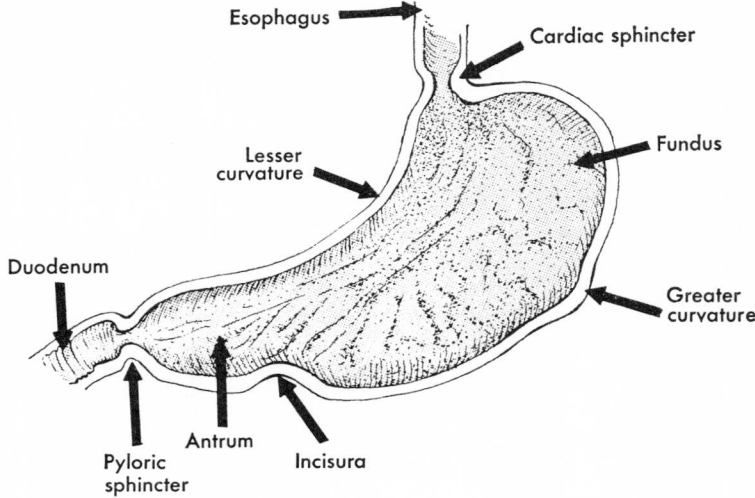

Fig. 8-3. Major parts of the stomach. (From Stacy, R. W., and Santolucito, J. A.: Modern college physiology, St. Louis, 1966, The C. V. Mosby Co.)

The fundus, or upper part of the stomach, receives the food mass first. Muscles in the stomach wall provide three basic muscle functions: storage, mixing, and slow-controlled emptying. Since the food mass lies against the stomach walls, it can cause the stomach to stretch outward to store as much as 1 liter, or approximately 1 quart.

Gradually local tonic muscle waves increase their kneading and mixing action as the mass of food and secretions moves on through the middle portion of the stomach toward the region of the pyloric antrum at the small end of the stomach. Here waves of peristaltic contractions reduce the food mass to a semifluid *chyme.*

Finally, with each peristaltic wave small amounts of chyme are forced through the pyloric valve into the small intestine. Thus this "pyloric pump" controls the emptying of the stomach contents into the duodenum (the first section of the small intestine) by constrictive action of the sphincter muscle (the pyloric valve) and by controlling the rate of propulsive peristaltic activity in the antrum. This finely coordinated control releases the acid chyme slowly enough so that it can be buffered by the alkaline intestinal secretion.

Chemical or secretory digestion

TYPES OF SECRETIONS. About 2,000 ml. (approximately 2 quarts) of gastric secretion is produced daily by special cells; they are of three basic types:

1. *Acid.* Hydrochloric acid is produced to aid in digestion and prepare certain enzymes and materials for digestion and absorption by creating the necessary degree of acidity for given enzymes to work.

2. *Mucus.* The special mucous secretions protect the stomach lining from the eroding effect of the acid. It also binds and mixes the food mass and helps move it along.

3. *Enzymes.* The main enzyme in the stomach is *pepsin*, which begins the breakdown of protein. It is first secreted in the inactive form pepsinogen, which is then activated by the hydrochloric acid present. A small amount of gastric lipase works on emulsified fats such as butterfat. This enzyme is called *tributyrinase* because it acts on the fat in butter, which is named *tributyrin*. This is a relatively minor digestive activity, however. In childhood an enzyme called *rennin* is also present in gastric secretions, aiding in the coagulation of milk. However, in adults this enzyme is absent.

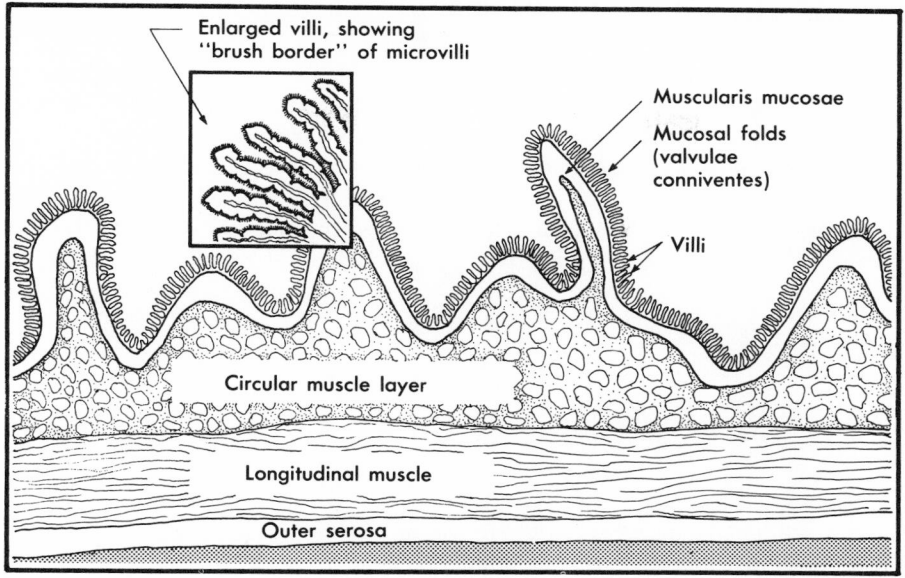

Fig. 8-4. Intestinal wall. Note the arrangement of muscle layers and the structures of the mucosa that increase the surface area for absorption—mucosal folds, villi, and microvilli.

CONTROL OF SECRETIONS. Stimuli for all these secretions are twofold:

1. *Nerve stimulus* in response to sensations of food taken in and to emotions. For example, in response to anger and hostility secretions increase. Fear and depression decrease secretions and hinder blood flow and muscular action as well. There is much truth to the saying "It's not what he eats that's bothering him, but what's eating him."

2. *Hormonal stimulus* in response to the entrance of food into the stomach. For example, certain stimulants, especially coffee, alcohol, and meat extractives, cause a hormone to be released in the antrum, which in turn stimulates the secretion of more hydrochloric acid. This is the reason for the elimination of these substances when a peptic ulcer is present—to cut down the secretion of hydrochloric acid.

Food remains in the stomach for varying lengths of time, depending on the type of food. Carbohydrates leave the stomach quickly. Protein leaves more quickly than fat. Small amounts of food leave the stomach in less time than a large meal.

Digestion in the small intestine

Up to this point, the digestion of food has been mainly mechanical, delivering to the small intestine a semifluid chyme made up of fine food particles mixed with watery secretions. Little chemical digestion has occurred thus far. The major task of digestion and of absorption, which follows, occurs in the small intestine. Its structural parts, synchronized movements, and array of enzymes are highly developed for this all-important final task of mechanical and chemical digestion.

Mechanical digestion. The exquisite structural arrangement of the intestinal wall is shown in the diagram in Fig. 8-4.

TYPES OF MUSCLES. Finely coordinated intestinal muscle action is achieved by the three basic layers of muscle: (1) a thin layer of smooth muscle in the inner lining of the intestine (mucosa) with fibers extending up into the villi, (2) the circular muscle layer, and (3) the longitudinal muscle next to the outer wall of the intestine (serosa). Under the control of the network of nerves in the intestine and also of pressure from food present or from hormonal stimuli, these muscles produce the movement necessary to aid mechanical digestion.

TYPES OF MUSCLE ACTION. The action of the circular muscles (segmentation rings) pro-

gressively chops the food mass into successive boluses. Then the rotation of the long muscle rolls the slowly moving food mass in a spiral motion, continuing to mix it and expose new surfaces for absorption. Other muscle contractions sweep back and forth, stirring the chyme at the mucosal surface. Peristaltic waves continue to move the food mass slowly forward, and sweeping motions of the surface

Table 8-1. Summary of digestive processes

NUTRIENT	MOUTH	STOMACH	SMALL INTESTINE
Carbo-hydrate	Starch $\xrightarrow{\text{Ptyalin}}$ Dextrins		Pancreas Starch $\xrightarrow{\text{Amylase}}$ (Disaccharides) Maltose and sucrose Intestine Lactose $\xrightarrow{\text{Lactase}}$ (Monosaccharides) Glucose and galactose Sucrose $\xrightarrow{\text{Sucrase}}$ Glucose and fructose Maltose $\xrightarrow{\text{Maltase}}$ Glucose and glucose
Protein	Protein	Protein $\xrightarrow[\text{Hydrochloric acid}]{\text{Pepsin}}$ Poly-peptides	Pancreas Proteins, polypeptides $\xrightarrow{\text{Trypsin}}$ Dipeptides Proteins, polypeptides $\xrightarrow{\text{Chymotrypsin}}$ Dipeptides Polypeptides, dipeptides $\xrightarrow{\text{Carboxypeptidase}}$ Amino acids Intestine Polypeptides, dipeptides $\xrightarrow{\text{Aminopeptidase}}$ Amino acids Dipeptides $\xrightarrow{\text{Dipeptidase}}$ Amino acids
Fat		Tributyrin (butterfat) $\xrightarrow{\text{Tributyrinase}}$ Glycerol Fatty acids	Pancreas Fats $\xrightarrow{\text{Lipase}}$ Glycerol Glycerides (di-, mono-) Fatty acids Intestine Fats $\xrightarrow{\text{Lipase}}$ Glycerol Glycerides (di-, mono-) Fatty acids Liver and gallbladder Fats $\xrightarrow{\text{Bile}}$ Emulsified fat

villi constantly stir the chyme that is in contact with the intestinal wall and expose additional nutrient material for absorption.

Chemical digestion. Since the major burden of chemical digestion falls on the small intestine, this portion of the alimentary tract secretes a large number of enzymes, each of which is specific for one of the fundamental types of nutrients. These important specific enzymes are secreted from the intestinal glands and from the pancreas. They are summarized in Table 8-1.

Thus four basic types of digestive material are secreted in the small intestine and aid in this final process:

1. *Enzymes.* As indicated, specific enzymes act on specific materials to bring about the final breakdown of the nutrient materials in food to a form in which the body can absorb and use them.

2. *Mucus.* In addition to enzymes, large quantities of mucus are secreted by intestinal glands located immediately inside the duodenum. This secretion protects the mucosa from irritation and digestion by the highly acid gastric juices that enter the intestine at this point. Emotions inhibit these mucous secretions and are an important factor in the production of duodenal ulcers. Additional mucous cells on the intestinal surface continue to secrete mucus as they are touched by the moving food mass. This provides continued lubrication and protection of tissues. The combined secretions of the mucous glands of the intestine and pancreas total about 4,200 ml. daily, or approximately 4 to 4½ quarts.

3. *Hormone.* A hormone called *secretin* is produced by the mucosa in the upper part of the small intestine. The presence of acid in the entering food mass causes this secretion. Its purpose in turn is to cause the pancreas to send pancreatic juices into the duodenum and buffer the acid chyme. The unprotected intestinal mucosa alone at this point could **not withstand this high degree of acidity.**

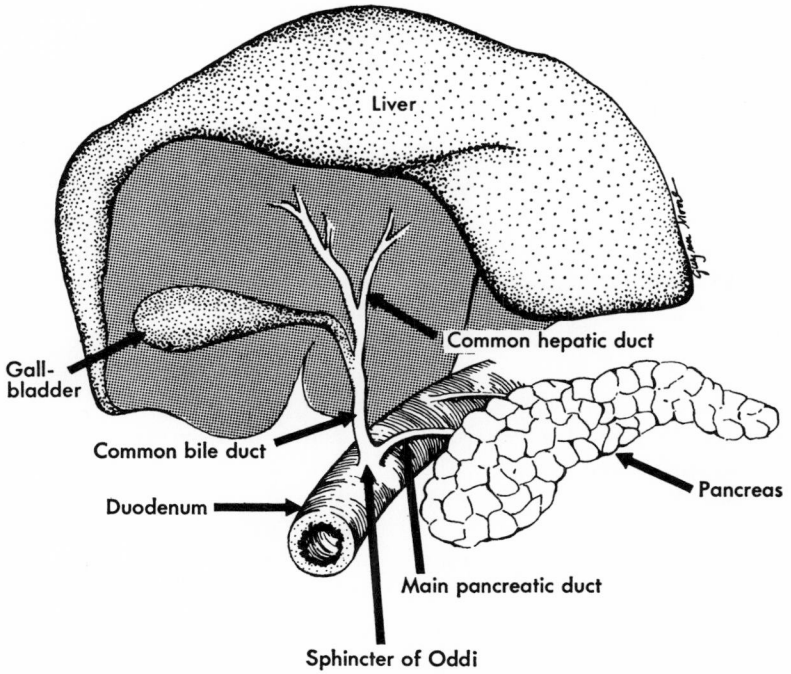

Fig. 8-5. Organs of the biliary system and the pancreatic ducts. (From Stacy, R. W., and Santolucito, J. A.: Modern college physiology, St. Louis, 1966, The C. V. Mosby Co.)

4. *Bile*. Another important aid to digestion and absorption in the small intestine is bile, since it is an emulsifying agent for fats. Bile is produced by the liver and is concentrated and stored by the gallbladder. When fat enters the duodenum, the hormone *cholecystokinin* is secreted by the glands of the intestinal mucosa. This hormone in turn stimulates the gallbladder to contract and release the needed bile. From 600 to 700 ml. of bile is produced daily.

Accessory organs

In addition to the gastrointestinal tract itself, important accessory organs lie adjacent to the small intestine and secrete their necessary materials to aid digestion through special ducts into the small intestine. These important accessory organs are the liver, the gallbladder, and the pancreas. The relative arrangements of these organs and their ducts to the small intestine are illustrated in Fig. 8-5. A summary of these combined digestive processes is given in Table 8-1.

ABSORPTION

After digestion of the food nutrients is complete, the simplified end products are ready to be absorbed. These include monosaccharides from carbohydrates such as glucose, fructose, and galactose; fatty acids and glycerides from fats; and amino acids from proteins. Also liberated are vitamins and minerals. Finally, there is a water base for solution and transport plus some necessary electrolytes.

Small intestine

Surface structures. Viewed from the outside, the intestine appears smooth, but the inner mucosal surface lining is quite different. Three types of convolutions and projections greatly enhance the absorbing surface area. These are illustrated in Fig. 8-4. First, the *mucosal folds* like hills and valleys in a mountain range are easily seen by the naked eye. Second, the *villi* are fingerlike projections on these folds, which can be seen by a simple microscope. Third, the *microvilli* are

extremely small projections on each villus and can only be seen with an electron microscope. This vast array of microvilli covering the edge of each villus is called the *brush border* because they look like bristles on a brush. Each villus has an ample network of blood capillaries as well as a central lymph vessel called *lacteal*. This is the special name given to these lymphatic vessels in the small intestine because the material that fills them during digestion is mainly fat substances, which gives it a creamy milklike appearance.

Absorbing surface area. These three structural elements of the intestine—mucosal folds, villi, and microvilli—increase the inner surface area some 600 times over that of the outside serosa! These special structures, plus the contracted length of the live organ (21 to 22 feet), combine to produce a tremendously large absorbing surface. The remarkable potential of this inner surface of the small intestine is a total absorbing surface area as large as or larger than half a basketball court!

All three of these mucosal surface structures function as a unit for the absorption of nutrients. Although the small intestine is popularly thought of as the lowly "gut," it is actually one of the most highly developed, exquisitely fashioned, specialized tissues in the human body!

Mechanisms of absorption. Absorption is accomplished by the small intestine by means of a number of processes, including passive diffusion, active "ferrying"—a carrier-mediated diffusion, energy-driven active transport, and penetration by engulfment—pinocytosis (p. 82).

Routes of absorption

CARBOHYDRATES AND PROTEINS. After their absorption by any of these processes, the nutrient components from carbohydrates and proteins enter the portal blood system directly and travel by way of the liver to the body tissues.

FATS. Only fat is unique in its route. After enzyme processing in the cells of the intestinal lumen, fat is largely converted to a complex with protein as a carrier and is transported by way of the lymph vessels in the center of the villi—the lacteals. From these vessels the fats flow into the larger lymph vessels and finally enter the common portal blood flow through the thoracic duct. Exceptions are the medium- and short-chain fatty acids, which are absorbed directly into villi blood circulation. However, most commonly consumed fats are made up of long-chain fatty acids, which travel the lacteal and lymphatic route.

Large intestine (colon)

The main absorption task remaining for the large intestine is that of taking up water. However, related factors are involved, such as the absorption of sodium and other minerals, absorption of some vitamins and amino acids, the action of intestinal bacteria, the collection of nondigestible residue, and the formation and elimination of feces.

Water absorption. Within a 24-hour period about 500 ml. of the remaining food mass leaves the ileum (the last portion of the small intestine) and enters the cecum (the pouch at the start of the large intestine). Here the *ileocecal valve* exerts important control over passage of the semiliquid chyme. Normally the valve remains closed. With each peristaltic wave, however, it relaxes briefly to allow a small amount of chyme to squirt into the cecum. This control mechanism holds the food mass in the small intestine long enough to ensure adequate digestion and absorption of vital nutrients. Such timing is vital and necessary because no digestive enzymes are secreted by the colon.

The chyme now moves slowly through the large intestine, aided by mucous secretion from glands in the colon and by muscle contraction. Studies with test meals indicate that the food residue mass moves through the large intestine at a gradually slowing pace. Usually the test meal, having traversed the 21 to 22 feet of small intestine, starts to enter the cecum about 4 hours after it is consumed. About 8 hours later it reaches the sigmoid colon, having traveled through the large

intestine for a distance of about 3 feet! In the sigmoid colon the mass descends still more slowly toward the anus. Even 72 hours after the meal has been eaten, as much as 25% of it may still remain in the rectum. It is evident that residue such as bran is an important food factor to help provide bulk and aid movement of the food mass along the tract.

The major portion of the water in the chyme (350 to 400 ml.) is absorbed in the first half of the colon. Only 100 to 150 ml. of water remains to form and aid in elimination of the feces.

Mineral absorption. Electrolytes, principally sodium, are transported into the bloodstream from the colon. From 20% to 70% of ingested calcium is eliminated in the feces, as is from 80% to 85% of ingested iron and a considerable amount of phosphates and some carbonate.

Bacterial action. Bacteria in the colon are closely associated with a number of vitamins. The colon bacteria synthesize vitamin K and some vitamins of the B complex (especially biotin and folic acid), which are absorbed from the colon in sufficient amounts to meet the daily requirement. Although vitamin B_{12} is also synthesized by intestinal bacteria, it is not absorbed from the large intestine because the necessary intrinsic factor for its absorption is not present at this point in the gastrointestinal tract (p. 61).

Intestinal bacteria also affect the color and odor of the stool. The brown color represents bile pigments, which are formed by the colon bacteria. Thus, when bile flow is hindered, the stools may become clay colored or white. The characteristic odor of the stool results from amines, formed by bacterial enzymes from amino acids. Gas, or flatus, formed in the large intestine contains hydrogen sulfide or methane produced by the bacteria. Gas formation, however, is caused not so much by specific foods as by the state of the body that receives them. Many foods have been labeled *gas forming*, but in reality such classifications have little or no scientific basis.

Residue. Since man has no microorganisms

or enzymes to break down cellulose, this plant product remains after digestion and absorption as residue. It contributes important bulk to the diet and helps form the feces. The increasing refinement of foods through various processing methods has generally reduced much more of the necessary dietary residue. More whole grains with intact bran layers are needed.

METABOLISM

The various absorbed nutrient components, including water and electrolytes, are now carried to the cells as ready-to-use materials to produce a myriad of substances needed by the body to sustain life. Metabolism encompasses the total continuous complex of chemical changes that determine the final use of the individual nutrients.

Each of these chemical processes is purposeful, and all are interdependent. The processes are designed to fill two essential needs: (1) to produce energy and (2) to maintain a dynamic equilibrium between the building up or breaking down of tissue. The controlling agents in the cells for these processes to be carried on in orderly fashion are the cell enzymes, their coenzymes, many of which involve the vitamins and minerals, and hormones.

All in all, it is an exciting biochemical system. Through it, the human body works to develop, sustain, and protect its most precious possession—life itself. Throughout the marvelous wonders of growth and the constant revelations of human existence can be seen.

PART

TWO

COMMUNITY NUTRITION: THE LIFE CYCLE

CHAPTER **9** # THE FOOD ENVIRONMENT

As was indicated in the beginning of this study of nutrition and health, health care is changing in method, in setting, and in the needs of the people. It is also changing in the nature of the health workers providing the care. Some form of community outreach from a central hospital or medical center is increasingly becoming an integral part of any health care system. This is inevitable if the real needs of people are to be learned and met, since care that is truly helpful must be based on these human life needs. Nutrition is basic to such health care.

Concerned health workers have a unique opportunity—indeed even a responsibility— to apply the knowledge of nutrition to the care of patients and families. In the first part of this book, you have studied some basic principles of human nutrition, but these can only come alive in terms of *personal need*. They cannot be applied abstractly in a vacuum —eating behavior or any other human behavior simply does not develop that way.

Thus health workers will be concerned at the core of their practice with *people*—people in families, people in communities, people in various work situations, people in financial distress, people with housing problems, people with deeply ingrained habits and customs, people with differing religious and cultural backgrounds, young people, old people, fat, thin, ill, well, discouraged, happy, clean, not so clean, educated, and illiterate people. There are many kinds of people in many

places with many needs. Each is a human being with unique dignity, pride, and worth.

Therefore knowledge alone is not enough. Human compassion and concern are needed, as well as practical guides, insights, appreciations, and some skills to be able to apply knowledge in a useful and helpful manner. The chapters in this section of your study will provide a background on which you may build as you help to fill these human needs.

THE ECOLOGY OF HUMAN NUTRITION

Ecology is almost a common household word today because the human environment is changing so rapidly. As a result, problems of balance in our environment, for example, pollution and malnutrition, and threatening health and causing disease.

The word "ecology" comes from a Greek word meaning "house." Just as many factors and forces within a family interact to influence the members, so an even more vast complex of interrelated forces in our physical and social system produces disease. Many factors work together to produce malnutrition. Some of these many related causes of malnutrition can be classed under the headings of agent, host, and environment.

Agent

The agent that is the fundamental cause of malnutrition is *lack of food*. Because of this, certain nutrients that are essential to cell activity are missing. Various factors may cause or modify this lack:

1. *Food quantity.* The total quantity of food eaten may be below the level required to maintain body tissues. The food deficiency may be partial or complete, seasonal or constant.

2. *Imbalance between need and community food supply.* The amount of food available for each person may be reduced by natural disasters, such as drought or flood, or by manmade disasters, such as war, overpopulation, poor distribution, or poverty.

3. *Food quality.* The food available may be of poor physical quality or nutritional value.

4. *Food timing.* The food may not be present in proper balance when needed (as in infant and child feeding for growth needs).

Host

The host is the person—infant, child, or adult—who suffers from malnutrition. Various characteristics in the host may influence the disease:

1. *Presence of other diseases.* Infections, allergies, metabolic disease, gastrointestinal diseases, and other such problems compound the course of malnutrition.

2. *Increased dietary needs.* Any physiologic cause of stress, such as growth, pregnancy, lactation, injury, illness, or physical labor, increases the demand for nutrients.

3. *Congenital defects.* Premature birth or defects such as cleft palate influence food intake.

4. *Personal factors.* Ignorance of food needs or food values, carelessness, lack of education, emotional problems, poor habits, or lack of appetite influences the kind and amount of food consumed.

Environment

Many environmental factors influence malnutrition. Some are close at hand and may be controlled by the individual, but many are more far-reaching ones. They seem too enormous, too powerful, or too remote in their source to be influenced by a single person. Mass action and extensive study are needed to deal with these problems. Following are some of the environmental problems:

1. *Sanitation.* Food contamination causes food loss and produces disease, thus compounding malnutrition.

2. *Culture.* Traditional food habits and customs may hinder nutrition.

3. *Social factors.* Interrelated social problems, such as poverty, racial discrimination, inadequate housing, and family disintegration, may contribute to lack of food and to malnutrition.

4. *Psychologic factors.* An example of the many psychologic problems that may contribute to malnutrition is maternal deprivation, which may lead to actual or felt rejection of a child by the mother and inadequate feeding.

5. *Economic and political structure.* The economic and political system of a region controls the power structure. It governs administrative policy and controls forms and channels of food supply.

6. *Agriculture.* Geography, climate, food technology, and methods of agriculture influence food supply. What food can and will be produced is determined by the natural resources available in a region and their degree of development.

Hunger in the United States

The interaction of some of these factors leading to malnutrition may be visualized in the diagram in Fig. 9-1. For example, kwashiorkor and marasmus are extreme states of malnutrition caused by protein and calorie deficiences (Figs. 9-2 and 9-3). Although one may not encounter such extreme states in everyday practice, nonetheless they exist in the United States. The findings of the U. S. Senate Select Committee on Nutrition and Human Needs and the National Nutrition Survey have indicated far more incidence of varying degrees of malnutrition than had been imagined. Such nutritional deficiency states should not exist in a nation with our degree of wealth and medical science and

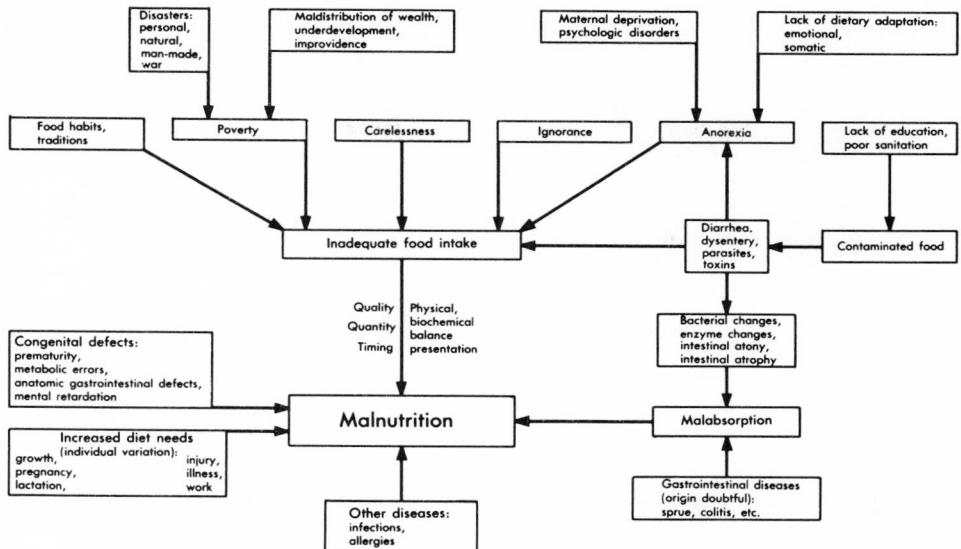

Fig. 9-1. The multiple etiology of malnutrition. (Modified from Williams, C. D.: Lancet **2:**342, 1962.)

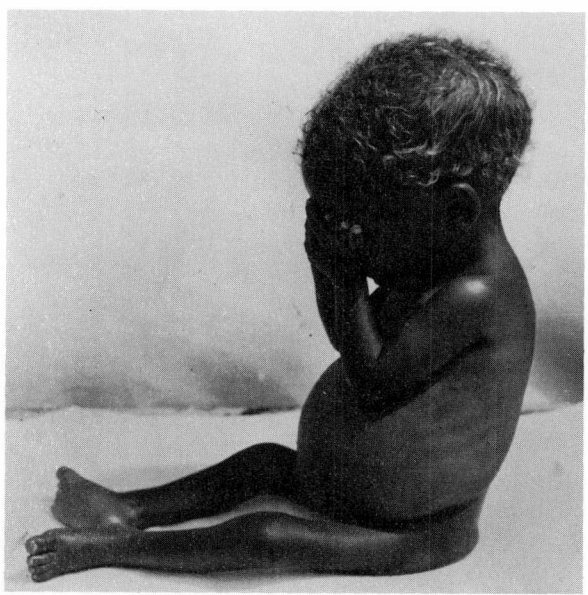

Fig. 9-2. A little African child suffering from kwashiorkor. Note uncurled, graying hair, edema, and skin lesions. (FAO photograph by M. Autret.)

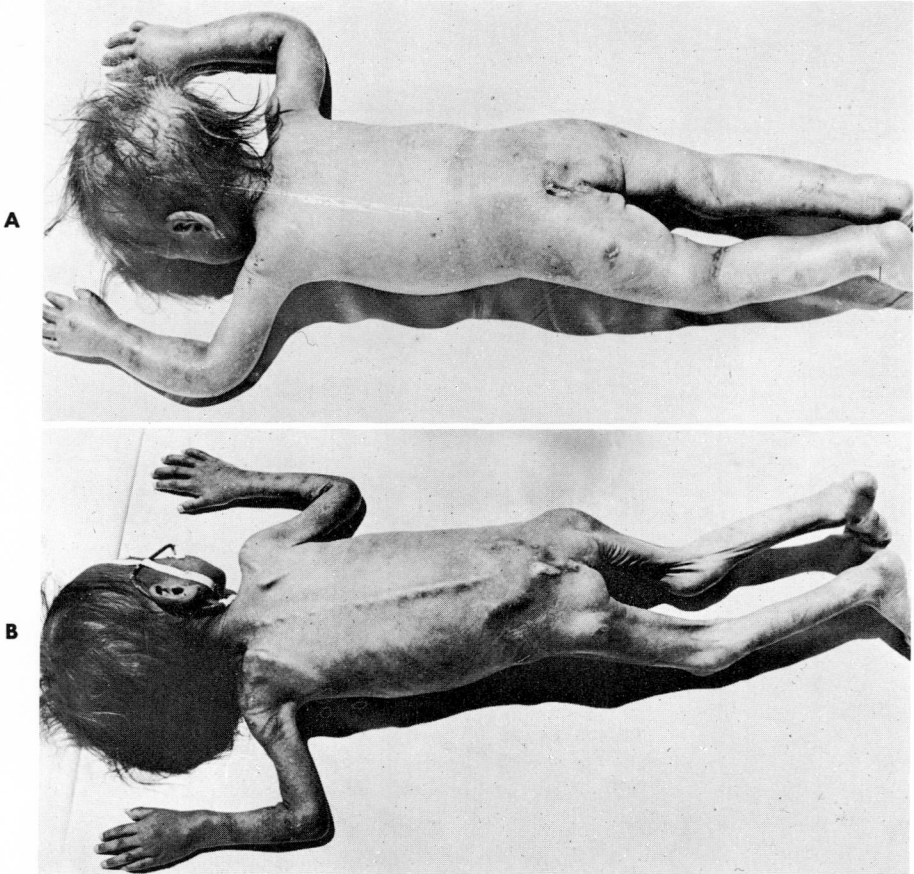

Fig. 9-3. A, Two-year-old child being treated for kwashiorkor. **B,** Two weeks after beginning treatment edema has disappeared, and skin lesions have improved. Note the muscular wasting, which had been concealed by edema. (Courtesy Pan American Sanitary Bureau, Regional Office of The World Health Organization.)

technology. The purpose of this chapter is to look at the imbalance between these environmental factors that cause varying degrees of malnutrition, which is less than the optimum nutrition sought as a base for life fulfillment and quality. These factors are those that characterize our changing environment.

ECONOMIC AND POLITICAL ENVIRONMENT

At its most fundamental level, the nutritional status of individuals in a society involves *money and politics*. That money is a basic

necessity for getting adequate food is plainly evident. Perhaps the role of politics and government programs in nutrition may not be so evident. However, both are always intertwined in any country's nutritional state. Therefore, to be realistic a look must first be taken at the problem of poverty and governmental programs to meet these problems.

The problem of poverty

As a result of the national attention given to the amount of hunger and malnutrition in this country, the public by and large has awakened to the fact that ill-fed persons can no longer be ignored. These problems have tended to be masked by statistics that point to a steadily rising average income or an ever-increasing gross national product. Despite protests to the contrary, scarcely any redistribution of income in the United States has occurred over the past 30 years. Now, as 30 years ago, 20% of our population possesses only 5% of the total wealth, and half of these possess no more than 1% to 2%.

Tremendous problems exist among the poor, at times seeming almost insurmountable. It is small wonder that a "culture of poverty" develops among the poor and is reinforced and perpetuated by society's values and attitudes. Too often they are walled off from the rest of society more completely by such attitudes than by physical barriers. They are poor not only in income but also in other aspects of their lives. They live in ill-kept, overcrowded buildings. Their education is usually inadequate in quality and quantity, and they have little or no access to educational opportunities. As a result, they are poorly prepared for jobs and often must make a day-to-day living at unskilled labor. Often their lives are barren with little beauty and even less hope.

Characteristics of the poor. As a result of these extreme pressures from their living conditions, poverty-stricken persons develop attitudes and characteristics that influence their use of community health services. Health workers must understand and appreciate these characteristics if they are to work *with* these families and avoid imposing directives *on* them.

The traits that characterize the discouraged poor manifest themselves in many ways and in many individual forms, but experienced, sensitive workers identify them essentially as feelings of *isolation, powerlessness,* and *insecurity.*

ISOLATION. Strong feelings of alienation are common among the poor. In many communities few if any channels of communication are open between the lowest income groups and the rest of society.

One of the values of the recent 1969 White House Conference on Hunger and Malnutrition was that just such needed dialogue was initiated. Among the 4,000 delegates were hundreds of poor persons. Other delegates involved students, social workers, executives of food companies, consumer advocates, government officials, academic nutritionists, and many concerned citizens. For the first time for many of these persons, they were forced to listen to points of view that they had never listened to before.

In most instances a poor person responds to his feelings of alienation by further withdrawal. He feels isolated and alone and concludes that no one is really concerned about his situation. The hazards to his health are inherent in poor housing and poor nutrition and are compounded by his distance from the sources of help that would be available to him in his community if he were able to make use of them.

POWERLESSNESS. It is ironic that often those persons most exposed to risks and emergencies have the fewest resources and the least power to cope with them. Extreme frustration is inevitable, and the poor person becomes overwhelmed. Why try, he concludes, if he has no control over the situation? Why plan, if he has no future different from today? In such a day-to-day struggle to exist, the poor person often sees little value in long-range preventive health measures.

INSECURITY. Subjected to forces outside his control, the poor individual has little or no security. A large proportion of the poor population work by the day, if at all. Their unskilled labor is highly expendable. If such a person is sick and cannot work, he usually faces loss of employment rather than sick leave. In his effort to supply his family needs, he is often vulnerable to schemes that can lead him into legal and still deeper financial problems. The impact of these pressures of insecurity and anxiety may incapacitate him. Often, when he appears detached and slow, it is only a defense mechanism to cope with intolerable personal situations. He may become frozen with concern, so that he may appear to care about nothing. Others may respond with hostility. The openly hostile poor strike out at the helping source because they see it as a part of the power structure, which they have come to view as towering and intolerable. As part of this power structure, the source of help appears to them to be an enemy to distrust rather than a friend to whom to look for help.

In such a setting, in which hunger may be a constant companion, food—which has for the poor the same deep psychologic and emotional meaning that it has for all people—assumes even greater meaning than it has for persons who rarely know hunger. For those in a chronic state of insecurity, food can be a serious matter involving the total person.

Role of the health worker. The question may well be asked at this point, how may a concerned health worker help individuals and families conditioned by years of poverty? In the face of such overpowering feelings of isolation, helplessness, and insecurity, what attitudes are necessary to help them? What methods and approaches are most likely to reach patients and clients and supply their needs? Some basic principles can be helpful.

SELF-AWARENESS. First, we must explore our own feelings about the poor. We must be aware of our own class values and attitudes. If we are to be agents of *change*, true "helping vehicles," we must first have some understanding of poor persons and their broad social setting. We must also understand ourselves better and our own cultural conditioning and biases.

RAPPORT. Genuine warmth, interest, friendliness, and kindness grow from the inside out and cannot be put on from the outside as one would put on a cloak. *Rapport* is that feeling of relationship between persons, which is born of mutual respect, regard, and trust. This sense of relationship gives both helper and helped a deep feeling of working *together*. Its most basic ingredient is concern for people and for persons—a positive orientation toward the human race in general and a love and concern for individuals in particular.

ACCEPTANCE. Acceptance is another way of stating the principle that one must begin where the patient is. To begin to help, a person must be accepted as he is in his existing situation. *His* concerns are important. It may be necessary to work with other team specialists to cut through the maze of factors involved in a given situation before the patient is ready to accept or even to consider the health practice or the diet counsel that he needs and that is desired for him. Much time may have to be spent, for example, in coming to understand the meaning of food to this person, before practical dietary matters can begin to be explored.

LISTENING. Here more than elsewhere, the art of listening—positive, active, creative listening—is vital. The patient must tell his story in his own way with no interruptions with distracting statements or questions and no deflecting of the conversation to another's problems. This listening must also be observant. Sequence of statements, subjects introduced, areas of intense feeling, and areas ignored give clues to needs. Throughout, we must guide with sensitivity and create a relaxed, nonthreatening atmosphere in the setting, in which the patient feels free to talk —*and we must listen.* The reason that some frustrated persons finally take their problems to the streets may well be that *no one listens to them unless they do.*

Areas of need. The Department of Agriculture in 1969 estimated that a minimum income of $106 a month was required to provide a sound diet for a family of four. At the same time, however, at least 20 to 30 million Americans do not have $106 a month for food. They live in a variety of geographic areas and come from a number of different ethnic and cultural backgrounds. These areas of need include many Mexican-Americans, both in the rural areas of the southwest and in the barrios of the larger Texas cities; American Indians on a number of reservations; persons in Appalachia; and unemployed agricultural workers in the deep south.

In addition, there are some 400,000 migrant and other seasonal farm workers. They are primarily blacks in the east and Mexican-Americans and blacks in the west. Generally these laborers do not have the benefits of most social and economic legislation to protect their rights as do other types of workers. Also they are ineligible for the food stamp program because they fail to meet residency requirements. Often private hospitals will admit them only if they can pay their bills in cash. Their health needs are high. For example, the net result of this lack of adequate diet is an infant mortality rate of 63 per 1,000 and a stillbirth rate of 70 per 1,000. These statistics are comparable to those for the inhabitants of underdeveloped countries. The average annual income of these migrant workers may be as low as approximately $1,800 to $1,900 per family.

Government programs

The Donated Food Commodities Program. The Donated Food Commodities Program originated in 1935 as a compromise piece of legislation. It was designed to subsidize the farmer by paying him for surplus foods to keep farm prices up. These commodities are then distributed by the government to the poor, sold overseas, or exported to underdeveloped countries. Since the early 1960s the Donated Food Commodities Program has offered eight to twenty of the following items each month:

Apple juice	Grits, corn	Peas, canned
Beans, dry	Lard/shortening	Potatoes, white,
Butter	Meat, canned	dehydrated
Cheese	Milk, evaporated,	Raisins
Corn, canned	instant, or dry	Rice
Cornmeal	Oats, rolled	Syrup, corn
Egg mix	Orange juice	Tomato juice
Flour	Peaches, canned	
Grapefruit juice	Peanut butter	

Today the program operates in approximately 1,000 counties of the nation's 3,100 counties. There is no tight administration from the federal level. As a result, many variations exist in the program's administration on the local level. A number of problems exist with this program.

TYPE OF FOOD. Because of the lack of variety, quality, and availability of foods offered, there is no nutritional balance. Of the supposedly twenty-three items in the program, at many distribution centers only a small number are, in fact, available from time to time. On occasion no more than six or eight of the items may be available. How, for example, is a family to have a balanced diet on bulgur wheat, corn flour, and lard? Yet some 3.8 million individuals rely on this program to gain a good part of their food supply from warehouses established to store and distribute the country's excess farm food items. With the priority of underwriting price supports for the farmer, these foods seem frequently to offer only "government-mandated malnutrition."

MODE OF PACKAGING. Another problem is the manner in which the foods are packaged for the recipients—often in large bags or containers, such as 30- to 100-pound sacks, or in the case of canned meat, a 3- to 5-pound can. How is an older person living alone with no refrigeration to handle such a meat item?

METHOD OF DISTRIBUTION. Often only one warehouse exists within an area of 100 square miles, requiring much travel to procure the foods and difficulty in getting them carried home. For example, rural poor persons have to collect promptly a complete month's supply of food a number of miles away from home. In other situations city poor, usually elderly women or those with small children, have to carry their allotment from the local welfare office, in many instances to a high-rise tenement apartment.

SOCIAL STIGMA. Since these foods often bear little resemblance to those purchased by the consumer at the supermarket, the commodity program often stigmatizes the poor. It serves further to widen the gap between the haves and the have-nots in our society. To many of these persons the certification experiences are humiliating barriers. For adequate nutrition they need other foods—fruits, vegetables, and meat—and a *person-centered* approach.

Food Stamp Program. In contrast to the Food Commodities Program, the Food Stamp Program offers greater convenience and more variety in the selection of foods. However, much of its effectiveness has been hampered by unrealistic and unreasonable methods of operation. The Food Stamp Program began in 1964 as a means of extending the purchasing power of money in low-income families. The food stamps may be used only to purchase domestic foods. The program was originated for the poor; yet it requires them to *purchase* these federal benefits. Often this has been the main difficulty or barrier to its use—the necessity for a lump outlay of cash for initial purchase. Many poor families simply do not have such a lump sum to spend.

PROGRAM IMPROVEMENTS. Since the 1969 White House Conference on Hunger and Malnutrition, the program has been improved. As a result it now serves the needs of more persons—about 10 million in 1971 and 13 to 14 million in 1973-1974. In general, in the revised program the price of stamps has been reduced, and free stamps are offered to those in the lowest income brackets. Table 9-1 gives examples of the general 1972 schedule of food stamp benefits per month.

The newly enacted food stamp amendments offer some valued reforms:

1. For the first time national standards of eligibility have been created: this causes more uniform administration of the program rather than dependence on the social values or ineptness of local officials.

2. No more than 30% of one's income can be paid out at one time for participating. Previously it had been as high as 50%.

3. If family income is under $30 a month, stamps for a family of four are free.

4. Self-certification of families on welfare is permitted.

5. A 60-day carry-on clause extends benefits for mobile families moving to new certification jurisdictions.

6. Allowable deductions permit payment of stamps from welfare checks.

7. Stamps can be used for meals for the elderly if the meals are delivered to their homes.

PROGRAM PROBLEMS. Although the overall program has been improved, some difficulties still exist. Eligibility proves a problem in some instances because of the definition of the word "household" as family members of blood relation under 60 years of age. This effectively deprives an elderly person living alone or with another family of assistance. Also methods of distribution often pose barriers. Some people lack money for transportation or are disabled. Alternative methods such as use of the mails would be helpful in such instances.

Nonetheless, the program has aided a large number of low-income families to improve their diets substantially by the addition of more milk, meat, fruits, and vegetables than they could otherwise purchase. The stamps are freely exchangeable in most food markets. The only stipulation is that they cannot be spent for imported foods or for nonfood items such as soaps, cleansers, paper goods, and other items necessary to personal hygiene and sanitation.

School Lunch Program. At its beginning the School Lunch Program was also agricul-

Table 9-1. 1972 schedule of food stamp benefits per month (abbreviated)

| | PURCHASE REQUIREMENT | |
| | FOUR PERSONS IN HOUSEHOLD (COUPON ALLOTMENT: $112.00) | EIGHT PERSONS IN HOUSEHOLD (COUPON ALLOTMENT: $192.00) |
MONTHLY NET INCOME (AFTER DEDUCTIONS)		
$ 0 to 29.99	$ 0.00	$ 0.00
30 to 39.99	4.00	5.00
40 to 49.99	7.00	9.00
50 to 59.99	10.00	12.00
60 to 69.99	13.00	16.00
150 to 169.99	45.00	45.00
170 to 179.00	47.00	51.00
360 to 389.99	88.00	108.00
390 to 419.99	Ineligible	117.00
630 to 659.99	Ineligible	152.00
Over 659.99	Ineligible	Ineligible

ture oriented. It was started in 1946 to use up war-inflated food production that had supplied world needs during World War II and afterward resulted in a surplus. In 1967 it was still meeting, in the main, the needs of children from middle-income families. It was helping the desperately poor scarcely at all.

In 1970, however, the Child Nutrition Act liberalized the program, which has been broadened to include preschool children and a breakfast program. Together these two meals supply one third to one half the recommended dietary allowances for these children. However, one of the problems still remaining is the barrier of a degrading and injurious "means test," which stigmatizes the poor children in many instances. Its administration has been somewhat erratic, varying among school districts and individual schools under local control. Sometimes difficulties are due to lack of funds, incompetent administration, or disinterest.

White House Conference recommendations. As a result of the 1969 White House Conference, several recommendations for change to improve the administration of these programs were suggested:

1. The Donated Food Commodities Program should be eliminated, since it fails to meet nutritional needs and is unrealistic.

2. The Food Stamp Program should minister also to the former recipients of the commodities program and continue to be strengthened.

3. The Food Stamp Program and the School Lunch Program, now called Child Feeding Program, should be removed from the Department of Agriculture and placed under the Department of Health, Education, and Welfare. A conflict of interest is built into a department that, on the one hand, is committed to support the farmer and agribusiness and, on the other, attempts to meet nutritional needs of people. National feeding programs should be separated from agricultural subsidy programs. As one specialist at the White House Conference said, "We talk too much about the cost of good nutrition and too little about the cost of bad nutrition!" We cannot afford, the conference concluded, *not* to feed *all* our children and feed them well. The highest priority should be given to the development of policies that will somehow enable every family to have an income that will allow for the purchase of a nutritionally adequate diet.

CHANGING FOOD ENVIRONMENT
Food channels

The number of food channels provides wide variety as a means of obtaining food. The rapid changes that are taking place in them mirror the changes in the overall food environment.

Supermarkets. The total food stores in the United States number some 208,000. Of these, 18% are supermarkets; however, this 18% does three fourths of the business in food sales. The supermarkets stock over 8,000 items, but even now the problem of shelf space is rapidly becoming acute with the increasing flow of new food items. It is predicted that by 1980 the stock will include over 10,000 items. The supermarket is largely a suburban shopping center development; hence such markets are few in inner-city areas, especially in poor, ghetto neighborhoods. It is predicted that within the next decade the middle-sized market will have become obsolete. Only the giant supermarkets with greater automation and small neighborhood stores will remain.

Small independent grocery stores. These small stores in neighborhood areas or rural communities often must sell their items for higher costs because they have a lower volume of sales. Often, however, the poor in city neighborhoods prefer these small markets because they are more comfortable where they are known and may obtain needed credit, or they may prefer them because the language barrier does not exist as in an ethnic neighborhood, or because cheaper small sizes of items are more available. Hence cost is often sacrificed for convenience, speed, and the human factor.

Community cooperatives. These cooperatives include large stores and small "food conspiracies." The principle is one of pooling resources for volume buying to make individual items cost less to participating individuals and families.

Farmers markets. Often seasonal produce is sold in markets that allow purchasers to obtain fresh produce at lower costs.

"Natural," "organic," or "health food" stores. The word "natural" is a generalized team covering all foods that are sold without artifical colorings, preservatives, or any kind of synthetic additives. The term "organic," as used by the followers of the natural food movement, has a more specialized meaning: it refers to a method of agriculture in which no chemical fertilizers have been used. Instead food has been fertilized with compost, manure, seaweed, or any kind of vegetation that can be incorporated into the soil; pesticides, herbicides, fungicides, fumigants, or hormones must not have been used; weeds and insects are controlled through nonsynthetic methods. The followers of these movements patronize their own stores. Many fad items are stocked.

"Fast foods" chain stores. A number of stores have grown around a single main item of prepared, ready-to-eat food such as chicken, fish, hamburger, or pizza.

Restaurants. A wide variety of restaurants exist, from those providing quick eating in a short-order coffee shop or cafeteria to more leisurely dining in fine restaurants. For many this food channel is their main food source.

Vending machines. An ever-increasing phenomenon is the vending machine. Through this spreading food channel numerous snack foods are dispensed, many with questionable nutritional contributions.

Food forms

Another characteristic of the changing food environment is the increasing variety of food forms available for purchase. Basically the two main food forms are primary and processed foods.

Primary foods. Fresh produce—single items of food as naturally grown—are called primary foods. Previously this formed the bulk of the food environment. Today, however, primary food is becoming an increasingly smaller percentage of the total food forms sold.

Processed foods. The number of new food forms is rapidly increasing and changing the nature of our food environment profoundly. These processed foods have developed for a number of reasons and produced the following food types.

CONVENIENCE FOODS. These foods include a number of items that are mainly time and work savers, such as dry packaged mixes or frozen dinners. They are increasingly demanded by an active and mobile population.

VARIETY FOODS. Many new foods have developed to meet widening tastes and desires of consumers or to win new markets for producers. Much of this stems from the nature of the food marketing industry, a highly competitive one in which many food items compete for consumer markets and in which the margin of profit is extremely small.

TEXTURED FOODS. A number of new foods are "textured," that is, a substitute food item is developed to replace a standard one. For example, textured vegetable proteins using largely soybean preparations have been developed to supply protein substitutes for meat items.

SNACK FOODS. A multitude of snack foods have developed around an increasingly informal life-style, which includes much eating "on the run." Also the sedentary life around the television set has been an influence. This increase in the use of snack foods has been largely stimulated by the impact of television advertising.

The extent of television's influence on the increased use of snack foods can easily be determined by watching a Saturday morning spate of children's television programs. Within a single hour a child may have been subjected to as many as twenty seven individual advertisements, each trying to tempt him to eat their products, which vary from breakfast cereals, many of which are sugar coated, to cookies, candy, gum, popcorn, sugar-coated vitamins, beverage mixes, canned desserts, frozen dinners, and drive-in restaurants. To an informed viewer the total impact is obviously *antinutritional*.

Council on Children, Media, and Merchandising. In response to this impact of television advertising on the snack habits of children, with its effect on dental caries and general health, the Council on Children, Media, and Merchandising has been formed. A child with moderate television watching habits sees over 5,000 commercials a year advising him what to eat. Advertisements of most of these products mislead the unsuspecting child to equate sugar with nutrition and energy and happiness with a food snack whose nutrient contribution is low. Thus the council's code includes mandatory identification of ingredients and nutrients in foods advertised over the nation's airways; reduction in the advocacy of sugar; elimination of toys, gimmicks, and bonuses to make a child select one food over another; restriction of the number and timing of advertisements; separation of advertisements from program content; and establishment of a research center to maintain surveillance over television's impact on children. This Council on Children, Media, and Merchandising was formed in late 1970. Its members represent recognized consumer groups and professionals in the health and nutrition fields.

Food additives

The advances in American agriculture and the increasing number of new food forms have largely been made possible by the addition and use of many agricultural chemicals and artificial food additives. These intentional food additives include agricultural chemicals and processed food additives.

Agricultural chemicals. America's present food supply is largely the result of many chemicals that are used in scientifically con-trolled amounts to accomplish many tasks. These chemicals include pesticides to control a wide variety of destructive insects and materials to kill weeds, control plant diseases, stop fruit from dropping prematurely, make leaves drop so that the harvesting will be easier, make seeds sprout, keep seeds from rotting before they sprout, and for many other purposes related to increased yield and improved marketing qualities. Additional chemicals are used during the storage phase to prevent the growth of molds and kill destructive insects, thus preventing costly food spoilage. Also agricultural chemicals are used in animal feed and to regulate plant growth.

Some questionable hormones, however, have been used in the meat industry shortly before cattle are slaughtered to increase their yield. One hormone, for example, used for this purpose was diethylstilbestrol (DES), a synthetic form of estrogen, to increase the production of fat in the tissue. Currently, however, DES has been banned by the Food and Drug Administration.

Processed food additives. The rapidly advancing technology of food processing has made use of an increasing number of food additives to produce new food forms. These food additives serve a variety of purposes:

1. *To add specific nutrients.* Much of our enrichment process has added nutrition to foods otherwise low in specific nutrients. For example, the addition of iodine to salt has largely eliminated goiter, the addition of vitamin D to milk has largely eliminated rickets, and the enrichment of grains with niacin has reduced pellegra.

2. *To produce uniform sensory properties.* Some food additives enhance such properties as color, flavor, aroma, texture, and general appearance. An example is the bleaching agent used in freshly milled wheat flour to make it white. Recently, however, several color additives have been banned by the FDA.

3. *To standardize functional properties.* A number of additives enhance and standardize functional properties of foods. In this class are

emulsifiers, stabilizers, moisture retainers, thickeners, binders, dough conditioners, anti-caking agents, jelling agents, and others.

4. *To preserve food.* Antioxidants prevent discoloration of fruits and rancidity of fats. Mold inhibitors and bacterial control agents preserve bread and other baked products.

5. *To control acidity or alkalinity.* The acidity or alkalinity of foods often affects their flavor and texture and the cooked product. Various acids, alkalies, buffers, and neutralizing agents are used to achieve the desired balance or flavor.

The role of FDA

The major government agency charged with the responsibility of maintaining the safety of food is the Food and Drug Administration (FDA). It is an agency within the U. S Department of Health, Education, and Welfare.

General purpose of FDA. The FDA was established in 1938 by the initial federal Food, Drug, and Cosmetic Act of that year. It is a law enforcement agency charged by Congress to ensure, among other things, that the food supply is safe, pure, and wholesome. It seeks to carry out its responsibility through scientific research and public education, as well as by surveillance and law enforcement. Section 401 of the federal Food, Drug, and Cosmetic Act is designed "to promote honesty and fair dealing in the interest of consumers." It seeks to carry out these responsibilities in three areas.

AGRICULTURAL CHEMICALS. The use of agricultural chemicals brings hazard as well as gain. The FDA seeks to control the use of such chemicals and prevent pesticide residues in food crops. It directs a pesticide control program in two phases: (1) requiring initial approval of use of the chemical and (2) continued surveillance of its use by sampling field produce. FDA also carries on a program of public education with producers, growers, county agents, insect-control specialists, pesticide dealers, and agricultural stations. An attempt is made to control the use of pesti-cides to prevent intolerable residues in food.

PACKAGING OF FOODS. The FDA also establishes regulations governing the definitions and standard of identity, reasonable standards of quality, and standards of fill of containers. For any food not having a standard of identity, the law requires that the ingredients in the product must be listed on the label in the order of predominence in the product. In other words, the ingredient in largest amount must be listed first and so on in descending order. The food label must indicate these standards and tell what is in the package. It must not be false or *misleading* in any particular.

FOOD ADDITIVES. The Food Additives Amendment to the federal Food, Drug, and Cosmetic Act of 1938 was passed on September 6, 1958. This amendment, which took effect on March 6, 1960, completely altered the government's method of regulating the use of additives in food. The law provided for the first time that no additive could be used in food unless the FDA, after a careful review of the test data, agreed that the compound was safe at the intended levels of use. An exception was made for all additives that, because of years of widespread use, were "generally recognized as safe," (GRAS) by experts in the field. This approach was a compromise between giving blanket approval to all additives then in use or banning all untested food additives until several years of laboratory safety studies could be conducted.

The Delaney clause to the Food Additives Amendment was attached in the final hours of congressional debate on the legislation. It states that "No additive shall be deemed safe if it is found to induce cancer when ingested by man or animal, or if it is found after tests which are appropriate for the evaluation of the safety of food additives, to induce cancer in man or animal." It was under this clause, for example, that cyclamates were banned in 1969.

GRAS list. The result of the food additives amendment has been to establish what is now known as the GRAS list. This list is a large number of food additives "generally recognized as safe" but not having undergone rigid testing requirements. The list includes several thousand food additives such as salt, sugar, baking powder, spices, flavorings, vitamins, minerals, preservatives, emulsifiers, nonnutritive sweeteners, and many others. All are considered harmless as commonly used in foods. Some are restricted to uses in certain foods and at certain levels, but most are limited only to "intended use" and to "good manufacturing practice."

Problems with the GRAS list. Problems, however, exist with the GRAS list. First, the number of GRAS items is uncertain, and no single compilation of them exists. Quoted statements concerning the number range from approximately 600 to several thousand. Second, in the decade since the GRAS list was formulated two developments have had direct bearing on the soundness of the original concept: (1) Sophistication about toxicity testing has greatly increased, and the inadequacy of relying on a lack of reported human adverse effects as the sole measure of safety has been recognized and (2) the demands of modern technology increase the uses of certain GRAS items well beyond the exposure patterns considered in the original development of the GRAS list. In short, the total food environment has changed radically, creating new problems.

As a result, the United States government has directed the FDA to reevaluate all the items on the GRAS list for safety. However, this directive also poses problems with the present limited allocations of funds and personnel to accomplish it. Herein lies the basis of our present dilemma. Food additives in general are facing increasing public scrutiny.

New nutrient-labeling regulations. In response to the rising consumer awareness of the nutritional needs in foods, the FDA has formulated new nutrient-labeling regulations for foods. The food industry has until 1974 to comply with these regulations. In essence the regulations have two major provisions.

CHANGE OF MDR (MINIMUM DAILY RE-QUIREMENTS) TO RDA (U. S. RECOMMENDED DAILY ALLOWANCES). The MDR was established in 1940 as the FDA's first regulation governing nutrients in foods. However, the standard was, as the name implies, only a minimal requirement, which did not involve a margin of safety to meet a variety of needs and has not been evaluated since its beginning. On the other hand, the RDA, which was established by the National Academy of Sciences in 1943, has been systematically upgraded and expanded over the years to reflect new knowledge. The RDA also is a standard based on a margin of safety to cover a variety of needs. Hence the standard in these new regulations uses the RDA as a point of reference rather than the previous stagnant and increasingly less relevant MDR.

REGULATION OF DIETARY SUPPLEMENTATION. To control the addition of nutrient supplements to foods and subsequent advertising claims, three classes of foods were described:

1. If a food contains less than 50% of the U. S. RDA for the nutrient it claims, it is not a dietary supplement, and only regular nutritional labeling is needed.

2. If a food product contains 50% to 150% of the U. S. RDA for the nutrient it claims, it must be considered a dietary supplement and must meet the standard for supplements. Furthermore, it must be so advertised.

3. If the item exceeds 150% of the RDA for the nutrient it claims, then it cannot be sold as a food or a supplement but must be labeled and marketed as a drug, subject to all the regulations that control them.

Nutritional labeling for most other foods is voluntary, although market competition will probably increase its use. However, if a food is enriched or fortified with any nutrient or if any nutritional claim is made about it (such as "high in vitamin A" or "low in calories"), then it must carry a full nutritional label as described above. These labels always have to follow the same format and appear to the right of the brand name display, so that a shopper will not have to hunt all over the can or package to find the information.

The regulations also provide for labeling of cholesterol and fat content of products. For example, if any product such as a vegetable oil or margarine is advertised as being low in saturated fats, then it must provide the detailed labeling on fat content according to saturated and polyunsaturated fatty acids.

Although there are, of course, some problems in working out these guidelines, most manufacturers in the food industry are working to solve these difficulties. Nutritional labeling is here. As indicated by numerous leaders in the field, a nutrition revolution has begun. Once people begin to understand the relationship between sound nutrition and good health, they will demand nutrition labeling and education, just as they demand responsible environmental policy to control pollution.

FOOD-BORNE DISEASE AGENTS

A number of agents in foods may be disease-causing organisms, including parasites, bacteria, viruses, and fungus toxins.

Parasites

A number of parasites inhabit man's intestinal tract. Some are disease producing and may be carried in foods, including worms and amebas.

Worms. Two types of worm are a serious concern in conjunction with food. One is the roundworm trichina found in pork. Another is a flatworm, the beef or pork tapeworm, which is found in animals that have eaten polluted garbage. If one eats the infected meat raw or rare, the adult tapeworm matures in the intestine and continues its reproductive cycle. It is important, therefore, that pollution control measures be rigidly enforced and that persons avoid eating rare beef or underdone pork.

Amebas. Although numerous harmless amebas normally inhabit man's intestinal tract, some are highly disease producing. The most widely known of these is the ameba that causes dysentery. The organism is ingested as a cyst in contaminated food or water. In the intestine the cyst grows and produces tissue-destroying enzymes that enable the organism to burrow into the intestinal lining and cause ulcers. Transmission is entirely by the human fecal-oral route: man is the carrier and the reservoir. Fecal contamination of food or water may be caused by soiled, unwashed hands and by flies. Carriers who are food handlers contaminate food and utensils. Leaking sewers may pollute water supplies. Control obviously centers on strict sanitation measures and personal hygiene.

Bacteria

Two terms that relate to bacterial sources of food-borne disease need to be distinguished: *food infection* and *food poisoning*. They are among the leading causes of food-borne disease.

Food infection. Food infections result from eating food that has large amounts of living bacteria in it. They multiply inside the digestive tract and cause infectious disease. Each specific disease is caused by a specific bacterium. Because incubation and multiplication of the bacteria take time, food infections develop relatively slowly. Symptoms appear usually 12 to 24 hours or more after the infected food has been eaten. Two of the most common among the food infections are those caused by *Salmonella* organisms or the agent causing cholera.

Food poisoning. Food poisoning is caused by eating food in which bacterial toxins have been produced by the growth of specific kinds of bacteria before the food is eaten. The powerful toxin is ingested directly; thus symptoms of food poisoning develop rapidly usually within 1 to 6 hours after the food is eaten. The most common food poisoning is caused by staphylococci. One fourth of all the outbreaks of food poisoning are in this category. The manifestations occur suddenly, with severe cramping, abdominal pain, nausea, vomiting, and diarrhea, usually accompanied by sweating, headache, and fever. There may be prostration and shock. Recovery is fairly rapid, however, and the symptoms subside within 24 hours. The amount of toxin in-

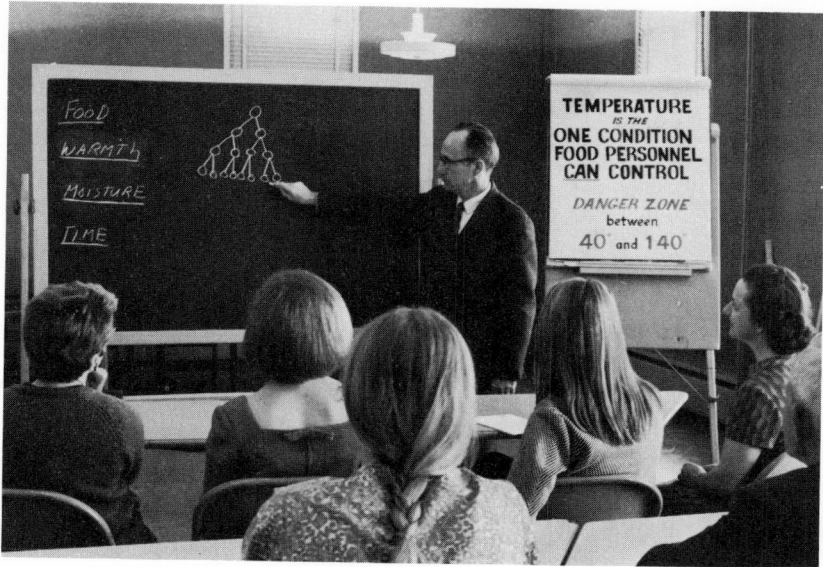

Fig. 9-4. Food handlers' class taught by sanitarian in a city health department. Instruction is provided for personnel involved in preparing and serving food for public use as a means of maintaining a safe food supply.

gested and the susceptibility of the individual eating it determine the degree of severity.

The source of contamination is usually some type of staphylococcal infection on the hands of a worker preparing the food. Custard or cream-filled bakery goods are particularly effective culture beds and hence common carriers of the toxins formed during their growth. Other foods that often support the development of staphylococci are processed meats, ham, tongue, cheese, ice cream, potato salad, sauces, chicken and ham salads, and combination dishes such as spaghetti or casseroles. Since the toxin causes no change in the normal appearance, odor, or taste of the food, the victim is not warned. The education and strict control of food handlers, an ongoing activity of many public health departments, is vital to the prevention of food poisoning incidents in the community (Fig. 9-4).

BOTULISM. Serious, often fatal food poisoning results from ingestion of food containing toxins produced by the bacterium *Clostridium botulinum*. Depending on the dose of toxin taken and the individual response, the illness may vary from mild discomfort to death within 24 hours. Mortality rates are high. Since boiling for 10 minutes destroys the toxin, all home-canned food, no matter how well preserved it is considered to be, should be boiled *at least* 10 minutes before eating.

Viruses

Illnesses produced by viral contamination of food are few in comparison with those produced by bacterial contamination. These include common upper respiratory tract infections such as those transmitted by colds and influenza. Acute viral hepatitis, an inflammatory disease of the liver, is also transmitted in this manner. It may be carried through infected food or water supplies or by blood through intravenous transfusion of infected blood or injection with a contaminated needle.

Fungus toxins (mycotoxins)

Crop damage by molds has long been an economic problem. For example, stored materials such as peanut meal or grains may become contaminated with mold growth and then be fed to animals such as poultry or pigs. Then persons eating such animals become infected and develop severe damage to the nervous system: paralysis or mental retardation may follow. Apparently these toxins are produced shortly after harvesting of the material and early in the storage period. Rapid drying, improved storage conditions, and possible use of fungicides are important control measures.

Natural food poisons

Certain plants and animals contain poisonous substances that occasionally cause human illness or death. Some organisms, for unknown reasons, are toxic at one season of the year and not at others. Some plants produce toxic substances at one point in their growth cycle and not at others. For centuries man has learned through painful experience which plants and animals are poisonous. Only recently, however, have others been recognized and their toxins isolated.

Poisonous plants. A number of poisonous plants exist, usually containing in a portion of their structure some kind of toxic material.

COTTONSEED. A toxic pigment, *gossypol*, is contained in cottonseed and has created problems in preparing protein-rich food supplements with the material. However, procedures for removing the toxin have been developed, and efforts are underway to develop strains of the plant that do not contain gossypol.

SOYBEANS. A trypsin inhibitor in *raw* soybeans is responsible for a toxic substance contained in them. Fortunately this substance is destroyed by heat and is therefore inactivated by cooking.

POTATOES. The green part of sprouting white potatoes contain sufficient amounts of the toxic substance *solanine* to cause gastroenteritis, jaundice, and prostration. Usually it is removed with the peel before the potato is cooked.

MUSHROOMS. Certain species of mushrooms belong to a poisonous variety. Wild mushrooms should be strictly avoided as food: a number of edible species, however, are grown commercially.

RHUBARB LEAVES. The large amount of oxalic acid contained in rhubarb leaves may cause illness. These leaves should not be used as leafy greens for cooking and eating.

FAVA BEANS. *Favism* is a severe form of hemolytic anemia produced by eating (or inhaling pollen) of fava beans (horsebeans) in persons sensitive to them. This sensitivity is a genetic condition in certain population groups and was first observed in certain members of the Mediterranean (Sicilian and Sardinian) and African populations. More recently it has been observed in about 10% of blacks in the United States.

Poisonous animals. Several animals may cause poisonous reactions.

PUFFER FISH. The puffer fish is so named because it can inflate its body with water or air until it forms a globe. It has a gland containing powerful poison to the nervous system, which causes death soon after eating it. Nonetheless the puffer fish is considered a delicacy in the Orient, and chefs take pride in their ability to remove the gland with great care before cooking the fish. This game of chance, however, brings death from poisoning each year to a number of persons whose chefs' knives slipped.

CLAMS AND MUSSELS. During the summer months certain species of clams and mussels in waters along the Pacific coast from Alaska to California feed on marine organisms—plankton—which infect the fish and produce a toxin. At this season the eating of these fish can be fatal.

HERRING. At different seasons in various locations herring apparently become poisonous as human food. Poisonings have been observed from herring caught in the waters around Cuba and Tahiti from May to October and around the New Hebrides Islands in the South Pacific from April to July. Just what accounts for these seasonal changes is not known.

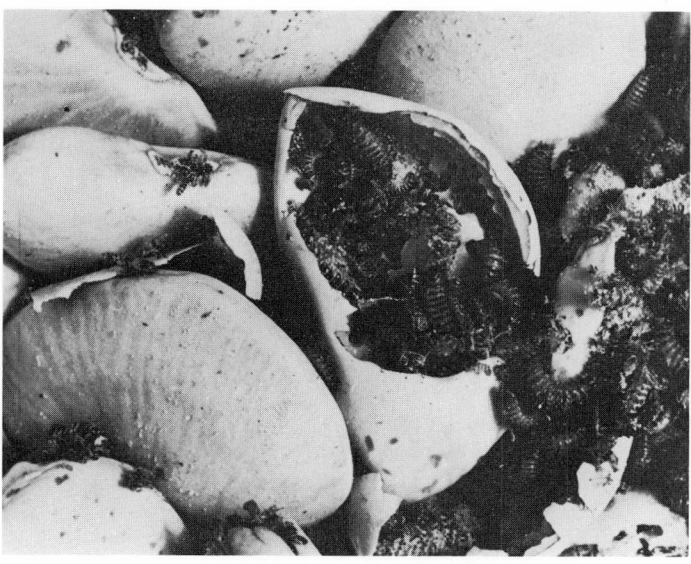

Fig. 9-5. Food spoilage in lima beans by insects. Protecting stored food against insects, molds, and rodents is a constant activity of agricultural experts. (USDA photograph.)

Food spoilage

Food-borne disease and economic waste may also be caused by general food spoilage. Food may deteriorate or become contaminated by chemical or physical changes, microbial growth, or contact with insects or rodents (Fig. 9-5). This is a common problem in food storage.

CHAPTER **10** FOOD HABITS

Important as a sound knowledge of the science of human nutrition is, it is not enough to provide health workers with the means needed to carry out their function in relation to *persons*. It is only the beginning. Unless knowledge is applied realistically to persons in their unique life situations with their particular cultural conditioning, they are not helped. Indeed, barriers and problems may even be created rather than solutions found.

Traditionally medical care has been based on the physical and biologic sciences. A knowledge of these is essential, of course, if one is to understand disease and care for persons who are ill. However, complexity is increasing from two points of view. Throughout the world, societies are becoming more complex with the intermingling of cultures and exchange of health workers across cultural boundaries. The study of disease processes and the growing concept of preventive medicine and health care prove increasingly the need to understand the social and cultural aspects of human behavior and especially to analyze human responses to health care.

This need is strikingly evident in the area of nutrition. Of course, patients' basic nutritional needs or deficiencies must be discovered, but differences in their ways of eating and their strong emotional responses to proposed changes in habits must also be observed.

DEVELOPMENT OF FOOD HABITS

Food habits do not develop in a vacuum. Like other forms of human behavior they are the result of many personal, cultural, social, and psychologic influences. Perhaps everyone tends to be somewhat *ethnocentric*—centered in his own culture. We tend to view our own way as the best or right one. The habits of another who differs from us are often looked on as foreign, or wrong, or superstitious, or stupid. However, if we are honest enough to recognize our own biases, many misconceptions that prevent understanding other people can be cleared away. Such misconceptions hinder our ability to give patients sensitive, constructive care.

In the last analysis, therefore, food habits are an integral part of a person's total life and personality. They result from the whole of one's life experiences and personal development from birth to death. Thus it is unrealistic to approach problems related to feeding a hospitalized patient or to helping the members of the family learn how to improve their diet without first asking the basic question "Why do we eat what we eat?" Only then can we go on from that beginning understanding to ask two follow-up questions: "What food habits, if any, need to be changed? How can we help this particular person make these habit changes?" The second question is the difficult part. In each patient, these factors are interwoven into a behavioral complex. He is a whole individual. To study these influences on food habits, however, we will look at each one of them separately.

SOCIAL INFLUENCES ON FOOD HABITS

Man's group behavior is molded by the numerous activities, processes, and structures by which his social life goes on. Largely such factors as class structure, value systems, and life-styles influence his habit patterns.

Class structure

The structure of a society is formed by groupings formed according to such factors as economic status, education, residence, occupation, or family. Within a given society many of these groups exist, and their values and habits vary. Smaller subgroups within a larger culture are often called *subcultures*. They may be established on the basis of region, religion, age, sex, social class, occupational group, or political party.

Social class especially influences value systems, responses, and behavior patterns. Social classes may be considered as comprising those persons having similar community status, responsibilities, and privileges. In America, although social classes are less distinct and rigid than in some countries, they tend to develop around three basic levels: upperclass, middleclass, and lowerclass. Variations exist within each one of these classes, and the class lines are often blurred, but movement from class to class is possible. Essentially the distinctions are based on the related factors of income, occupation, education, and residence.

The democratic philosophy of American society and the humanitarian ideal underlying the health professions combine to make the reality of class differences difficult to accept. Yet the differences do exist. They probably influence our approach to patients, relationships with them, and the outcome of those relationships more than we may be aware or care to admit.

Value systems

A society's social organization is bound up in its value system, which develops as a result of its history and heritage. For example, values held in America stem largely from its relatively recent pioneer history. The majority of American settlers were from rigidly puritan backgrounds. Their highest values were placed on industry, self-control and self-denial, work, willpower, cleanliness, honesty, responsibility, and initiative. These values became intensified because the survival of the settlers often depended on the exercise of these characteristics. Pleasure and entertainment were considered to have secondary value at best and in most instances were held by the settlers who lived through the most difficult pioneer periods to be unworthy or even evil. In general, the American value system has been based on four main factors: equality, sociality, success, and change. These basic values have largely shaped our personal goals and at the same time contributed to our frustrations in the face of inequality and rigidity.

Life-styles

Life-styles, however, are gradually changing along with the rapid changes that are occurring in the total society. Largely as a result of our devastating experiences with such profound social issues as war, poverty, and malnutrition, many persons have begun to reexamine basic values. As a result, new and varied life-styles are emerging as young people, especially, react against some of the less human applications of our rapidly expanding technology and seek less emphasis on material values and more emphasis on human values. Perhaps the measure of a nation's worth is not so much based on its gross national product, but on the quality of life that it produces in its individual citizens. Continual examination of one's life values is always constructive and growth producing. Socrates said, "The unexamined life is not worth living." New strength can come from such a reasoned and *human* look at ourselves.

Food and social factors

The food habits of people in any setting are highly socialized and perform significant social functions.

Social relationships. Food is a symbol of sociability, warmth, friendliness, and social acceptance. The breaking of bread together binds a group. From the earliest Christian era such custom enriched fellowship and became the symbol of the Communion meal. "And they, continuing daily with one accord, breaking bread from house to house, did eat their meat with gladness and singleness of heart" (Acts 2:46).

A similar use of food for binding fellowship is seen in the honor reception, the wedding breakfast, the political party banquet, and the serving of food to visitors. From the first hours of life, eating is not a solitary experience. It is a matter of two people—a feeding adult and an eating newborn.

People tend to accept food more readily from those persons viewed as friends or allies; people most enjoy eating with those persons to whom they feel close. New foods or advice about foods tends to be accepted from persons who are trusted and respected.

Maternal role. Food is symbolic of motherliness. In the family the early feeding process is the vehicle of much conscious and unconscious learning between mother and child. The mother teaches what is acceptable as food, when to eat, how much to eat, and why it is eaten. Many mothers are unaware that they impart their own likes and dislikes to their children.

A mother's self-esteem is deeply involved in feeding her family. She must feel that she has done the right thing for them as a mother.

Status foods. Status is often thought of in terms of food. A person may build a reputation as a gourmet by eating exotic foods (which he secretly may not enjoy) simply as a means of gaining prestige among his peers. High prestige foods such as roasts or steaks are usually served for dinner guests. Lower prestige foods such as hamburger or liver are rarely served to guests. For some social groups forms of bread vary in status; for example, white bread is preferred to dark. In some groups purchased bread has higher status than homemade biscuits; in others the reverse is true.

Family relationships. Eating together as a family group builds closeness and family solidarity. Food habits that are most closely associated with family sentiments are the most tenacious throughout life. The role of each family member is most clearly illustrated to the child as the family eats together. Long into adulthood certain foods trigger a flood of childhood memories, and these foods are valued for reasons totally apart from any nutritional value.

Increasingly, however, families tend not to eat together as much as in the past. We are becoming a society of individual "snackers," often eating rapidly while engaged in other activities. In many families, dinner is the only meal that may be eaten together.

Economic factors

People tend to eat foods that are readily available to them and that they can afford. Family income, community sources of food, and market conditions influence food habits and ultimate food choices.

Social problems and food habits

Among the many effects of rapid social change, with the uprooting and displacing of persons and families, are changes in the food habits of millions of persons.

Poverty. As has been discussed in the previous chapter, growing numbers of persons in large urban centers are caught in the grip of poverty. Many are members of minority groups who live in slums where they are often disregarded by the mainstream of a sophisticated, affluent society. Many are unprepared for earning a living in industry's automated age and are often frightened, insecure, and lonely. Many persons from such nearby places as Puerto Rico, Cuba, and Mexico or from some areas of the United States such as the rural South have made their way to the cities where they hoped to find a new life. Instead many found obstacles that they cannot surmount. As a result, they live a marginal existence at best. Inadequate housing is attended by problems related to cooking, refrigeration, storage, and sanitation. Malnutrition, broken spirit, and hostility often result.

Family disintegration. Abject poverty for some workers and increased affluence for others has resulted from industrialization and changing urban and suburban living patterns. Family patterns and values are changing. An increasing variety of "family" groups live in a variety of life styles. An increasing number of families seldom gather for meals. In such families the reinforcement of group unity and stability that was formerly felt from eating together is lost. Children are often left to shift for themselves and develop erratic eating habits. They tend to fill their stomachs with a diet that is nutritionally inadequate. The increased number of teen-age marriages often between young people with limited means of support and little knowledge of food preparation or of child feeding may lead to poor food choices and eating habits.

Alcoholism. Alcoholism is frequently associated with poor nutrition. Both the problem drinker and his family may be affected. The wage earner may spend a great portion of the family's small income for alcohol with inadequate funds remaining to feed the family. The alcoholic, even though not depriving others of food, frequently damages his own health by obtaining in alcohol the mere calories that he needs for direct energy. He neglects to eat a proper diet that would supply the many other nutrients that his body needs, and malnutrition results.

Food misinformation and fads

Reasons for food fads. Certain food fads develop as a means of meeting human needs. A person such as an entertainer or an athlete, whose physique or appearance is important to his position, may take up food fads that promise vigor, beauty, or weight control. An aging person may clutch at a food or preparation that promises potency or longer life. A teen-ager may adopt peer group fads to secure his acceptance by the group. All these personal needs and life pressures have to be considered in helping persons find alternative means of improving nutrition while at the same time meeting human need.

False claims by food faddists. Food faddists make exaggerated claims for certain types of food. These claims fall into four basic classifications:
1. Certain foods will cure certain specific conditions.
2. Certain foods are harmful and should be omitted from the diet.
3. Special food combinations are effective as reducing diets and have special therapeutic effects.
4. Only "natural" foods can meet body needs and prevent disease.

If these claims are examined carefully, it will be noted that each one of them focuses on foods per se, not on the chemical components in them—the nutrients, which are the actual physiologic agents of life and health. *The nutrients, not specific foods as such, have specific functions in the body.* Each of these nutrients may be found in a number of different foods. People require specific nutrients, never specific foods.

Examples of food fads. A number of food fads have flourished from time to time. Following are a few examples and the false ideas that they represent:

1. Milk and fish form a harmful combination and should never be eaten together.
 FACT. *Both milk and fish are excellent foods alone or together. Only if either milk or fish is contaminated or spoiled by improper handling or lack of refrigeration may difficulty be encountered.*
2. Pasteurized milk is a "dead milk" and should be replaced by raw milk.
 FACT. *The process of pasteurization may destroy a small amount of vitamin C, but the quantity of it in cow's milk is so small that it makes no significant contribution to the human diet, and its destruction by pasteurization is therefore not important. Control of microorganisms by pasteurization and the prevention of the spread of disease by this means far outweigh any imagined dietary loss.*
3. Citrus fruits, such as oranges and lemons, make the body acid or produce "acid stomach."
 FACT. *Hydrochloric acid, secreted by special cells in the stomach, forms the naturally acid medium of the stomach. Citrus fruits have no influence on this secretion. Since they are oxidized by the body, almost all fruits form an alkaline, not an acid residue.*
4. Onion and garlic will cure a cold or purify the blood.
 FACT. *No such powers are in either food–unless, of*

course, large use of them isolates one socially. Extension of this superstition that garlic has an effect on the blood is the basis on which the quack is able to sell "garlic pills" to cure high blood pressure.

5. Yogurt, blackstrap molasses, honey, and other such "wonder foods" assure good health.

   FACT. *Yogurt is merely a fermented cultured form of milk. It has no mysterious additional properties. It costs more than plain milk. Blackstrap molasses is a syrup formed in the process of refining sugar. It contains vitamins and minerals, but so do many other foods in more common use. Honey is simply a form of sugar (fructose). Some have claimed any number of unfounded curative properties for honey combined with vinegar.*

6. Oysters, olives, lean meat, and raw egg enhance sexual potency and fertility.

   FACT. *Perhaps the notion that there is a connection between lean meat and potency had its origin in the primitive belief that eating certain foods gave persons the characteristics of what was eaten. Hence lean meat (animal flesh) was supposed to arouse animal passion. Such folklore has no basis in fact. No food has any effect on sexual potency. This same notion of strength and virility associated with meat is the basis for the high status position that meat holds in today's diet. A man tends to feel that dinner is incomplete or inadequate unless it is centered around some kind of meat.*

7. Grape juice, tomato juice, and beets are strong blood builders.

   FACT. *The nutrients necessary to the promotion of red blood cells are protein and iron, neither of which are supplied by these foods. This superstition probably arises from the color of these foods: like blood, they are red.*

8. Fish, celery, and nutmeg are good brain foods; raw beef juice is good nerve food.

   FACT. *No food as such builds any specific tissue. Again, it is the specific nutrients in foods that are required for the building of special tissue.*

9. Gelatin in large amounts builds strong fingernails.

   FACT. *Gelatin is an incomplete protein, which alone builds nothing. Nail formation is influenced by many other factors, such as general body nutrition, health environment, and local nail care.*

10. Seaweed, or kelp, products are important dietary supplements that prevent iodine deficiency.

    FACT. *The small amount of iodine needed by the body is supplied in iodized table salt, which is commonly used in the American diet and in seafood. To spend money on seaweed because it provides additional iodine is sheer waste.*

11. Special food combinations are highly effective as reducing diets. Examples of such odd combinations are bananas and skim milk, lamb chops and pineapple, steak and spinach, or just eggs and more eggs.

    FACT. *A weight-reduction program is successful only when caloric intake is less than output (energy expenditure). For optimum nutrition during such a program, the diet must contain a wisely balanced group of nutrients. These faddish reducing combinations do not.*

12. Special foods influence pregnancy and lactation by marking the child, by tainting breast milk, or by increasing milk production. Examples of such taboos or unfounded notions about the need for special foods follow:

    a. Strawberry birthmarks on infants are caused by strawberries eaten by the mother during her pregnancy.

    b. Cravings for special foods or for clay or cornstarch indicate physical needs of the gestating woman.

    c. Beer increases lactation.

    d. Foods such as cabbage, chocolate, and onions taint breast milk and produce gastrointestinal upsets in the nursing infant.

    FACT. *It is not specific foods that are needed for optimum maternal nutrition. It is increased amounts of specific nutrients that are required. No food can mark the developing fetus. No food taints breast milk. The lactating mother does not need beer, although she may well need to increase her total daily fluid intake. Each of the beliefs listed here is unfounded.*

PSYCHOLOGIC INFLUENCES ON FOOD HABITS

Many psychologic meanings are associated with food. Food feeds the psyche as well as the body; hence food plays a large part in meeting emotional needs.

Food behavior

Basic human needs. Such basic physiologic needs as hunger and thirst must be met before higher needs for security, love, status, and self-fulfillment or creative growth can be met. Food plays a part in all these needs, especially the basic ones. In the person existing in a state of basic hunger or semistarvation, the whole existence is concerned with food. Such a person thinks, talks, and dreams about food. Under less severe circumstances, however, the concern for food may be on a relatively higher abstract level and involve symbolism that is associated with meeting these other human needs.

Food and psychologic factors

Factors that are particularly pertinent to the shaping of food habits are motivation and perception.

Motivation. People are not the same the world over. People of differing cultures are not motivated by the same needs and goals. Even primary biologic drives such as hunger and sex are modified in their interpretations or expression by many cultural, social, and personal influences. The kinds of foods sought, prized, or accepted by one individual at one time and place may be violently rejected by another individual living in different circumstances.

Perception. Perception is the way of looking at things. It is the process of adding meaning to what is taken in through the senses. It is perception that enables one to create a relatively stable environment out of an otherwise chaotic assortment of sensory impressions, but perception also limits understanding. A host of subjective elements such as hunger, thirst, hate, fear, self-interest, values, and temperament influence responses to the various phenomena that are presented by the outer world. These responses are called behavior. We look at the world through our own special set of lenses or spectacles. But we must learn to look *at* our own spectacles and not just *through* them. At the same time we must also look *at* and *through* the spectacles of our patients. They are also constantly perceiving their world in terms of their own "filter" or lenses. This takes skill, but we must care enough to work at it. Individual food behavior is constantly being influenced by such unique perceptions of individual life situations. We cannot be of real help to another person unless we try to see his situation as he sees it and understand his behavior on that basis.

Food symbolism

Several areas of psychologic significance give symbolic meanings to food.

Milk. Of all commonly used foods milk perhaps has more psychologic meaning than any other. To many persons milk symbolizes security and comfort. This is especially likely to be true if the individual's early relationships with the mother figure were satisfactory. At the same time milk may mean dependence and helplessness, particularly in periods of stress. For example, ulcer patients on prolonged treatment of milk every few hours may find in such routine a socially accepted form of symbolic regression.

Sex-related attitudes. Certain foods carry masculine meanings, including meat and bread, which carry a meaning of the paternal role of hunter and provider. Meat in primitive tribal cultures was often considered the only food that would make a warrior strong and courageous. Many traditions about the magic power of meat and blood are known to students of anthropology. In America the tradition that strong men eat meat has been fostered until modern times by frontier history. The survival of the pioneers depended on their physical energy, strength, activity, and aggression. Meat has been the center of the meal both in terms of menu planning and money expended. For example, eggs are nutritionally equal to meat (actually better in ideal amino acid combination); but eggs never quite make the grade as a meat substitute, being offered only as a last resort.

Vegetables and fruits, on the other hand, carry feminine meanings. They connote the maternal role of the one who feeds and gives. This symbolic concept has a fascinating history. When early human beings first settled down after a purely nomadic and hunting existence to an agricultural life, women tilled the fields, whereas men continued to hunt and fight. The supremacy of the male is bound up with his belief in the "feminine weakness" represented by "mere" fruits and vegetables. The less educated (and the less psychologically developed) a man is, the more likely he is to scorn fruits and vegetables on emotional grounds, although he usually is totally unaware of the reason for his preference and attributes it simply to the taste of the food itself.

Fruits are most feminine in meaning. The apple for the teacher, the gift basket, grapes, and peaches and cream symbolize love, beauty, sexuality, exteem, and luxury. The reproductive notion is basic in the word "*fruition*," the bearing of fruit. Vegetables bear ideas related to even more primitive and earthy aspects of femininity—vegetate, vegetation. Fruits and vegetables are seasonal, ripe, bright colored, and pleasantly shaped.

Age. Milk and strained foods, sometimes necessary components of a therapeutic diet for the adult, are considered infant foods and may be rejected, particularly by the person who is uncertain that he has genuinely attained adult status. Such a person may be of any chronologic age.

As the child grows older, his food horizon widens. When he leaves home for school, he encounters new foods and is given greater freedom of choice. He also compares his family food to that of his friends and begins to learn the social status of foods. Certain foods such as peanut butter become labeled as child food and are promoted as such by advertisers.

During adolescence, the struggle for selfhood ensues. Not only clothes, late hours, driving, and dating, but also foods become battlegrounds between the generations. The teen-ager periodically adopts food fads, exhibits intense likes and dislikes, and displays enormous appetite. His obsession with his body image is basically a sexual problem. It may take the form of muscle-building foods for boys or figure-control diets for girls.

Adulthood brings certain ideas of food privileges. Foods such as olives, shrimp, and gourmet dishes may be considered adult. Drinks such as coffee, tea, or alcohol are reserved in most groups for adults.

Reward foods. Sweets are often used to bribe children—given as rewards for good behavior and withheld for bad behavior. Sometimes unusual foods, special methods of preparation, or rare delicacies become rewards or punishments.

Illness. Illness is a period of psychologic stress. At this time some degree of regression usually manifests itself. The patient may become picky about his food and make frequent special demands. Poor appetite may compound feeding problems. The patient, more than the well person, needs to be involved in the selection of his food.

CULTURAL INFLUENCES ON FOOD HABITS

Margaret Mead states that culture involves not only the more obvious and historic aspects of man's communal life, such as his language, religion, politics, and technology, but it also involves all the little habits of everyday life, such as preparing and serving food and caring for children—feeding or lulling them to sleep. Often the most significant thing that can be known about a culture is what it takes for granted in daily life.

These many facets of a person's culture are *learned*. Gradually as a child grows up within a given society, the slow process of conscious and unconscious learning of values, attitudes, habits, and practices takes place through the conscious and unconscious influence of parents, teachers, and other enculturating agents of his society. Whatever is invented, transmitted, and perpetuated—his socially acquired knowledge and habits—he learns as part of his culture. These, then, become internalized and deeply entrenched.

Function of culture

The culture of a people develops over a long period of time. It is partly the result of this people's *adaptation to environment*, which often makes survival possible. Sometimes the changing of these habits by an outsider who does not understand these adaptations may upset this balance with nature as has been the case when some health workers have tried to impose Western culture and habits on people in other parts of the world without prior study and appreciation of established customs. Such programs have failed for this reason.

The culture of a people also develops as a means of *interpreting common (and sometimes terrifying) life experiences*, such as birth, death, illness, disease, sex, and natural phenomena. Rituals, taboos, totems, habits, and practices develop to explain, placate, or protect and to establish human environmental relationships. A certain poisonous plant, for example, may have become taboo in a society as a food because the tribal ancestors observed that it caused death.

Food in a culture

Food habits are among the oldest and most entrenched aspects of many cultures. They exert a deep influence on human behavior. In spite of considerable variation, food habits are largely based on food availability, economics, or symbolism. Included under these influential factors are the geography of the land, the agriculture practiced, economy and market practices, and history and traditions.

Cultural determination of what constitutes food. Items considered to be food in one culture may be regarded with disgust or actually cause illness in persons of another culture. In American milk is valued as a basic food, whereas in many other cultures it is regarded with disgust as an animal mucous discharge. Some cultures consider insects such as dragonflies and locusts, which they boil, dry, and grind into a powder, and crickets, flying and red ants, beetles, and water bugs, which are fried in lard, as delicacies. These are items that would not be accepted as food in this country. Bread is another example. Many a diet-obsessed American rejects bread, but in a Greek home bread is the main food—*the* meal. All other foods are considered accompaniments and are eaten between bites of bread.

Religious aspects of culture also control food rejection and acceptance. Pork, for example, is unacceptable as food for a Moslem or an Orthodox Jew. Any meat is unacceptable to the Seventh-Day Adventist. The strict Hindu or Buddhist eats no meat. In his youth Ghandi is said to have intellectually agreed that beef was a good food for human use and therefore to have eaten some, but his Hindu culture and rejection of beef was so deeply ingrained and internalized that the food made him violently ill and he never used it again.

Politics. Food use has had political as well as religious significance in man's history. In India the fasts of Ghandi wielded tremendous political power and contributed enormously to that country's achieving independence from Great Britain. The Boston Tea Party was concerned with important interrelationships between food, economics, and a budding nation's political views. Tea was considered to be an almost essential commodity by the American colonies, and English taxes on tea stimulated the politics of American independence.

Major life experiences. The birth of a child is observed in many cultures by a meal that symbolizes a general celebration of the beginning of life. It is an occasion for feasting or in some cultures for offering special foods to one or more deities. Soon after birth a baptism or dedication ceremony may be followed by a special family meal. Birthdays are celebrated with special foods. Stages of the young person's development are often observed by special food uses. For example, at a coming-of-age ceremony, such as the Bar Mitzvah for Jewish boys at the age of 13 years, honeycake, wine, canapés, and strudel are generally served.

Weddings are especially surrounded with symbolic foods. The bride's cake and the wedding reception are common in Western culture. Family feasting often lasts for several days in other cultures in which the eating of special foods together seals the marriage pact.

Pregnancy is also attended by many food symbols, taboos, and practices. Certain foods may be avoided in the belief that they will mark the infant. Other foods may be denied the pregnant woman in the belief that she will contaminate the food supply.

In many cultures the death of a member of the group involves food use symbolizing the general fact that each individual life has its end. In one group food may be buried with the body to sustain the departed on the journey to the hereafter. In another group food may be the main expression of sympathy, sorrow, or support for the bereaved and many offerings of food brought to the house by neighbors. A special funeral supper may be a part of the mourning or wake prescribed in still another group.

Cultural food patterns

A number of different cultural food patterns are represented in American community life. Many have contributed characteristic dishes or modes of cooking to American eating habits, and, in turn, many food habits of the subcultures have been Americanized. Traditional foods tend to be used more consistently by the older members of the family, whereas the younger ones may use such foods only on special occasions or holidays. Nonetheless, these traditional food patterns have strong meanings and serve to bind families and cultural communities in close fellowship. A few representative cultural food patterns will be presented here. However, among persons of all cultures, individual tastes vary, geographic patterns within a country vary, and economic factors cause wide differences, as does the educational level. In various food patterns the type of food may be unique and there may be special dishes and methods of preparation. These special food patterns may relate to certain ethnic or regional groups and make use of foods that are easily available in that region. Other food patterns may develop in relation to religious beliefs or festivals. Whatever the origin, such food practices are usually deeply ingrained in the lives of the people and are important to respect.

Jewish food pattern. Jewish dietary food laws vary among the three basic groups within Judaism: Orthodox—strict observance; Conservative—nominal observance; and Reform—less ceremonial emphasis and minimal observance of the general dietary laws.

This body of dietary laws is called the *Rules of Kashruth*, and foods selected and prepared accordingly are called *kosher* foods. Both words come from the Hebrew word *"kashar,"* meaning right or fit. The basis of these laws is primarily self-purification and a means of service to God, although they probably also had some hygienic or ethical foundation in the beginning. Most of these rules relate to ordinances given the ancient Hebrews, as recorded in the Old Testament books of the law (Leviticus and Deuteronomy), and to the Jewish traditions accumulated over the centuries. These traditions were collected and interpreted in the Talmud, a body of laws set down in the fourth to the sixth centuries B.C. Since the original Hebrew religion was centered in practices of animal sacrifice and the blood had special ritual significance, the present Jewish dietary laws apply specifically to the slaughter, preparation, and service of meat; to the combining of meat and milk; to fish; and to eggs.

FOOD RESTRICTIONS

1. The only meat allowed is the meat of cloven-hoofed guadrupeds that chew a cud (cattle, sheep, goats, and deer). Only the forequarters of these animals may be used. The hindquarters may be eaten only if the sinew of Jacob (hind sinew of the thigh) is removed (Lev. 11:1-8).

2. Chickens, turkeys, geese, pheasants, and ducks may be eaten (Lev. 11:13-19).

3. Ritual slaughter follows rigid rules based on minimal pain to the animal and maximum blood drainage and involves several steps. The meat is water soaked in a special vessel, then rinsed, and thoroughly salted with coarse salt. It is placed on a perforated board, tilted to permit blood to flow off, and left to stand for an hour. After draining thoroughly, it is washed three times before being cooked.

4. No blood may be eaten as food in any form. Blood is considered synonymous with life (Gen. 9:4; Lev. 3:17).

5. No combining of meat and milk is allowed. This prohibition is based on the oft-repeated Old Testament command, "Thou

shalt not seethe a kid in its mother's milk" (Exod. 23:19). Milk or food made with milk, such as cheese and ice cream, may be eaten just before a meal, but not for 6 hours after eating a meal that contains meat. In the Orthodox Jewish household the custom is to maintain two sets of dishes, one for serving meat and the other for serving dairy meals.

6. Only those fish with fins and scales are allowed. No shellfish or eels may be eaten (Lev. 11:9-12). Fish of the type permitted may be eaten with either dairy or meat meals.

7. No egg that contains a blood spot may be eaten. Eggs may be taken with either dairy or meat meals.

8. No special restrictions apply to fruits, vegetables, or cereals.

FOODS FOR SPECIAL OCCASIONS. Many of the traditional Jewish foods are related to festivals of the Jewish calendar. These festivals, or holidays, commemorate events in Jewish history. Often special Sabbath dishes are used. In Orthodox Jewish homes, no food is prepared on the Sabbath, which begins at sundown on Friday and ends when the first star becomes visible Saturday evening. Foods are prepared on Friday and held for use on the Sabbath. A long-honored custom is that of inviting a guest to share the Sabbath meal as a remembrance of the biblical statement, "For you were once strangers in the land of Egypt" (Exod. 22:20). A few representative Jewish foods follow:

1. Challah—a special Sabbath loaf of white bread, shaped as a twist or a beehive coil, used at the beginning of the meal after the kiddush (the blessing over wine)
2. Gefüllte (gelfilte) fish—from a German word that means stuffed fish, usually the first course of the Sabbath eve meal and made of fish filet, chopped, seasoned, and stuffed back into the skin or minced and rolled into balls
3. Bagels—doughnut-shaped, hard yeast rolls
4. Blintzes—thin filled and rolled pancakes

5. Borscht (borsch)—soup of meat stock and beaten egg or sour cream with beets, cabbage, or spinach (served hot or cold)
6. Kasha—buckwheat groats (hulled kernels), used as a cooked cereal or as a potato substitute with gravy
7. Knishes—pastry filled with ground meat or cheese
8. Lox—smoked, salted salmon
9. Matzo—flat unleavened bread
10. Strudel—thin pastry, filled with fruit and nuts and rolled, then baked

Mexican food pattern. A blending of the food habits of the Spanish settlers and native Indian tribes forms the basis of the present food patterns of persons of Mexican heritage, sometimes called Chicanos, who now live in the United States, chiefly in the southwest. Three foods are basic to this pattern—dried beans, chili peppers, and corn. Variations and additions may be found in different localities or among those of different income levels.

FOOD GROUPS

1. *Milk.* Little milk is used. A small amount of evaporated milk may be purchased for babies.

2. *Meat.* Because of its cost, little meat is taken: beef or chicken may be eaten two or three times a week. Eggs also are used occasionally and fish, rarely.

3. *Vegetables.* Corn, fresh or canned, and chili peppers are the main vegetables. Chicos is steamed green corn dried on the cob. Pasole is similar to whole-grain hominy (limetreated, hulled whole kernels). Chili peppers provide a good source of vitamin C; they are usually dried and ground into a powder. Pinto or chalice beans are used daily; they may be reheated by frying (refried beans) or cooked with beef, garlic, and chili peppers (chili con carne).

4. *Fruits.* Depending on availability and cost, oranges, apples, bananas, and canned peaches are used.

5. *Bread and cereals.* For centuries corn has been the basic grain used as bread and cereal by the Mexican people. Masa (dough)

is made from dry corn that has been heated, soaked in lime water, washed, and ground wet to form a mass with the consistency of putty. This dough is then formed into thin, unleavened cakes and baked on a hot griddle to make the typical tortilla. Wheat is now replacing corn for making some tortillas. Unless the wheat flour is enriched, however, the calcium in the treated corn is lost to the Mexican diet. Cornmeal gruel, or atole, is served with hot milk. Rice cooked in milk may be used as a desert. Oatmeal is a popular breakfast cereal.

6. *Beverages.* Large amounts of coffee are generally used. In some families coffee is given to young children also.

7. *Seasonings.* Chili pepper, onions, and garlic are used most frequently; occasionally other herbs may be added. Lard is the basic fat.

Puerto Rican food pattern. The Puerto Rican people share a common Spanish heritage with the Mexicans. A large part of their food pattern is similar. However, the use of tropical fruits and vegetables that grow on the island have formed the base of the Puerto Rican food pattern. Some of these habits are carried over to Puerto Ricans living in this country, when the foods are available in local neighborhood markets. Almost everyone eats the main food, viandas, which are starchy vegetables and fruits, such as plantain and green bananas. The two other staples of the diet are rice and beans. Milk, meat, yellow and green vegetables, and other fruits are used in limited quantities.

FOOD GROUPS

1. *Viandas.* The many kinds of viandas eaten every day include green bananas, green and ripe plantain, white and yellow sweet potatoes, white yams, breadfruit, and cassava. These foods are cooked in many ways. Usually codfish and onion are added. If income permits, some avocado and hard-boiled eggs are also added. This dish is called *serenata.* A soup containing vianda and meat is called *sancocho.*

2. *Rice.* A large portion of daily calories is obtained from rice. Most Puerto Ricans eat about 7 ounces daily, usually cooked in salted water and seasoned with lard. Other rice dishes include rice stewed with beans and sofrito (a sauce of tomatoes, green pepper, onion, garlic, salt pork, lard, and herbs); rice with chicken, seasoned with olives, red pepper, and sofrito; a dessert made with rice, sugar, and spices; and a thick soup of chicken and rice.

3. *Other cereal grains.* Some wheat is used in the form of bread, noodles, and spaghetti. Oatmeal and cornmeal mush may be added if income permits.

4. *Beans.* Legumes used include chickpeas (garbanzos), navy beans, red kidney beans (preferred), and dried peas. Usually they are boiled until tender and cooked with sofrito.

5. *Meat.* Most families cannot afford meat, although pork and chicken are used when income allows. The only animal protein that the majority can buy is dried codfish.

6. *Milk.* Low-income groups can afford little milk. Most of what is taken is boiled and used with coffee; some cocoa and chocolate are used in the same way.

7. *Vegetables and fruits.* Small amounts of other vegetables are used by the Puerto Rican people. Many tropical fruits are available in the island. Puerto Rico is the home of the *acerola,* the tiny, sour West Indian cherry, which looks like a miniature apple and has the highest quantity of ascorbic acid known to be contained in any food (about 1,000 mg./100 gm.). Other fruits include oranges, pineapples, grapefruits, papayas, and mangoes.

MEAL PATTERN. In most households a typical day's food pattern would include coffee with milk for breakfast; a large plate of viandas with codfish for lunch; and rice, beans, and viandas for dinner. If income permits, egg or oatmeal may be added to the breakfast, some meat to dinner, and fruit between meals. This simple daily diet contrasts with a holiday meal such as that enjoyed at Christmas time. This feast would include whole pig roasted on a spit, blood sausage, green bananas or plantains cooked in the ashes, rice, pasteles (plantain dough filled with chopped pork, sofrito, olives, raisins, and boiled peas), rice pudding, and wine, beer, or brandy.

An effort is being made by the Puerto Rican government to improve the diet of their people. The basic foods that everyone eats are listed (rice, beans, viandas, codfish, lard, sugar, and coffee); then suggestions are made for items that need to be added, such as either dry or goat's milk, meat and eggs, yellow and green vegetables, and fresh native fruit.

Chinese food pattern. Traditional Chinese cooking is based on three principles: (1) natural flavors must be developed; (2) texture and color must be maintained; and (3) undesired qualities of foods must be masked or modified. Like the French, Chinese cooks believe that refrigeration lessens natural flavors. They select the freshest possible foods, hold them the shortest possible time, and then cook them quickly at a high temperature in small amounts of liquid or fat. This is called *stir-frying*. By these means natural flavor, color, and texture are preserved. Vegetables are cooked just before serving, so that they are still crisp and flavorful when eaten. The only sauce that may be served with them is a thin, translucent one, usually made with cornstarch. A thick gravy is never used. To mask some flavors or textures or to enhance others, foods that have been dried, salted, pickled, spiced, candied, or canned may be added as garnishes or relishes.

FOOD GROUPS

1. *Milk.* Little milk and limited amounts of cheese are used.

2. *Meat.* Pork, lamb, chicken, duck, fish, and shellfish are used in many ways. Usually they are cooked in combination with vegetables, thus extending the amount of meat. Eggs and soybeans in the form of soybean curd and milk add to the protein content of the Chinese diet. Some characteristic dishes include egg roll—a thin dough spread with meat and vegetable filling, rolled and fried in deep fat; egg foo yung—an omelet of egg, chopped chicken, mushrooms, scallions, celery, and bean sprouts; and sweet and sour pork—pork cubes fried and then simmered in a sweet-sour sauce of brown sugar, vinegar, and other seasonings. Chow mein or chop suey is purely an American invention. It is a mixture of meat, celery, and bean sprouts, served over rice or noodles and seasoned with soy sauce.

3. *Vegetables.* Cooked by the characteristic method just described—stir-frying—vegetables such as cabbage, cucumbers, snow peas, melons, squashes, greens, mushrooms, bean sprouts, and sweet potatoes are made into many fine dishes.

4. *Fruit.* Usually fruits are eaten fresh. Pineapple and a few others are sometimes used in combination dishes.

5. *Bread and cereals.* Rice is the staple grain used at most meals.

6. *Seasoning.* Soy sauce is a basic seasoning. Almonds, ginger, and sesame seed are also used. The most frequently used cooking fats are lard and peanut oil.

7. *Beverage.* The traditional beverage is unsweetened green tea.

Japanese food pattern. Japanese food patterns are in some ways similar to Chinese. Rice is a basic constituent of the diet, soy sauce is used for seasoning, and tea is the main beverage. However, some characteristic differences occur. The Japanese diet contains more seafood, especially raw fish. A number of taboos prohibit certain food combinations or the use of certain foods in specific localities or at specific times. Some of these taboos are associated with religious practices such as ancestor veneration.

FOOD GROUPS

1. *Milk.* Little milk or cheese is used. Some evaporated or dried milk may be added in cooking or given to babies.

2. *Meat.* The main animal protein source is seafood. Many varieties of fish and shellfish such as raw squid or octopus are served.

Other unusual saltwater fare are eels, abalone, and globe fish (puffer fish) (p. 112). More familiar to the Westerner are crab, shrimp, mackerel, carp, and salmon. Families living inland especially may also eat rabbit, chicken, and occasionally beef or lamb. Eggs are a source of additional protein.

3. *Vegetables.* Japanese menus include many vegetables, usually steamed and served with soy sauce. Pickled vegetables are also well liked.

4. *Fruit.* Fresh fruit is eaten in season, a tray of fruit being a regular course of the main meal.

5. *Bread and cereals.* Although rice is the staple grain, some corn, barley, and oats are served, and white wheat bread is coming into increasing use in Japanese cities.

MEAL PATTERN. A specific sequence of courses is usually followed at most traditional Japanese dinners: green tea, unsweetened; some appetizer, such as soy cake or red bean cake, a raw fish (sashimi) or radish (komono) relish; broiled fish or omelet; vegetables with soy sauce; plain steamed rice; herb relish; fruits in season; a broth-base soup; and perhaps more unsweetened green tea. Typical dishes include tempura (batter-fried shrimp) and aborakge (fried soybean curd). Sukiyaki, a mixture of sautéed beef and vegetables served with soy sauce, is as American as chow mein. Soybean oil is the main cooking fat.

Italian food pattern. The sharing of food and companionship is an important part of the Italian life pattern. Meals are associated with much warmth and fellowship, and special occasions are marked by the sharing of food with families and friends. Leisurely meals are customary, with a light breakfast, dinner in the middle of the day, and a small evening meal. Bread and pasta are the basic Italian foods. On religious fast days, such as Fridays, Lent, and the period of Advent before Christmas, pasta is prepared with meatless sauces or with fish.

FOOD GROUPS

1. *Milk.* Milk is seldom used alone as a beverage but is frequently consumed with coffee in a mixture of about half and half. Cheese, however, is a favorite food. Parmesan and Romano are hard grating cheeses used in cooking; ricotta and mozzarella are two soft Italian cheeses used in cooking or with bread.

2. *Meat.* Chicken baked with oil or in tomato sauce is often used. Beef and veal are eaten as meatballs, meat loaf, cutlets, stews, roasts, and chops. Roasted or fried Italian pork sausages is common. A number of Italian cold cuts are famous—salami, mortadella (bologna-type sausage), coppa (peppered sausage), and prosciutto (Italian cured ham). Many kinds of fish are used. Fresh fish are preferred, but some canned fish such as tuna, sardines, anchovies, and special salted codfish are used also. Some characteristic meat dishes are chicken browned in olive oil, then simmered in wine and tomato sauce and thin floured strips of veal browned in olive oil and simmered in a sauce flavored with wine and herbs. Italian meatballs are served with spaghetti, and dry salted codfish, soaked several days and browned in olive oil, is simmered with tomato sauce and herbs.

3. *Vegetables.* Favorite vegetables include zucchini and other types of squash, broccoli, spinach, eggplant, salad greens, green beans, peppers, and tomatoes. The latter are used in many ways—in sauces, either whole or as paste, or pureed. Vegetables are usually cooked in water, drained, and seasoned with olive oil or with oil and vinegar. Combination salads of salad greens, with a simple dressing of olive oil, vinegar, garlic, salt, and pepper is called *insalata.*

4. *Fruit.* Fresh fruit in season is eaten for dessert.

5. *Bread and cereals.* Bread is present at every Italian meal as a highly regarded principal food. It is made into loaves of many shapes, each one characteristic of a different Italian province. All Italian breads are made of wheat flour and are white, crusty, and substantial. Some rice and cornmeal are used in special dishes; for example, polenta is a thick, yellow cornmeal mush, sometimes made into

a casserole with sausage, tomato sauce, and cheese.

A basic item in the Italian food pattern is pasta. This term is used for all the wheat products made into various forms such as spaghetti, macaroni, and egg noodles. Pasta is served in many ways. Spaghetti is commonly used with a characteristic tomato sauce and cheese or with meatballs or fish. Special dishes of pasta of various kinds filled with meat mixtures are served on holidays—ravioli, lasagna, manicotti, tortellini, and cannelloni. A dry red or white wine is usually served also.

6. *Soups*. Thick soups often serve as a main food for lighter meals. Minestrone is made with vegetables, chick-peas, and pasta. Often a substantial bean soup is used.

7. *Seasonings and basic cooking method*. Herbs and spices characteristically used in Italian dishes include oregano, rosemary, basil, saffron, parsley, and nutmeg. Garlic is used often, as are wine, olive oil, tomato puree, salt pork, and cheese. The basic process of Italian cooking of main dishes is the initial browning of the seasonings in olive oil, adding of meat or fish for browning also, then covering with liquid such as wine, tomato sauce, or broth, and simmering slowly on low heat for several hours.

Greek food pattern. In the close-knit, traditionally organized life of the Greek family, food and ceremonial aspects of meals constitute primary values. In many Greek homes the meal is a family ritual. A blessing is said or sung, and hospitality is extended to guests. Everyday meals are simple, but holiday ones are the occasion for serving a great variety of delicacies. Bread is always the center of every meal—indeed it *is* the meal—with other foods considered accompaniments to it: bread is eaten between bites of other food. During religious holidays such as Lent, there are fast days of meatless meals, with large use of vegetables.

FOOD GROUPS

1. *Milk*. A relatively small amount of milk is used as a beverage by adults, who usually take this food in the form of yogurt. Children drink hot boiled milk sweetened with sugar. Cheese is a favorite food, however. Varieties include feta, a special white cheese made from sheep's milk and preserved in brine, and two hard, salty cheese, caceri and cephalotyri.

2. *Meat*. Lamb is the favorite meat. Little beef and some pork and chicken are eaten. Frequent use is made of organ meats or fresh fish. Eggs are sometimes used as a main dish, but not at breakfast.

3. *Vegetables*. Vegetables are usually cooked until soft and are seasoned with meat broth or tomato with onions, olive oil, and parsley. Vegetables are often the main dish. Large amounts of many varieties are eaten with fresh ones preferred. Combination salad of thinly cut raw vegetables with a simple dressing of olive oil and vinegar or lemon juice is often used. Many legumes (beans, peas, lentils, and chick-peas) are eaten. Often a meal consists of cooked dried beans served with olives and pickles. A characteristic dish is dolmathes, a meat and rice mixture rolled in cabbage or vine leaves, steamed, and served with egg sauce.

4. *Fruits*. Large amounts of fruit are eaten. Peeled raw fruit is an everyday dessert.

5. *Bread and cereals*. Bread is made of plain wheat flour, water, salt, and yeast. An indispensable part of every meal, it is preferred plain without butter, jam, or jelly. Dark breads are used by some families. Wheat products such as noodles, macaroni, and sphaghetti may be used plain or with meat and tomato sauce. Rice is commonly served. A characteristic rice dish is pilaf, which is rice, first browned in butter, covered with broth or water, and simmered until the liquid is absorbed.

6. *Desserts*. Desserts other than raw fruit are usually served on special occasions such as holiday meals. Such a characteristic dessert is baklava, made of many layers of very thin pastry, brushed with butter, sprinkled with nuts, sugar, and spices, cut in diamond shapes, baked, and then served with syrup.

FOOD HABIT CHANGES

Food habits, therefore, are deeply significant in every person's life. In considering whether any particular change in habit may be desirable from a health and nutrition standpoint, it is important to include variety and an appreciation for habits already established and to build on these.

Variety in food patterns

It is plain that there is no one way of eating. Variety in food patterns is desirable as a means of building a broader nutritional intake, as well as meeting a variety of personal needs. Consider such variety in the following food factors: number of meals, type of foods, method of preparation, and place of eating.

Number of meals. Good nutrition does not demand any specific number of meals a day— only specific nutrients. Given meal patterns relate to cultural habits and physical activities, not biologic necessity. A given amount of specific nutrients and energy value (calories) over a 24-hour period is the important factor. How this food is distributed over the day is purely individual choice, determined by practical life situations, cultural background, or personal preference.

Type of foods. An increasingly large variety in types of food is apparent in any food market. There are "convenience foods," processed foods, and food combinations, as well as primary foods—single fresh foods as they are grown. As indicated, the total food environment is rapidly changing as the result of rapidly changing food technology. To ignore these changes in discussing food needs with persons is unrealistic. Also the deeply ingrained cultural food patterns must be respected.

Method of preparation. Much interesting variety in foods can be introduced by using differing methods of preparation. Such adventure and creativity may be encouraged with various seasonings, combinations, modes of cooking, and methods of serving.

Persons who have an ethnic food pattern should be encouraged to experiment and introduce food items of another ethnic pattern. Such "international dinners" are becoming increasingly popular.

Place of eating. Where and with whom food is eaten also adds variety to the diet. Group eating may be a picnic in the park or the backyard, a fish cookout by the river, or a family meal around the table. Perhaps a variety of ethnic dishes may be introduced by occasional family visits to different types of restaurants.

Principles of approach

Three main guides are important principles for approaching any possible change in food habits:

1. Carry out an intensive study of the cultural practices, especially food habits as related to health and nutrition.

2. Analyze these habits in an *unprejudiced* manner in light of scientific nutritional principles and consideration of local conditions.

3. Relate habit change to need:

a. *Beneficial habits.* Encourage those traditional practices that are healthful.

b. *Harmless habits.* Do not interfere with those that are harmless.

c. *Habits that need change.* Habits that may be harmful or result in inadequate nutrition may be improved by means of persuasion and demonstration. When it is necessary to introduce a treatment or a needed food item that is unacceptable on cultural grounds, ways of neutralizing it or presenting the essential aspect of the food in a culturally acceptable form may be devised.

In any event, nutrition education and desirable habit change must be done within the individual life situation. Social, personal, and cultural habits of eating and food use must be considered. All nutrition education must be based on personal goals and individual life-style.

CHAPTER 11 DIET COUNSELING: FOOD NEEDS AND COSTS

THE PATIENT AND HIS HEALTH NEEDS

Health care that is helpful and useful to the patient must always be based on his particular health needs. For this reason finding out what his needs are and planning with him the best way of meeting these needs is a necessary beginning and continuing part of patient care and education. Health counseling in its broad sense involves this type of activity—helping the patient to meet his health needs.

Good health, however, as seen, depends on good nutrition. Therefore a basic part of meeting a patient's health needs always involves meeting his nutritional needs. Thus in a variety of situations health workers will be closely involved with the health team—the general health team, the nursing team, or the nutritional care team—in helping to meet the patient's nutritional care and education needs.

In general, to accomplish these goals, you will be helping the physician, the nurse, or the nutrition specialist in several ways: (1) to obtain basic information about the patient and his living situation that relates to his health needs; (2) to provide some basic health teaching to help him meet these needs; and (3) to support the patient in his efforts to meet his needs, through encouragement, reinforcement, and general concern and caring.

Therefore a basic skill all health workers must learn is that of talking with patients in a helpful manner. This means two things: we must *hear* and *see* what the patient is saying, but, more than this, we must understand what he *means* by what he is saying. Overuse of the worn phrase, "Do you know what I mean?" indicates the constant struggle to be understood by others. Skills in *interviewing*, therefore, are essential in health care.

INTERVIEWING

Interviewing does not necessarily mean only the more formal or structured diet history or other history-taking activity. More often, perhaps, it means the purposeful "planned conversation" either in the hospital or clinic setting or the telephone call to the home to determine ongoing needs or progress. Several general principles of interviewing should constantly guide such activity.

Focus

As indicated, the focus of all health care activity is the individual patient and his health needs. The central concern is *person-centered* care.

Purpose

The purpose of the health worker is to provide whatever help the patient may need to determine his health needs and personal goals and to provide the means of meeting these needs and goals. Several skills help to accomplish this purpose:

1. Encourage the patient to talk about his ideas, desires, and feelings to help identify both his immediate and long-term needs. Often he must be allowed to "tell his own story in his own way."

2. Let the patient know of your genuine desire to understand his ideas, desires, and feelings so that together you may identify his particular health needs.

3. Provide the kind of information (facts, knowledge, resource people, services, and facilities) that will help the patient meet his needs.

4. Allow the patient an opportunity to explore and discuss the information you present and thus arrive at his own solution for the best way of meeting his needs. This means that often you will be acting as a "sounding board" for the patient to test his ideas and practical means of solution.

Means

Several means are used by health workers to accomplish these purposes. This refers to factors that health workers create and are responsible for: they include key matters such as the nature of the relationship established with the patient, the kind of climate created, and the attitudes displayed, both toward the patient and toward self.

Relationship. The most important means of helping persons is a relationship of mutual trust and respect. The most significant tool we ever have in existence for helping others is *ourselves*. Our role is that of a "helping vehicle." Within this kind of a relationship true healing can take place.

Climate. The kind of climate that we create involves both the physical setting and the psychologic feelings involved. The circumstances surrounding the interview should be as comfortable as possible with regard to the physical conditions of ventilation, heating, lighting, and sitting or lying down. Other influences include providing sufficient time

for the interview in a quiet place free from interruptions and with sufficient privacy to assure confidentiality.

Attitudes. Several attitudes are necessary components of a health worker's capacity to help meet patients' needs, including the following:

1. *Warmth.* A genuine concern for the patient is displayed in interest, friendliness and kindness. We convey warmth by being human and thoughtful.

2. *Acceptance.* We must meet the patient "as he is, where he is." To accept a patient does not necessarily mean approval of his behavior. It does mean a realization that the patient's behavior is purposeful to him, that it has meaning to him, and that by it he is trying to accomplish something as a means of handling his stress. An attitude of acceptance simply conveys to a person that his thoughts, ideas, and actions are important and worth attention because they are his and he is a person, a human being with the right to be treated as a person of worth and dignity.

3. *Objectivity.* To be objective is to be free from bias. It is a nonjudgmental attitude. Of course, complete objectivity is impossible, but reasonable objectivity is certainly a goal that can be attained. We must be aware of our own feelings and biases and attempt to control them. Evaluation of a situation must be based on what is actually happening, the facts as we perceive them. It cannot be based on mere opinions, assumptions, or inferences.

4. *Compassion.* Compassion means to feel with and for another person or oneself. It means the acceptance of the impact of an emotion, holding it long enough with sufficient absorption to accept its meaning, and entering into a "fellowship of feeling" with the person who is moved by that emotion. There is nothing soft or easy in developing the attitude of compassion. It requires emotional maturity.

The word "attitude" refers to that aspect of personality that accounts for consistent behavior toward persons, situations, or objects. Our attitudes are *learned*. Hence they are the result of total life experiences and influences. But, because they are learned, they can be examined. We can become more aware of them. We can try to strengthen those attitudes which are desirable, such as the ones listed previously, and at the same time seek to change those which are less desirable.

Measure

Continuous and terminal evaluations of our interviews must always be a part of our activity. Evaluation is a measure of behavior changes in the patient and in ourselves as related to the needs and goals that were originally identified.

In summary, therefore, the health worker will always be dealing with this sequence of questions in interviewing:

1. What is wrong? What is the health problem or need of the patient?

2. What does the patient want to do about it? What is his immediate goal? What is his long-range goal?

3. What information do I need to know to help the patient? What does the patient need to know to help take care of his needs? What knowledge and skills are necessary to solve the health problem?

4. What has to be done to help meet the need? What plan of action is best for solving the health problem and meeting the patient's personal goals?

5. What happened? What was the result of the action planned? Did it solve the problem or meet the need? If not, why not? What change in plan is indicated?

Important actions of the interview

Several important actions of the interview can be identified and deserve study and development of skills.

Observation. Ordinarily we do not deliberately and minutely look at all the persons that we meet. However, in the care of persons with health needs the helping role requires different behavior. Our purpose is to gather information that will guide us in understanding the patient and his environment. Observation is a skill that is developed through concentration, study, and practice. Areas of observation include physiologic functioning and physical features, behavior patterns, and environment.

PHYSIOLOGIC FUNCTIONING AND PHYSICAL FEATURES. In Table 1-1, p. 7, a list of clinical signs of nutritional status is given. Such features as these may be used as a basis for making detailed observations concerning the patient's physical features. Learning to take an organized look at the person—starting at the head and moving downward—may help develop greater accuracy and objectivity. It is true that we see what we have "mind set," sensitivity, or awareness to see. We need to develop antennas, therefore, to pick up many details that may provide important clues to help identify needs.

BEHAVIOR PATTERNS. Observe closely not only the physical features of the patient but also his immediate behavior in the health care situation. Attempt to look at this behavior in terms of its meaning to him and to his concept of himself and his illness. From these observations of patient behavior, certain assumptions—"educated guesses"—concerning immediate and longterm needs and goals can be made, always recognizing that these are assumptions and will have to be clarified with the patient to determine whether they are indeed factual. This action helps us to understand our own feelings and to rule out our own biases, prejudices, or distortions of the situation.

ENVIRONMENT. Observing the patient's immediate environment in an organized manner is also helpful. This may be the home environment on a visit or the immediate environment in the hospital.

Listening. Listening and hearing are not the same thing. Hearing is only the first phase of the listening process. The function of listening is to hear, to identify the sound, to understand its meaning, and to learn by it.

Although the senses have amazing powers of perception, they are limited. For example, the eye can handle about 5 million bits of information per second, but the resolving power of the brain is only about 500 bits per second. So the nervous system must constantly select and discriminate among those bits of information it confronts. Listening is also limited. A large part of communication time is spent in listening, but the average person without special training has only a 25% listening efficiency. In other words, he only "hears" a small percent of the total communication surrounding him.

The task of the health worker is to learn the art of "creative listening"—listening with a sincere effort to see matters from the patient's point of view. First of all, we must learn to be comfortable as a listener. Usually our lives are so filled with activity and *noise* that to sit and listen quietly is often difficult. Moreover, we have had little experience during our own development of being listened to, so that listening to others must be learned. We practice "how to listen," however, by staying close by, assuming a comfortable position, and giving our full attention to the person who is speaking. We show genuine interest by indicating agreement or understanding with a nod of the head or making such sounds as "uh-huh," "I see," or "and then?" at the appropriate moments in the conversation. We must learn to remain silent when the other person's comment jogs some personal memory or parallel experience. We learn to listen not only to the words the patient uses but also to the repetition of key words, to the rise and fall in the tone of his voice, to hesitant or aggressive expression of words and ideas, and to the softness or harshness of tone. We listen to the overall content of what is being said, to the main ideas being expressed, and to the topics chosen for discussion. We listen for the feelings, needs, and goals that are expressed. We also listen for clues, sometimes not so openly expressed, to these feelings, needs, and goals. We learn to listen to the silences and to be comfortable with them, giving the patient time to frame his thoughts and express himself.

Responding. The responses that we give to the patient may be verbal or nonverbal. Nonverbal responses include signs and actions, such as gestures and movements, silences, facial expressions, and touch. Verbal responses make use of language—words and meanings—but we must remember that we give our own meanings to the words that we use. A word is only a symbol, not the thing itself. Thus we must give attention to our choice of words—we must "begin where the patient is." We must watch the level and pace of our speaking. Questions should be clear, concise, free from bias, and nonthreatening. Sometimes a verbal response may be a simple restatement of the patient's statement. This enables him to hear what he has said so that he can reinforce, expand, or correct it. At other times, the response may be a "reflection" of what the expressed feelings seem to be. This will enable the patient to respond, to verify or deny that this was indeed his feeling. We must never act on assumptions about the patient's feelings without verifying them with him first.

Terminating the interview. The close of the interview should meet several needs. It may be used to summarize the main points covered or to reinforce learning. If contact with the patient is to continue, it can include plans for the follow-up appointments or activities. It should always leave the patient with a sense that the health worker's concern has been sincere and that the door is always open for further communication, should the patient so desire.

Recording. Some means of recording the important points of the interview should be planned. This should be as unobtrusive as possible with little note-taking during the interview itself and completion of the record afterward. If some mechanical device is used, such as a tape recorder, the patient's permission must always be obtained before the tape is started. He may need to be assured that his identity will be erased and that the recording is to be used for a specific purpose, such as to help the health worker to improve his interviewing skills or to learn the health needs of a particular group of people.

Various members of the health team contribute information about the patient in a system of written reports: this is the patient's legal chart. There is an obligation to the patient to respect the confidentiality of his communication and to screen what and how much information is shared and with whom. At the same time, health workers have a responsibility for relaying to other members of the health team pertinent information to aid in the total planning of care for this person.

What aspects of the patient interview have to be recorded then? Data from two basic areas of communication should be recorded: (1) a description of the patient's general physical and emotional status, followed in some instances by judgment of the immediate and the ongoing care needs and (2) whatever care and teaching was administered, with a description of the results. In addition, we may sometimes wish to include appointments made for the patient or notes of information concerning the patient's needs that were passed on to other members of the health team or to other agencies. Similar information is often communicated through oral team reports and various case conferences.

NUTRITION HISTORY AND ANALYSIS
Personal life situation

The initial principle of all counseling follows from the previous discussion of interviewing. Begin where persons are. The first step, therefore, is to learn the person's situation and values and then to identify his nutritional needs. In determining the personal life situation of the patient and hence the basis for planning his care, two central questions will be used: Who is he? and Where is he? The latter question means not only where he is in terms of space—housing or care facility—but also where he is in terms of his acceptance of his disease, his knowledge of its care, and his attitude toward it. Tool A (p. 134) and Tool B (pp. 134 to 136) provide guides for determining nutritional needs of

patients and helping to plan their care. The first sections of these two aids give an outline of points to be considered in gathering information concerning the living situation of the patient.

Food habits

A number of means may be used to obtain information about the food habits of the patient. Such knowledge is necessary if a realistic food plan is to be developed that will meet the patient's needs. Some of the following are examples of methods that may be used.

Twenty-four hour recall. The patient is asked to recall every item of food or nutrient taken during the preceding 24 hours. This method is not particularly useful with a hospitalized patient because the food that has been served is already known and the patient played a relatively small part in its control. However, it may occasionally be useful in clinic or home care as one means to compare with others for actual food intake.

Food use lists. A list of commonly used foods may be given to the patient to check frequency of use of each item. This may give some indication of general food patterns.

Food records. The patient may be asked to keep for 24 hours, 3 days, 1 week, or longer a record of all food items used during that period of time. So that the record may be as accurate as possible, the manner in which the request is presented is important. Discuss openly with him the reasons for keeping it, explaining that it is not for any kind of "grading," but for help in planning.

Activity-associated general day's food pattern. Perhaps one of the simplest and most helpful methods for both the interviewer and the patient is the activity-associated general day's food pattern (p. 136). Since for most persons, eating is related to activity or work schedule throughout the day, making use of the association between the two gives a structure—a beginning, a middle, and an ending—and provides memory jogs for the patient to enable him to give greater detail about his

Tool A. Guide for assessment and care of nutrition needs

I. Assess nutrition needs
 A. The person
  1. Who he is: age, sex, family, occupational role, culture, socioeconomic status, personal characteristics, limitations, strengths
  2. Where he is: physical setting—place of care, its possibilities and limitations; personal setting—mental, psychologic, emotional, and physical, in relation to health or disease, adaptation
  3. His nutritional status: food habits and general nutritional analysis (pp. 133 to 139), clinical observations and signs (Table 1-1, p. 7)
 B. The disease or normal physiologic stress (such as pregnancy and growth)
  1. The general disease or physiologic process: anatomy and physiology, signs and symptoms, general treatment or management, pathology, course, prognosis
  2. Patient's unique experience with the disease or physiologic stress: duration, intensity, medical management, prior diet therapy, adaptation, problems and solutions, knowledge of disease and its care—source, form, attitude, behavior response
II. Identify and define problems and develop plan of care
 A. Explore present needs
  1. Day-to-day nutritional support: maintenance, optimum intake, basic nutritional requirements
  2. Nutritional therapy: treatment by modified diet
  3. Teaching: basic nutrition knowledge or principles of special diet modifications
 B. Explore future needs
  1. Continuity of care: home, responsible significant others, extended-care facility
  2. Plan for medical management: health team conferences, nursing team conferences
  3. Plan for nutritional care: diet modifications, practical food management (family situation, living alone, degree of disability, etc.), follow-up diet counseling and nutrition education, community resources
III. Carry out plan of care
 A. Physical, psychosocial responses: diet and its meaning
 B. Teaching plan: materials needed, content, sequence, methods, approaches, plan for evaluation
 C. Records of action for study
IV. Check results
 A. Follow-up care: planned with patient, family, and health team
 B. Reinforcement to strengthen learning
 C. Revision: as needed

Tool B. Stages of nutrition interview

I. The patient as a person
 A. Introduction
  1. Developing a relationship — Establishing rapport; putting the patient at ease; gaining the patient's confidence and trust; mutual trust
  2. Defining roles — Selling health worker's role as helper, health counselor, teacher; determining patient's role as learner and active participant in taking increasing responsibility for own learning and care according to individual capacity

Tool B. Stages of nutrition interview—cont'd

3. Determining the patient's health need or problem and related personal goals

Discovering whether the patient's goals are different than expected; deciding whether underlying objectives exist other than those concerning the immediate dietary problem

4. Redefining objectives in light of patient's goals

Seeing counseling goals in terms of those of patient

B. Patient profile

Who and what kind of person is the patient

1. Gathering physical data
   a. Age
   b. Height
   c. Weight—present and past history
   d. Experience with disease or weight problem

How do these affect the dietary problem? How long has the problem existed? Has the patient known anyone with a similar problem?

2. Understanding the patient's setting

The patient's environment: social and economic factors involved

   a. Family

Identity of family (ethnic); number in family; who cooks, markets, etc.

   b. Work

Hours; extent of activity; effect on eating habits; education

   c. Social activity

Recreation: physical exercise

3. Interpreting the patient's attitudes toward his disease or weight problem

How has the patient's experience with the problem influenced his belief about it? Have family members or friends influenced him? Fears, misconceptions, understanding

II. The patient's food habits

A. Nutrition history

1. Determining present food intake

What does the patient usually eat? Flavorings, seasonings, condiments, beverages, other relevant additions

2. Learning place and time

Where and when does the patient eat? How do these affect what he eats? Can any times or places be changed or eliminated?

3. Referring to checklist of various food groups and some individual foods

Keeping some form of reminder for the counselor to make sure that relevant foods have been covered

4. Determining who prepares the food and how

Possible consultation with the wife or mother

B. Physical exercise and recreation: activities associated with the patient's food habits

Work, school, social gatherings, travel

C. Food reactions: patient's likes, dislikes, intolerances, allergies

Could food be accepted in a different form or using another method of preparation? Possible substitutes?

III. Diet counseling

A. Choosing the diet

What is the diet ordered by the physician or the nutritionist? What form will be best understood by the patient?

B. Explaining the reasons for the diet

Why the increases in certain foods or restrictions on others; the effect of the disease on food; the effect of food on the disease

C. Planning a daily food pattern with the patient

Considering the patient's likes and dislikes, his usual habits, and the restrictions because of his dietary problem; developing a dietary plan that fits into his daily activity

Continued.

Tool B. Stages of nutrition interview—cont'd

D. Reviewing the diet and answering questions	Answering inquires throughout interview but asking specifically for questions or feedback toward the end
	Does the patient understand?
IV. Termination of the interview	
A. Planning for follow-up	When will the patient be seen again? Encouraging him to record questions or problems that may develop to discuss next time
	Should he keep food records of any kind?
B. Recording the interview	Completing any needed charting of the interview
	Keeping any needed notes in records

Tool C. Nutrition history: activity-associated general day's food pattern

Name _____ Date _____

Ht. _____ Wt.(lb.) _____ (kg.) _____ Age _____

Ideal wt. _____

Referral
Diagnosis
Diet order
Members of household
Occupation
Recreation, physical activity
Present food intake

	Place	Hour	Frequency, form, and amount checklist
Breakfast			Milk
			Cheese
			Meat
			Fish
Noon meal			Poultry
			Eggs
			Cream
			Butter, margarine
Evening meal			Other fats
			Vegetables, green
Extra meals			Vegetables, other
			Fruits (citrus)
			Legumes
Summary			Potato
			Bread—kind
			Sugar
			Desserts
			Beverages
			Alcohol
			Vitamins
			Candy

food habits. A general form on which such an interview might be based is given in Tool C (p. 136).

Diet history and analysis

With an interviewing schedule such as the activity-associated general day's food pattern, three basic steps may be followed in performing a nutrition analysis: taking a diet history, using a food checklist, and making an analysis of food habits.

Diet history. A general pattern of the day's activity and food intake should be obtained. You may begin the interview with questions such as "About what time do you usually get up in the morning? After you get up do you usually have something to eat? Can you give me examples of what you might have?" When this phase has been fully explored, lead the patient slowly through the usual routine for the day with questions related to his routine of where, when, and what he might have to eat.

Sometimes labels for informal meals are omitted, so that the patient will remember to mention food that was eaten but was not considered a meal. For example, you might ask "In the middle of the day do you usually have something to eat? Can you give me some examples?"

Since family dinner is usually a more structured meal, review it more carefully, an item at a time, from the first dish served through the main dish, the dessert, and each of the various accompaniments. With respect to each item, ask questions in terms of general habit—food item, form, frequency, preparation, portion, seasoning—not in terms of any one day's food intake. Sometimes pictures or models of portion sizes may be helpful in arriving at a clear picture of the patient's general habits of food use.

Food checklist. The day's pattern should be checked by nutrient groups. Such a cross-check helps to tally the day's use by given types of food. By referring to a cross-list of food items that have been categorized according to nutrient groups, the general use of the

basic nutrients can be determined. Some examples follow:

1. *Protein foods*—milk, meat, fish, poultry, eggs, and cheese
2. *Fruits and vegetables*—vitamins C and A sources, citrus and substitutes, deep green and yellow vegetables, and raw and cooked fruits and vegetables, including manner of cooking
3. *Cereal grains and bread*—whole grain or enriched forms and frequency of use
4. *Desserts and beverages*—coffee, tea, soft drinks, and alcohol
5. *Miscellaneous snack items*—candy, chips, nuts, and cookies
6. *Nutrient supplements*—vitamins and minerals

As this cross-check is made, ask questions that will reflect back to the patient his original responses about the frequency of use of an item and the form in which it is consumed. For example, you might say, "Let's see now, tell me if this is about right. You mentioned drinking milk at dinner, but not at any other time. Would you say, then, that you usually drink one glass of milk a day?" Weighted phrases such as "only one" or "plenty of" and approving or disapproving tones or facial expressions should be avoided. They tend to imply judgments and prevent straightforward responses.

Throughout such an interview, you may gain important clues to food attitudes and values. Note these carefully and remember them for later thought and possible exploration. Remain interested and accepting, and the information that you receive should be fairly valid and straightforward. Avoid being judgmental or authoritarian, so that the patient will present the true situation and not only what he thinks will be found acceptable.

Analysis of food habits. The general food pattern thus obtained should be analyzed by some kind of dietary guide. Perhaps the most familiar guide is the list known as the Basic Four Food Groups outlined in Tool D (p. 138). This guide groups food according to major nutrient components contributed to the

Tool D. Daily food guide—the basic four food groups

FOOD GROUP	MAIN NUTRIENTS	DAILY AMOUNTS*
Milk		
Milk, cheese, ice cream, or other products made with whole or skimmed milk	Calcium Protein Riboflavin	Children under 9: 2 to 3 cups Children 9 to 12: 3 or more cups Teen-agers: 4 or more cups Adults: 2 or more cups Pregnant women: 3 or more cups Nursing mothers: 4 or more cups (1 cup = 8 oz. fluid milk or designated milk equivalent†)
Meats		
Beef, veal, lamb, pork, poultry, fish, eggs	Protein Iron Thiamine	2 or more servings Count as one serving: 2 to 3 oz. lean, boneless, cooked meat, poultry, or fish
Alternates: dry beans and peas, nuts, peanut butter	Niacin Riboflavin	2 eggs 1 cup cooked dry beans or peas 4 tablespoons peanut butter
Vegetables and fruits		4 or more servings Count as 1 serving: ½ cup vegetable or fruit or a portion such as 1 medium apple, banana, orange, potato, or ½ a medium grapefruit or melon
	Vitamin A	Include: 1 dark green or deep yellow vegetable or fruit rich in vitamin A, at least every other day
	Vitamin C (ascorbic acid)	1 citrus or other fruit or vegetable rich in vitamin C daily
	Smaller amounts of other vitamins and minerals	Other vegetables and fruits, including potatoes
Bread and cereals		4 or more servings of whole grain, enriched, or restored Count as 1 serving:
	Thiamine Niacin Riboflavin Iron Protein	1 slice bread 1 oz. (1 cup) ready-to-eat cereal, flake or puff varieties ½ to ¾ cup cooked cereal ½ to ¾ cup cooked pastes (macaroni, spaghetti, noodles) Crackers: 5 saltines, 2 squares graham crackers, etc.

*Use additional amounts of these foods or added butter, margarine, oils, sugars, etc., as desired or needed.

†Milk equivalents: 1 oz. cheddar cheese, 3 servings cottage cheese, 1 cup fluid skimmed milk, 1 cup buttermilk, ¼ cup dry skimmed milk powder, 1 cup ice milk, 1⅔ cups ice cream, ½ cup evaporated milk

Tool E. Nutritional analysis sheet

FOOD INTAKE (FAMILY MEMBER, CLINIC PATIENT)	DIETARY GUIDE (BASIC FOUR FOOD GROUPS AND MAIN NUTRIENT CONTRIBUTIONS OF EACH)	ANALYSIS OF FOOD INTAKE
Milk group		
Meat group		
Vegetable-fruit group		
Bread-cereal group		
Miscellaneous additions		

daily diet and gives the general quantities needed for nutritional adequacy in terms of numbers of servings for different ages or circumstances, such as pregnancy and lactation. A nutritional analysis sheet that may be used for this kind of analysis is provided in Tool E above. Using this analysis sheet, place the foods eaten by the patient in the respective food groups side by side with the recommended intake; thus they may be analyzed easily. You may wish to explore this analysis with the patient to point out possible additions or modifications that he needs and discuss a plan by which these nutrients may best be obtained.

Follow-through plans

After you have analyzed the patient's food habits with him, you may help him to develop a menu pattern and some suggested meal plans to guide his follow-up at home. You will make wise use of resources such as other

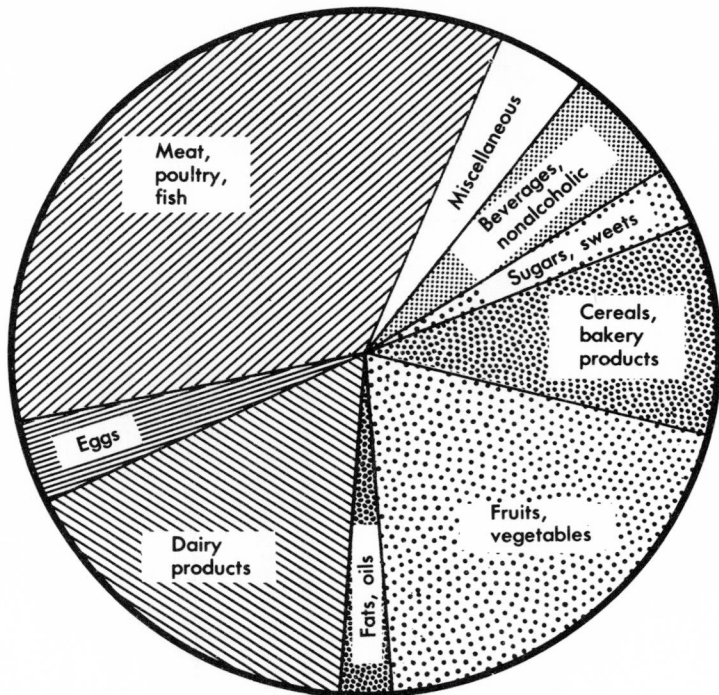

Fig. 11-1. The family food dollar, showing the relative amount of money spent on common food items. (Data from Nationwide USDA Survey, 1963 to 1966.)

Table 11-1. Market basket for lower-cost family food plan*

FOOD GROUP	FOOD ITEMS INCLUDED
Milk, cheese	Only nonfat dry milk, cheese
Meat, fish, poultry	Stewing beef, ground beef, salt pork, sausage, chicken, fish
Beans, peas, nuts	Dried beans, peanut butter
Flour, cereals, baked goods	Large proportion of flour and cornmeal; only cereals for cooking (no ready-to-eat cereals); rice and macaroni products; bread, crackers, and some sweet crackers
Citrus fruits, tomatoes	Canned orange juice, some fresh oranges, canned tomatoes
Potatoes	Only fresh potatoes (no processed)
Dark green and deep yellow vegetables	Sweet potatoes and carrots
Other vegetables and fruits	Cabbage, onions, bananas, apples; canned apples, corn, fruit juice; dried prunes
Fats, oils	Margarine, lard, and salad dressings
Sugars, sweets	Sugar, syrup, jelly
Accessories	A few seasonings; no soft drinks

*From Peterkin, B. B.: Low-cost food plan—choices influence cost, Family Econ. Rev., pp. 7-9, March, 1967.

members of the health team, especially the dietitian or nutritionist, nursing staff, physician, social worker, or other therapists. The patient may also need help with marketing, economical buying, and suggestions for preparation of specific foods. Continued work with the patient may take the form of return visits to the home, visits by the patient to the clinic or community health center, or use of other community resources, such as volunteer health or professional organizations or agricultural extension services.

Occasionally you may need to make a more detailed check of a particular nutrient, such as protein or sodium. In such cases food value tables such as the one included in Appendix A of this book may be used for reference and calculation.

FOOD NEEDS AND COSTS

The average family in the United States spends about 20% of its income on food. About one-third to one-half of this money is spent for such luxury items as expensive cuts of meat, out-of-season fresh fruits and vegetables, and other special foods. Nutritious attractive meals can be had for less. Diet counseling with a low-income family will have to involve guidance for the use of limited food dollars. Sometimes the financial need is even more pronounced, and the health worker must help plan for the family in circumstances of extreme poverty, using government food assistance such as the Food Stamp Program and the Donated Food Commodities Program (p. 103).

Although the amount of money spent for various foods varies according to availability or inflated food prices, the family food dollar is spent on the average according to the amounts shown in Fig. 11-1. This information results from a nationwide survey conducted by the U. S. Department of Agriculture. This government agency has made available several food plans according to family income level: a moderate-cost food plan, a low-cost food plan, and an economy family food plan.

The items listed in Table 11-1 give the food choices that would have to be used in a still lower-cost family food plan.

"Basic four" food bargains

A food plan may be based on the basic four food groups as a guideline (Table 11-2). Table 11-2 may help to find ways in which food bargains, nutritionally speaking, can be obtained with careful planning. The food choices in the less expensive column are compared with those in the more expensive one.

Food buying guides

A number of factors influence the way in which a family divides its food dollars:
1. Family income
2. Number, sex, ages, and general activities of the family members
3. Whether any part of the family food is produced or preserved at home (gardening, canning, freezing)
4. Likes and dislikes of family members; special family dishes
5. Special dietary needs of any family member
6. Time, transportation, and energy available for shopping and food preparation
7. Skill and experience that the family has in food management (planning, shopping, storing, preparing)
8. Storage and cooking facilities at home
9. Amount and kind of entertaining, if any, that the family does
10. Number of meals eaten away from home
11. Value the family places on food and eating

Economy buying suggestions. In each basic food group, suggestions for wise, economical buying may be explored with the patient and the family.

MEATS, FISH, POULTRY, AND EGGS. Since meat is commonly one of the more costly food items, considerable study should be given to how it is marketed. Excellent learning material is available through the local county home adviser of the agricultural exten-

Table 11-2. Bargains in the basic four food groups*

FOOD GROUP	USUALLY LESS EXPENSIVE, MORE FOOD VALUE FOR THE MONEY	USUALLY MORE EXPENSIVE, LESS FOOD VALUE FOR THE MONEY
Milk products	Concentrated, fluid, and dry nonfat milk, evaporated, buttermilk	Fluid whole milk, chocolate drink, condensed milk, sweet or sour cream
	Mild cheddar, Swiss, cottage cheese	Sharp cheddar, Roquefort or blue, grated or sliced cheese, cream cheese, yogurt
	Ice milk, imitation ice milk, imitation ice cream	Ice cream, sherbet
Meats and meat substitutes		
Meat	Good and standard grades	Prime and choice grades
	Less tender cuts	Tender cuts
	Home-cooked meats	Canned meats, sliced luncheon meats
	Pork or beef liver, heart, kidney, tongue	Calf liver
Poultry	Stewing chickens, whole broiler-fryers, large turkeys	Poultry parts, specialty products, canned poultry, small turkeys
Fish	Rock cod, butterfish, other fresh fish in season, frozen filets, steaks, and sticks	Salmon, crab, lobster, prawns, shrimp, oysters
Eggs	Grade A	Grade AA
Beans, peas, and lentils	Dried beans, peas, lentils	Canned baked beans, soups
Nuts	Peanut butter, walnuts, other nuts in shell	Pecans, cashews, shelled nuts, prepared nuts
Vegetables, fruits	Local vegetables and fruits in season	Out-of-season vegetables and fruits, unusual vegetables and fruits, those in short supply
Vitamin A rich	Carrots, collards, sweet potatoes, green leafy vegetables, spinach, pumpkin, winter squash, broccoli, and in season cantaloupe, apricots, persimmons	Tomatoes, Brussels sprouts, asparagus, peaches, watermelon, papaya, bananas, tangerines
Vitamin C rich	Oranges, grapefruit, and their juice, cabbage, greens, green pepper, cantaloupe, strawberries, tomatoes, broccoli in season	Tangerines, apples, bananas, peaches, pears
Others	Medium-sized potatoes, non baking types	Baking potatoes, new potatoes, canned or frozen potatoes, potato chips
	Romaine, leaf lettuce	Iceberg lettuce, frozen specialty packs of vegetables
Breads, cereals	Whole wheat and enriched flour	Stone-ground, unenriched, and cake flour
	Whole grain and enriched breads	French, Vienna, other specialty breads, hard rolls
	Homemade rolls and coffee cake	Ready-made rolls and coffee cakes, frozen or partially baked products
	Whole grain or restored uncooked cereals	Ready-to-eat cereals, puffed, sugar-coated
	Graham crackers, whole grain wafers	Zwieback, specialty crackers, and wafers
	Enriched uncooked macaroni, spaghetti, noodles	Unenriched, canned, or frozen macaroni, spaghetti, noodles
	Brown rice, converted rice	Quick-cooking, seasoned, or canned rice

*From Cook, F., Groppe, C., and Ferree, M.: Balanced food values and cents, Berkeley, Calif., 1970, University of California Agricultural Extension Service, Pub. HXT-42, pp. 6-7.

sion service. The following suggestions may be helpful:

1. Buy cuts of meat that give the most lean meat for the money: avoid paying large amounts for gristle, bone, and fat.

2. Check the meat grade. The lower grade provides good quality, less fat, and costs less. The six grades currently used for grading meat in the United States are prime, choice, good, standard, commercial, utility, cutter, and canner.

3. The less costly meats have just as much food value as the higher-cost cuts. They can be made equally tender and flavorful by using methods for cooking that involve water or steam, such as pot roasting or braising.

4. Grades of ground meat that sell at lower cost should be used, but the amount of fat should not be excessive.

5. Organ meats such as liver, kidney, and heart are nutritious bargains and should be used often. A good cookbook can easily supply appetizing ways of preparing them. Other variety meats include brains, tongue, sweetbreads (thymus gland), and tripe (the plain or smooth stomach lining, especially the pocket-shaped part from the end of the cow's second stomach).

6. Buy poultry whole, not cut up.

7. Fish is usually a good buy, since it is sold in cuts that contain little or no waste. Shellfish is more costly.

8. Less expensive pack styles of canned fish should be used.

9. Try using some textured vegetable protein products as meat substitutes or extenders.

10. Eggs are sold according to grade and size, neither of which are related to food value. Therefore buy the least expensive. Shell color (white, brown, or speckled) varies with species and breeds of poultry and has no effect on egg quality.

DAIRY PRODUCTS. Milk and milk products are bargains in nutrition. It is difficult to get enough calcium and riboflavin without including dairy products in some form in the diet.

1. Fluid skimmed milk, buttermilk, and canned evaporated milk cost less than fresh, whole, fluid milk. So-called low-fat milks are 2% butterfat (whole milk is 4%).

2. Nonfat dry milk is the best bargain of all forms. It may be reconstituted with water for use as a beverage or used in many ways in cooking to add valuable nutrition.

3. If family size permits, buy milk in large containers. Fluid milk sometimes costs less in the half-gallon or large bulk containers than in the quart one.

4. Also, if possible, buy cheese in bulk: it costs less and keeps better. The spread and imported cheeses are more expensive.

5. Cottage cheese is an unripened, soft-curd cheese (80% moisture) and hence is rather perishable. Buy it, therefore, only in the amount that will be used fairly soon.

VEGETABLES AND FRUITS. Vegetables and fruits are the main sources of vitamins A and C, two nutrients found in community surveys to be most often lacking in the average American diet.

1. Buy fresh vegetables and fruits in season. Except for unpredictable crop shortages or surpluses, prices go through seasonal cycles according to supply.

2. Avoid fancy grades of canned vegetables and fruits. Grading is based on shape, size, and perfection of pieces. Lower grades contain small, broken, or imperfect pieces that are equal to higher grades in food value and are therefore good buys.

3. If family size warrants, fruits and vegetables should be bought in large cans.

4. Dehydrated foods vary in price. Dried beans, peas, and lentils are excellent food buys. Specialty dried foods such as potatoes, however, are usually more expensive than the fresh product.

5. Frozen vegetables and fruits are usually more expensive than fresh or canned. However, specials and large family-size packages should be compared weight for weight with canned or fresh produce in season.

6. Cook vegetables with care. Excess cooking water and time destroys vitamins and

minerals and robs the vegetable of color and texture. Such unappetizing food then often goes uneaten by the family, causing costly waste.

7. If the family knows the person in charge of produce at the market, they can sometimes get good usable produce that has been discarded on certain days when the fresh supply comes in. It will require careful checking and much cutting away of defective parts but often it costs nothing except the time and effort in handling the crate and culling the material.

BREAD AND CEREALS. Cereals in general are bargains in nutrition. They are found in American markets in many forms and are usually an economy food.

1. Buy grains in bulk for cheaper costs. However, adequate storage should be planned (at room temperature or cooler in a tight container) to avoid the waste resulting from spoilage by dust, moisture, or insects.

2. Buy whole grain or enriched cereal products to ensure the content of B-complex vitamins, calcium, and iron.

3. Try unusual forms of grain. For example, bulgur is cooked, dried wheat with the outer bran removed, and the remaining kernels cooked to the desired size. Dry, cracked bulgur keeps well in a porous container in a cool place. It has a toastlike color, is rich in wheat flavor, equal in food value to whole wheat, and makes an economical addition to family menus for variety.

4. Buy regular enriched white rice: any processing or specialty preparation increases the cost. Use brown rice often for added nutrition and flavor.

5. Avoid costly waste from careless handling of breads and cereals. Dry cereals should be stored in a cool, dry place. The package should be closed tightly after each use. For long storage bread should be frozen or placed in the refrigerator.

Summary of good marketing and food handling practices

Planning ahead. Use market guides, plan general menus, keep a kitchen supply checklist, and make out a market list ahead, according to location of items in your regular market. Such planning helps to avoid impulse buying and extra trips. Completely unplanned purchases account for over half the items bought in supermarkets today! Also it is a good idea not to plan trips to the market when hungry.

Buying wisely. Learn the market items, packaging grades, brands, portion yields, measures, and food values in market units. Watch for sales and buy in quantity if it means a saving and if the material can be stored and used properly. Be cautious in selecting convenience foods. The added saving of time may not be worth the added cost.

Storing food carefully. The kitchen waste that results from food spoilage and misuse should be controlled. Conserve food by storing items according to their nature and use. Dry storage, covered containers, and refrigeration should be used as needed. After a food package has been opened and part of its contents consumed, the opened package with the remaining food should be kept at the front of the shelf for early use. Avoid plate waste: cook only the amount needed by the family and use leftovers intelligently.

Cooking food well. Retain maximum food value. Also prepare food with imagination and good sense. Zest and appeal can be given to dishes by using a variety of seasonings and combinations. However much the family may know about nutrition, people usually eat because they are hungry or because the food looks and tastes good—not necessarily because it is the most nutritious. Thus it is wise to "package" nutrition in appealing and imaginative dishes.

NUTRITION EDUCATION
Group instruction

As indicated throughout the discussion in this chapter, much of your nutrition work with patients will be on an individual basis; however, occasionally group instruction may be involved. A guide is given in Tool F (p. 145) to a teaching plan for group instruction.

TOOL F. Teaching plan for group instruction

I. Preparation

   A. Research the subject and make a careful study. Prepare an outline and finally reduce the kernel of the material to one sentence.

   B. Make out a teaching plan.

      1. *Aim.* Define the patient-learning goals. Make sure that this goal (a) relates to this patient's needs, so that he can identify with it, (b) suggests teaching procedure, and (c) is a realistic one that can be attained within the class period.

      2. *Approach.* Create a learning situation that will (a) secure attention and interest, (b) stimulate learning readiness, (c) be relevant and lead into the class topic, and (d) raise pertinent questions.

      3. *Answers.* Guide learning experiences and activities so that they (a) secure group involvement, (b) lead to the organization of concepts, (c) provide an opportunity to explore background and alternative answers, (d) provide resource material for analysis and discussion, and (e) allow for continuous feedback by a variety of methods.

      4. *Application.* To help each patient to apply the proffered material to his own needs (a) summarize key points, (b) bring the group to a decision concerning a plan of action if indicated, and (c) enable each patient to ask specifically, "What does this mean to me?" and to perceive the answer with clarity.

      5. *Assignment.* To secure carry-over into life situations (a) obtain any further needed information from sources in the community and, (b) if the program involves a series of classes, propose possible feedback for next class.

   C. Prepare and check out all aids and equipment ahead of time.

II. Presentation

   A. Arrange in advance for the room, chairs, speaker's desk, displays, materials, and equipment necessary.

   B. Carry out the teaching plan.

      1. *Timing.* Begin and end on time, and place the material for balance and interest.

      2. *Group involvement.* Maintain a relaxed and permissive atmosphere. Be flexible and allow for an adjustment of the original plan as the situation warrants. Use resource people as needed.

III. Purpose fulfilled?

   A. Evaluate class results in light of its objective.

   B. Plan follow-up activity.

Tests of the success of diet counseling or nutrition teaching

Health teaching involves dynamic interaction between teacher and learner, health worker and patient or family. From time to time, you will want to evaluate your own growth in increased sensitivity to the needs and perceptions of other persons. Such appraisals will help toward a realistic self-understanding. The following key questions may serve as a means of such examination:

1. *Do I listen when the patient talks?*

2. *Does the patient understand what I am saying?* Are the words and phrases that I use so related to his experience that he may identify with and build on them?

3. *Do I respect the necessity for cultural harmony?* Does my teaching conflict in any way with the patient's cultural values and conditioning? Do I have the imagination to find ways to integrate my knowledge with this patient's conditioning?

4. *Am I comfortable with silences that allow the patient to think through the idea raised?*

5. *Do I accept without approval or disapproval what the patient says?*

6. *Do I keep the conversation patient centered?*

7. *Do I reflect without interpretation key words and phrases expressed by the patient?*

8. *Am I genuinely interested?* Do I show my interest? Do I indicate my concern by looking directly at the patient and by my facial expression, nod of head, and tone of voice?

9. *Has my teaching been practical?* Will my suggestions prove workable for this patient in his special life situation? Does he have the resources to carry out such a plan?

10. *Has my teaching been important?* Does this teaching really matter to the patient's health? If he makes the changes agreed on, will they really make a difference in the outcome?

11. *Do I always respect the patient's presence?* If other persons are present and I must discuss the patient with them, do I keep all communications directed to and through him?

12. *At the end of the interview, do I leave the door open to further reflect and exploration as needed?*

Evaluate your diet counseling and nutrition teaching by applying these twelve tests to your daily work. As a result, your contacts with individuals and groups will be far more rewarding and helpful. Always the therapy for growth can be summarized in a simple formula: *explore more closely with the patient the patient's real needs.*

12 NUTRITION IN PREGNANCY AND LACTATION

LIFE CYCLE NEEDS FOR GROWTH AND DEVELOPMENT

Physical growth may be defined essentially as an increase in size. Biologic growth takes place through cell multiplication. Development is the associated process in which growing tissues and organs take on increased complexity of function. Food is an integral part of the developing life. Throughout, at each of its stages of growth and development, nutritional needs are intimately related to total physical maturation and psychosocial development. The *whole* process produces the *whole* person.

These nutritional needs may be considered in five basic stages of life:

1. *Pregnancy*, in which the human life begins and develops to birth
2. *Infancy*, the rapid first year of growth
3. *Childhood*, the period from the beginning of the second year through the child's elementary-school years
4. *Adolescence*, the turbulent teen years of rapid growth and sexual maturing
5. *Adulthood*, during which growth levels off and gradually declines in the final process of aging

Nutrition undergirds the quality of life throughout the human life cycle: it supports the right to be well born; it ensures optimum growth and development; it maintains productive adulthood; it cushions and enriches old age. Thus through all the successive stages of human development, food and feeding behaviors are intimately related to the whole of life—psychosocial needs as well as physical requirements. Aging is a *total life process* attended from birth to death by constant and dynamic change. Throughout, however, the overall aging process of the life cycle remains uniquely *individual*.

In this and the following two chapters the relation of nutrition to the life cycle will be discussed. Note that each age builds on the previous one. First of all, the story of life begins with conception and unfolds through the tremendous growth and development of the prenatal period. Because the health of body tissues is dependent on certain essential chemical nutrients in food, as has been shown, obviously the development of the infant during fetal life is directly related to the diet of the mother. Thus, to guide your study of maternal nutrition, consider carefully the following questions:

1. What influence does maternal nutrition have on the outcome of pregnancy?

2. How does the normal physiology of pregnancy and fetal growth relate to prenatal nutritional needs? How may these needs be met through food choices?

3. How may general dietary problems associated with pregnancy best be met?

4. How should the diet be managed in complications of pregnancy?

5. What are the nutritional needs of a lactating mother?

THE RELATION OF NUTRITION AND PREGNANCY
False assumptions and folklore

For centuries in all cultures a great body of folklore has grown up around pregnancy. Many traditional practices and diets have been followed, many of which have had little basis in fact. Maternal nutrition through the ups and downs of the past three decades has suffered from much ignorance and neglect. Early in the 1900s a German obstetrician, Ludwig Prochownick, initiated the teaching that "semi-starvation of the mother is really a blessing in disguise" and repeated it during World War I's strict food rationing. His rationale for this concept was that such a curtailment of food for the mother produces a small, lightweight baby, who would be easy to deliver. Thus he proposed a diet low in calories, carbohydrates, and protein and restricted in water and salt. Incredible as it seems now in retrospect, despite *any* scientific evidence to support such ideas, this general view became implanted in obstetric textbooks and practice and was passed on from one generation of physicians to the next.

Thus much of the present-day clinical advice given to prenatal patients in American obstetric practice has been based only on supposition, not scientific fact. As a result, two false assumptions have grown and formed the basis for wrong advice: (1) *the "parasite" theory* (whatever the fetus needs it will draw from the stores of the mother despite the maternal diet) and (2) *the "maternal instinct" theory* (whatever the fetus needs, the mother will instinctively crave and consume). Both these theories are false. On the contrary, the overwhelming scientific evidence for nutritional needs of pregnancy is becoming increasingly apparent.

Positive physiologic demands of pregnancy

In the past few years two main factors have led to reconsideration of prevailing practices of maternal care. The first is a growing awareness of the relatively high national maternal and infant morbidity rates, especially in "reproductive casualties" among infants. The United States ranks thirteenth among the nations of the world in infant mortality rates, despite its position of wealth and medical knowledge and skill. It ranks even lower—seventeenth—among the nations of the world in the broader and perhaps more significant statistic of low birth weight babies. Such premature, or poorly formed, infants have a much higher death rate than do well-formed ones.

A second factor that influenced a closer look at our practices has been the increasing number of studies reporting the effectiveness of optimum nutrition and nutrition education during pregnancy in reducing these rates. Much data have been gathered from clinic populations in America, Europe, and Canada, for example, that have demonstrated a remarkable reduction in reproductive casualty rates. In all these studies primary attention was given to vigorous programs of sound nutrition with adequate protein of high biologic value, sufficient calories to spare protein for tissue synthesis, and enough salt and other regulatory agents of vitamins and minerals, instead of the traditional priority given to weight control and salt restriction.

A number of leaders in the field of maternal care have commented that apparently the answer to the question of why the United States has failed to reduce its infant mortality rate and why its prematurity rate has been rising, factors of life in no other advanced nation in the world, may well be an *iatrogenic* one (caused by physician treatment). This is a direct challenge to the traditional European and American obstetric practice of demanding restraint of weight gain by calorie restriction (which always involves nutrient curtailment), a limitation on salt intake, and the use of saline diuretics. None of these restrictions has been used in the clinic population studies indicated. Thus the conclusions of these leaders are that the change desired in the alarming national statistics may well lie in prenatal care programs and that real progress can be made *merely by feeding pregnant women*.

National Research Council report

These concerns led a few years ago to the formation of the Committee on Maternal Nutrition of the National Research Council. After a 3-year study the committee issued a definitive report, *Maternal Nutrition and the Course of Human Pregnancy*. This report clearly shows the need for change in traditional practices of care—the abandonment of unscientific, unfounded notions of a new and positive approach to the dietary management of pregnancy.

From the overwhelming evidence involved in the committee's deliberations and report, several important considerations emerged as determinants of specific nutritional requirements during pregnancy:

1. *Age and parity of the mother*. Higher risk is involved in both ends of the age cycle in reproduction. The teen-age mother adds her own needs presented by her continuing growth to those introduced by her pregnancy. At the other end of the reproductive span, hazards increase with age. Also parity, number of pregnancies, and the intervals between them influence the needs of the mother and the outcome of pregnancy.

2. *Preconception nutrition*. The mother brings to her pregnancy all her previous life experiences, including her diet. Her general health, fitness, and state of nutrition at the time of her infant's conception are products of her lifelong dietary habits and possibly of generations before her own conception. The woman is the product of the growth that has preceded.

3. *Complex metabolic interactions of pregnancy*. Three distinct biologic entities are involved in pregnancy—the mother, the fetus, and the placenta. Together they form a

unique biologic *synergism*. Constant metabolic interactions go on among them. Their functions, although unique, are at the same time *interdependent*. Any number of variables, therefore, may combine in ways that make the determination of general needs difficult.

4. *Individual needs and adaptations*. Individual nutritional needs vary with time and circumstance. Homeostatic mechanisms appear to operate with special efficiency during pregnancy, but special conditions of stress add nutrient requirements to those for normal needs.

Changing concepts in maternal nutrition

As a result of this background study and growing awareness of need, concepts of maternal nutrition have begun to change. Several factors emerge as a basis for a more positive approach to prenatal care.

Perinatal concept. The prefix "peri" comes from the Greek root meaning about, around, or surrounding. As knowledge and understanding increase, we realize that the whole of an individual's life experiences surrounding the pregnancy must be considered. The nutritional status developed over previous years of living and establishment of reserves for possible future pregnancies are important. Throughout a woman's life she is providing for the ongoing continuum of life through the food she eats and thus the nourishment that she gives to her unborn child. She carries over the same nutritional principles in her feeding and teaching of the growing child, principles that she thus in turn passes on to her child. All these factors surrounding the total reproductive cycle must be considered, not merely the 9 months of an individual pregnancy.

Synergistic concept. The word "synergism" comes from two Greek roots, "syn," meaning with or together, and "ergon," meaning work. Thus synergism is a term used to describe biologic systems in which two or more factors *work together* to produce a total effect greater than and *different* from the sum of their parts. In short a new whole is created by the unified joint effort of blending the parts, in which each part strengthens the action of the other.

Of the many biologic and physiologic interactions providing examples of synergism, pregnancy is a prime case in point. The mother, the fetus, and the placenta all combine to create a new whole, which did not exist before. Together they produce a total effect greater than and different from the sum of their parts, all for the purpose of sustaining and nurturing the pregnancy and offspring. Measures of physiologic health change, therefore, during this synergistic response to the pregnancy. For example, blood volume, cardiac output, ventilation rate, and tidal volume of air increase. Therefore physiologic norms of the nonpregnant woman do not apply. Also normal physiologic adjustment to pregnancy cannot be viewed as abnormal or pathologic with application of treatment procedures for that same type of response in an abnormal state. For example, the physiologic generalized edema of pregnancy is a normal protective response and should not be confused with or treated as abnormal edema in other states, such as congestive heart failure. The protective response of general edema is associated with improved reproductive performance; thus such edema in late pregnancy is a benign, healthy phenomenon in the well-nourished woman.

Weight gain in pregnancy

QUALITY OF WEIGHT GAIN. The primary consideration lies in the quality of the weight gain, not in the quantity. Optimum weight gain of the mother during pregnancy makes an important contribution to a successful course and outcome. The concept of caloric restrictions to avoid large total weight gains and hence complications of pregnancy is without foundation, as has been shown. This concept has found its way into textbooks of obstetrics and been widely followed by the medical profession, despite lack of scientific basis. Not only has such a practice not proved healthful, but it has also imposed much harm.

Evidence has mounted from many sources that women produce healthy babies within a wide range of total weight gain. Depending on a woman's weight at conception, the range of weight change in pregnancy may vary from little or none to a gain of 60 pounds or more. A normal outcome may be found anywhere in that range.

Therefore the important factor is the quality of the gain and the foods consumed to bring it about, rather than a restriction on the quantity of weight gained. There has been a failure to distinguish between weight gained as a result of edema and that because of deposition of fat. This laying down of extra adipose fat tissue provides maternal stores for energy to sustain fetal growth during the latter part of pregnancy and lactation to follow. About 4 to 8 pounds of fat is commonly deposited for these stores, presumably as a result of stimulus by progesterone, acting centrally to reset a "lipostat," a fat-producing mechanism in the hypothalamus. When the pregnancy is over, the lipostat reverts to its usual nonpregnant level, and the added fat is lost.

The average weight of the products of a normal pregnancy are given in the following list:

Products	Weight (lb.)
Fetus	7.5
Placenta	1
Amniotic fluid	2
Uterus (increase)	2.5
Breast tissue (increase)	3
Blood volume (increase)	4 (1,500 ml.)
Maternal stores	4 to 8
	24 to 28

Clearly, therefore, severe caloric restriction is unphysiologic and potentially harmful to the developing fetus and to the mother. Usually it is accompanied by restriction of vitally needed nutrients essential to the growth process going on during pregnancy. Therefore weight reduction should *never* be undertaken during pregnancy. To the contrary, adequate weight gain should be encouraged with the use of a nourishing, well-balanced diet as outlined in this discussion.

RATE OF WEIGHT GAIN. About 2 to 4 pounds is an average gain during the first trimester. Thereafter about a pound a week during the remainder of the pregnancy is usual. There is no scientific justification for routinely limiting weight gain to lesser amounts. Only unusual patterns of gain, such as a sharp, sudden increase in weight about the twentieth week of pregnancy, which may indicate excessive, not normal, water retention, should be watched.

Sodium restriction in pregnancy. Just as with restriction of calories, routine restriction of sodium is unphysiologic and unfounded. Physicians who prescribe diets low in calories and in salt are placing pregnant women and their offspring at disadvantage and unnecessary risk. A number of studies have indicated the need for sodium during pregnancy and the harm to maternal-fetal health by restricting salt. Combined with the added injury of routine use of diuretics, such a program places the pregnant woman and her fetus in double jeopardy. The National Research Council report labels such routine use of salt-free diets and diuretics as potentially dangerous.

POSITIVE NUTRITIONAL DEMANDS OF PREGNANCY

The period of gestation is an exceedingly rapid growth period. The human life grows from a single fertilized egg cell (ovum) to a fully developed infant weighing about 7 pounds! In the previous part of this study of nutrition protein was discussed as the essential nutrient material for building tissues. Obviously, therefore, such a rapid growth period places the primary demand on larger amounts of protein in the diet of the mother. Other nutrient considerations center about sufficient calories and key minerals and vitamins to meet this increased growth demand. In considering each of these nutritional needs for pregnancy, three basic factors are vital: (1) the amount of increased intake of the nutrient demanded by the pregnancy, (2) why this increase is required, and (3) how it may be obtained in basic foods.

Protein

Amount of increase. The recommended allowances outlined by the National Research Council are guidelines, not rigid requirements. The need for individual counseling and for correct use of these recommendations is clearly stated by the council: "They are not called 'requirements' because they are not intended to represent merely literal (minimal) requirements of average individuals, but to cover substantially the individual variations in the requirements of normal people." The current NRC recommendations indicate a need of 85 gm. of protein daily. This represents an increase of about 50% over the normal diet. However, the recent studies discussed previously indicate that more protein is needed, especially for a large number of high-risk or active women. The need is nearer 100 gm. daily, or about double their previous intake.

Reasons for increased requirement. A number of reasons for increased protein reflect the tremendous growth period involved.

RAPID GROWTH OF THE FETUS. A study of fetal tissue composition indicates that the amount of nitrogen stored by the embryo rises from 0.9 gm. at conception to 55.9 gm. at delivery. The mere increase in size of the infant from one cell to multiple cells in a 7-pound child indicates how much protein is required for such rapid growth.

DEVELOPMENT OF THE PLACENTA. The mature placenta at term has stored about 17 gm. of nitrogen. Sufficient protein is required for its complete development during pregnancy as a vital organ to sustain, support, and nourish the fetus.

ENLARGEMENT OF MATERNAL TISSUES. Increased development of breast and uterine tissue is required to support pregnancy. An estimated 17 gm. of nitrogen is incorporated into the developing maternal breast tissue and nearly 40 gm. in the increased uterine tissue. In addition, a general maternal reserve tissue is required. About 200 to 350 gm. of nitrogen is stored for the approaching losses during labor and delivery. For example, 300 to 500 ml. or more of blood (protein tissue) may be lost during delivery. Also the increased tissue is required in preparation for the physiologic demand of lactation to follow.

INCREASED MATERNAL CIRCULATING BLOOD VOLUME. A particular increase of protein is demanded by the increase in the mother's circulating blood volume of 20% to 50% or more above her normal volume. With this increase comes need for increased synthesis of the constituents of blood, especially hemoglobin and plasma protein, both of which are proteins vital to the support of pregnancy. Increased hemoglobin is required to supply oxygen to the growing cells. Increased plasma protein (albumin) is required to keep the increased blood volume circulating (pp. 81 and 83). Plasma protein is necessary to maintain colloidal osmotic pressure and hence prevent accumulation of abnormal amounts of water in the tissues.

FORMATION OF AMNIOTIC FLUID. The fluid surrounding the fetus is designed to protect it from shock or trauma. The fluid contains protein, and hence its formation requires still more protein.

STORAGE RESERVES. Increased storage reserves are required in maternal tissue to prepare for labor, delivery, the immediate postpartum period, and lactation. About 200 to 350 gm. of nitrogen is stored thus as a maternal reserve.

Food sources. Milk, meat, eggs, and cheese are complete protein foods of high biologic value. The quantities of each used daily during pregnancy should increase. Protein-rich foods also contribute other nutrients such as calcium, iron, and B vitamins. Additional protein may be obtained from whole grains, legumes, and nuts. The amounts of these foods that would supply the quantities of protein needed are indicated in the recommended daily food plan (Table 12-1).

Calories

Calories should be sufficient to meet energy and nutrient demands and to spare protein for tissue building. Although the current

Table 12-1. Daily food plan for pregnancy and lactation

FOOD	NONPREGNANT WOMAN OR DURING FIRST HALF OF PREGNANCY	SECOND HALF OF PREGNANCY	LACTATION
Milk, cheese, ice cream, skimmed milk, buttermilk (food made with milk can supply part of requirement)	2 to 4 cups	4 cups	4 to 5 cups
Meat (lean meat, fish, poultry, cheese, occasional dried beans or peas)	1 serving (3 to 4 oz.)	2 servings (6 to 8 oz.); include liver frequently	2½ servings (8 oz.)
Eggs	1	1 to 2	1 to 2
Vegetable* (dark green or deep yellow)	1 serving	1 serving	1 to 2 servings
Vitamin C foods* Good source—citrus fruits, berries, cantaloupe Fair source—tomatoes, cabbage, greens, potatoes in skin	1 good source or 2 fair ones	1 good source and 1 fair one or 2 good ones	1 good source and 1 fair one or 2 good ones
Other vegetables and fruits	1 serving	2 servings	2 servings
Bread† and cereals (whole grain or enriched)	3 servings	4 to 5 servings	5 servings
Butter or fortified margarine	As desired or needed for calories	As desired or needed for calories	As desired or needed for calories

*Use some raw daily.
†One slice bread equals one serving.

allowances of the NRC represent only about a 15% increase over the usual intake of an adult woman, this amount is insufficient for many active or nutritionally deficient women, many of whom may easily need as much as 2,800 to 3,000 calories. The emphasis should be a positive one, on ample calories to ensure nutrient and energy needs, not a negative idea of restricting calories.

Minerals

The same minerals as those required for adult women should continue to be used, with special emphasis on two particular minerals: calcium and iron.

Calcium. The pregnant woman should increase her daily amount of calcium by about 0.4 gm., which means that the total daily intake, especially during the last half of pregnancy, should be about 1.2 gm.: this is a 50% increase.

REASONS FOR INCREASED REQUIREMENT. The importance of calcium to mother and fetus is clearly indicated by the size of the recommended increase. Calcium is needed for the increased construction and growth of bones as well as tooth buds in the developing fetus. It is also an important constituent of the blood-clotting mechanism (p. 66). It is used in normal muscle action and other essential metabolic activities, but, especially for the rapid mineralization of skeletal tissue during the final period of growth, more calcium is essential.

FOOD SOURCES. Dairy products are the primary source of calcium. Therefore some increase in milk or equivalent milk foods (cheese, ice cream or nonfat dry milk, used in cooking) is needed. Additional calcium may be obtained in whole or enriched cereal grains and in green, leafy vegetables. Occasionally a woman in the latter part of pregnancy may experience cramping of the leg muscles, induced perhaps by a transitory imbalance in the serum calcium to phosphorus ratio (p. 66). This may be caused by the relatively high phosphorus content of milk. As a result some health workers routinely advise pregnant women to drink no milk, but this is not indicated. To eliminate milk altogether from her diet would delete an excellent source of other important nutrients, including protein, riboflavin, and vitamin A. Thus to control this minor complaint of muscle cramping a more reasonable approach is simply to indicate to her the amount of milk (3 to 4 cups) or equivalent milk foods that would supply her needs, rather than removing milk altogether. Often the difficulty is caused by the *excessive* use of milk beyond these needs.

Iron. A woman should maintain a daily intake of 18 mg. of iron throughout her childbearing years. This amount will replenish menstrual losses and restore tissue and liver reserves after each pregnancy. To meet the iron needs of pregnancy iron supplements to dietary sources are usually recommended.

REASONS FOR INCREASED REQUIREMENT. The increased need for iron may be appreciated by computing the "iron cost" of a pregnancy.

Extra iron used in:	
Products of conception	370 mg.
Maternal blood increase	290 mg.
Total	660 mg.
Less iron saved by:	
Cessation of menstruation	120 mg.
Total	540 mg.
	(More with multiple births)

The increase in maternal circulating blood volume, as indicated in the discussion of protein needs, has been estimated to be from 20% to 50% above the usual nonpregnant level. Iron is essential to the formation of the hemoglobin required for the increased amount of blood. An adequate supply of this mineral is therefore important to maintain the mother's hemoglobin level. If low preconception stores are suspected, if there is a history of anemia, or if there is doubt concerning adequate dietary iron sources, iron supplementation is needed. The NRC report on maternity nutrition recommended a supplement of 30 to 60 mg. of iron daily. Iron is also needed for fetal development, especially for storage of reserve in the liver. About a 3- to 4-month supply of iron is stored in the developing liver to supply the infant's need after birth because milk, the first food given, lacks iron. Adequate maternal iron stores also fortify the mother against the blood losses at delivery.

FOOD SOURCES. Liver contains far more iron than any other food. Women who dislike liver may be encouraged to use it more frequently by being given suggestions for preparing and serving it in appetizing ways. Other meats, dried beans and fruit, green vegetables, eggs, and whole grain or enriched cereals are additional sources of iron.

Vitamins

Increased amounts of vitamins A, B complex, C, and D are required during pregnancy.

Vitamin A. A daily increase of 1,000 I.U. is needed for pregnancy, about a 20% increase over the usual adult intake. This increase of vitamin A is essential for the increased cell growth and development, maintenance of epithelial tissue in the developing skin and internal mucosal tissues lining body cavities, tooth formation, normal bone growth, and vision development. Good food sources that help supply this increased amount of vitamin A include liver, egg yolk, butter or fortified margarine, and dark green and yellow vegetables and fruits.

B vitamins. During pregnancy there is an especially increased need for B vitamins. These are usually supplied by the general increases indicated in the overall diet. The B vitamins are important during pregnancy as coenzyme factors in a number of metabolic activities, especially energy production, and in the function of muscle and nerve tissues. Therefore these vitamins, particularly folic acid, play key roles in the increased metabolic activities of the pregnancy. The NRC report on maternal nutrition recommends a folic acid supplement of 0.2 to 0.4 mg. daily to protect against megaloblastic anemia (p. 60).

Vitamin C. Special emphasis must be

Table 12-2. Recommended daily dietary allowances of some selected nutrients for pregnancy and lactation (National Research Council, 1973 revision)

NUTRIENTS	NONPREGNANT GIRL 11 TO 14 YR. 44 KG. 97 LB.	NONPREGNANT GIRL 15 TO 18 YR. 54 KG. 119 LB.	NONPREGNANT WOMAN 25 YR. 58 KG. 128 LB.	PREGNANCY ADDED NEED	PREGNANCY 11 TO 14 YR.	PREGNANCY 15 TO 18 YR.	PREGNANCY WOMAN 25 YR.	LACTATION ADDED NEED	LACTATION 11 TO 14 YR.	LACTATION 15 TO 18 YR.	LACTATION WOMAN 25 YR.
Calories	2,400	2,100	2,000	300	2,700	2,400	2,300	500	2,900	2,600	2,500
Protein (gm.)	44	48	46	30	74	78	76	20	64	68	66
Calcium (mg.)	1,200	1,200	800	400	1,600	1,600	1,200	400	1,600	1,600	1,200
Iron (mg.)	18	18	18		18+	18+	18+		18	18	18
Vitamin A (I.U.)	4,000	4,000	4,000	1,000	5,000	5,000	5,000	2,000	6,000	6,000	6,000
Thiamine (mg.)	1.2	1.1	1.0	0.3	1.5	1.4	1.3	0.3	1.5	1.4	1.3
Riboflavin (mg.)	1.3	1.4	1.2	0.3	1.6	1.7	1.5	0.5	1.8	1.9	1.7
Niacin (mg.)	16	14	13	2.0	18	16	15	4.0	20	18	17
Ascorbic acid (mg.)	45	45	45	15	60	60	60	15	60	60	60
Vitamin D (I.U.)	400	400			400	400	400		400	400	400

placed on the pregnant woman's need for ascorbic acid. A daily increase of 15 mg. has been recommended by the NRC, but high-risk mothers or active women may well require more. Ascorbic acid is exceedingly important to the growing organism: it is essential to the formation of intercellular cement substance in developing connective tissue and vascular systems; it also increases the absorption of iron that is needed for the increasing quantities of hemoglobin. The pregnant woman should be encouraged, therefore, to eat additional quantities of foods that are common sources of vitamin C, including citrus fruit, berries, melons, cabbage, potatoes, tomatoes, and leafy greens.

Vitamin D. The increased need for calcium and phosphorus presented by the developing fetal skeletal tissue requires additional vitamin D to promote the absorption and use of these minerals. The recommended amount for pregnancy is 400 I.U. daily. Frequently supplementary vitamin D may be ordered by the physician. Food sources include fortified milk, butter, liver, egg yolk, and fortified margarine.

Daily food pattern

A diet consisting of a variety of foods can supply needed nutrients and make eating a pleasure. Adequate amounts of nutrients during the early part of pregnancy and the increased quantities of certain substances needed during the latter half may be met by intelligent planning around the daily food plan. Key foods are presented in Table 12-1 in a daily food plan, which may be used with patients as a helpful guide for teaching. Additional food may be added according to individual energy and nutrient needs or lifestyles.

Also, for a review of these nutrient demands of pregnancy, a summary is given in Table 12-2.

GENERAL FUNCTIONAL GASTROINTESTINAL PROBLEMS

During pregnancy several gastrointestinal difficulties may be encountered. These are highly individual in form and extent and will require individual counseling or control. Usually the complaints are relatively minor; however, if they persist or become extreme, they will require medical attention.

Nausea and vomiting

Nausea and vomiting is usually a mild complaint limited to early pregnancy. It is commonly called *morning sickness* because it occurs more often on rising than later in the day. A number of factors may contribute to the condition. Some are physiologic, based on hormonal changes that occur in early pregnancy, and others may be psychologic, various situational tensions or anxieties concerning the pregnancy itself. Simple treatment usually improves food toleration. Small, frequent meals, fairly dry and consisting chiefly of easily digested energy foods such as carbohydrates, are more readily tolerated. Liquids are better tolerated between meals, instead of with the food. If the condition develops into *hyperemesis* (severe, prolonged, persistent vomiting), the physician will probably hospitalize the patient and feed her intravenously to prevent complications and dehydration.

Constipation

The complaint of constipation is seldom more than minor. The pressure of the enlarging uterus on the lower portion of the intestine, especially during the latter part of pregnancy, may make elimination somewhat difficult. Increased fluid intake and use of naturally laxative foods such as whole grains with added bran, dried fruits (especially prunes and figs), and other fruits and juices usually induce regularity. Laxatives should not be used except under medical supervision.

COMPLICATIONS OF PREGNANCY
Anemia

Anemia is common during pregnancy: about 10% of the patients in large prenatal clinics in the United States have hemoglobin concentrations of less than 10 gm./100 ml. and a hematocrit reading below 32. Anemia is far more prevalent among the poor, many of whom live on diets barely adequate for subsistence. However, anemia is by no means restricted to the lower economic groups. Several common types are encountered in pregnancy and require nutritional attention.

Iron-deficiency anemia. Iron-deficiency anemia is by far the most common cause of anemia in pregnancy. The cost of a single normal pregnancy in iron stores is large— about 500 to 800 mg. Of this amount nearly 300 mg. is used by the fetus. The remainder is utilized in the expansion of maternal red cell volume and hemoglobin mass. This total iron requirement exceeds the available reserves in the average woman; thus, in addition to including iron-rich foods in the diet, supplementation is recommended.

Hemorrhagic anemia. Anemia caused by blood loss is more likely to occur during delivery than during the pregnancy. However, blood loss may occur earlier as the result of abortion or ruptured tubal pregnancy. Most patients undergoing these "reproductive casualties" receive blood by transfusion, but iron therapy may be indicated in addition, to support the formation of hemoglobin needed for adequate replacement.

Megaloblastic anemia. The word "megaloblastic" comes from the Greek, meaning large embryo. Thus megaloblastic anemia is characterized by malformed red blood cells— large, immature cells containing little or no hemoglobin. This malformation in red cells is the result of folic acid deficiency. Manifestations include intensified nausea, vomiting, and anorexia. As the anemia progresses, loss of appetite is more marked, thus further compounding the nutritional deficiency. The folic acid requirement is greatly increased by pregnancy.

• • •

Additional nutrients are also essential in the formation of red blood cells, including ascorbic acid, vitamin B_{12}, copper, and zinc. Protein, of course, is the essential base for formation and must be in plentiful supply to provide the necessary essential amino acids.

Toxemia of pregnancy

Toxemia is the general term given to an acute hypertensive disorder appearing after about the twentieth week of pregnancy and accompanied by increased edema, protein in the urine, and, in severe cases, convulsions and coma. When it occurs, it is usually seen in the third trimester toward term. The term *preeclampsia* is given to the initial stages of the acute disorder. The term *eclampsia* is defined as being closely related to preeclampsia and in most cases is its end result in the convulsive stage.

Toxemia occurs in 6% to 7% of all pregnancies. It helps to account (along with hemorrhage and infections) for the majority of all maternal deaths (about 1,000 annually in the United States) and for the majority of deaths of all newborn infants (some 30,000 stillbirths and neonatal deaths per year). Toxemia is closely associated with poverty and resulting malnutrition, as is clearly shown by case distribution. The states with the lowest per capita income have the highest mortality rates. Most of the toxemia could be prevented by good prenatal care, which should always include attention to sound nutrition.

There is much controversy concerning the cause and treatment of toxemia. However, increasing clinical and laboratory evidence indicates that toxemia is a *disease of malnutrition* and that the malnutrition affects primarily the liver and its metabolic activities. The characteristic symptoms encountered in toxemia are decreased serum protein levels (hypoproteinemia) and the resulting decreased blood volume (hypovolemia). These symptoms closely resemble those encountered in liver disorders in protein deficiency diseases such as kwashiorkor. Moreover, cases of toxemia have responded to protein therapy, indicating an increased need for this nutrient. Several nutrient factors therefore seem to be involved.

Protein. Protein has a direct relationship, as you have learned, to the constant circulation of fluids from the vascular compartment (blood capillaries) into the tissue spaces surrounding the capillaries, and then back into the blood vessels (pp. 81 and 82). The decrease of plasma proteins observed in toxemia and the resulting decrease in vascular blood volume (hypovolemia) clearly indicate that protein is an essential nutrient in pregnancy to maintain the integrity of the increased blood volume and to protect against toxemia. It is also required in the many areas of tissue synthesis for support and maintenance of a successful pregnancy. In all cases inadequate protein seems clearly to contribute to the complex of malnutrition factors that surrounds the incidence of toxemia. The diet of the pregnant woman should therefore contain optimum quantities of protein of high biologic value to provide resources against toxemia.

Calories. The concept of calorie restriction to avoid large total weight gain and thus protect against toxemia has been largely refuted by overwhelming evidence. Reports increasingly indicate that weight gain per se is *not* a causative factor in toxemia. To the contrary, there is evidence that sufficient weight gain is imperative to support fetal development and to avoid low birth weight babies. Some confusion has resulted from failure to distinguish between weight gains as the result of abnormal edema and weight gain caused by normal accumulation of fat and extra tissue growth, preparing the body for sustaining the pregnancy and for lactation to follow. Thus it is clear that, rather than restriction of calories, the diet for pregnant women should have an ample amount of calories to meet the energy demands imposed on them and to conserve protein for tissue-building functions and the maintenance of optimum levels of plasma protein.

Salt. Another practice in the past treatment of toxemia has been that of salt restriction. Because of increased edema during pregnancy, salt was restricted on the assumption that the edema was caused by sodium retention. This is not the case, however. Instead the increased fluid accumulation in the tissue is directly related to the decreased plasma proteins and hence to the decreased vascular volume resulting from the movement of water from the plasma compartment into the tissue spaces. This is an excellent example of an imbalance in the capillary fluid shift mechanism as discussed previously (pp. 81 and 82). Thus the restriction of salt, especially when combined with the use of diuretics, only adds insult to injury by further reducing an already shrunken plasma volume. It is now recognized that salt is needed in pregnancy and a normal amount should be used, rather than being restricted.

Vitamins and minerals. The optimum diet for pregnancy includes increased quantities of vitamins and minerals. These regulatory agents are particularly needed to avoid the general state of malnutrition, which predisposes to toxemia. The pregnant woman has a special need for those nutrients that contribute to building of skeletal mass in the fetus (calcium, phosphorus, and vitamin D), for those that have direct influence on tissue synthesis and energy production (largely B vitamins and ascorbic acid), and especially for those intimately related to the formation of red blood cells (particularly iron and folic acid). Routine use of an adequate diet plus supplementation of these materials is indicated to ensure adequate red blood cell formation.

NUTRITION DURING LACTATION

The physiologic stress of lactation is even greater than that of pregnancy. The lactating mother consequently requires more dietary additions than does the pregnant woman. A comparison between the nutritional needs and optimum daily food patterns of women in these two states may be made in Tables 12-1 and 12-2.

Nutritional requirements

The basic nutritional requirements during pregnancy persist throughout lactation, with the additions discussed here.

Protein. An increase of protein is recommended for the woman during lactation, totaling an allowance of 65 to 100 gm. daily.

Calories. The greatest recommended increase is in calories. Five hundred to 1,000 calories daily more than the usual adult allowance is needed for lactation, making a daily total of 2,500 to 3,000 calories. This additional requirement of calories for the overall total lactation process (about 120 calories/100 ml. of milk) represents two factors:

1. *Milk content.* An average range of daily milk production of lactating women is 800 to 850 ml., or about 26 to 30 ounces. Human milk has a caloric value of about 20 calories per ounce. Thus this breast milk has a value of 500 to 600 calories.

2. *Milk production.* The metabolic work involved in producing this amount of milk requires from 200 to 400 calories.

In view of these two amounts the mother who desires to breast-feed her baby can be assured that these calories go into milk production—not into her own figure.

Minerals. The quantities of calcium and iron required by the lactating mother are the same as those needed during pregnancy. The increased amount of calcium that is required during pregnancy for mineralization of the fetal skeleton is now diverted into the production of the mother's milk. Iron, however, is not a principal mineral component of milk; thus it need not be increased for milk production per se.

Vitamins. The increased quantity of vitamin C recommended for the pregnant woman is also recommended for the lactating mother. No further increase is needed, since milk contains little vitamin C. An increase over the mother's prenatal intake of vitamin A, however, is recommended (2,000 I.U.). The B-complex vitamins riboflavin and niacin are important components of milk and hence have to be increased. These B vitamins are also important coenzyme factors in cell oxidation and energy metabolism.

Fluids. A practice sometimes neglected because fluids may not be considered a nutrient, but one that is highly important to adequate milk production, is increased intake of fluids. Water and beverages such as juices, tea, coffee, and milk all help to provide the fluid necessary to produce milk, since milk is a fluid tissue.

Rest and relaxation

In addition to increased diet, the mother who would breast-feed her baby requires rest, moderate exercise, and relaxation. Often the mother may be helped by being counseled about her new family situation and cooperatively developing plans to accommodate these needs.

SUMMARY

Throughout the experiences of pregnancy and lactation, intelligent care is clearly based on general nutritional fitness and attention to individual needs. These nutritional factors after all should be but a continuation of a woman's lifetime nutritional experience.

CHAPTER **13** NUTRITION FOR GROWTH AND DEVELOPMENT: INFANCY, CHILDHOOD, AND ADOLESCENCE

At birth the newborn infant demonstrates in form and function the tremendous growth and development that has already taken place during fetal life. He brings to the beginning of his life cycle the genetic inheritance of his parents and of generations before them and the physical resources provided him by his mother. On this heritage and these resources his total life experience now will make an indelible imprint. Therefore the molding of growth and development factors in these early impressionable years is of vital importance.

Physiologic growth is dependent on special chemical nutrients in the food a person eats and the biochemical processes of metabolism that supply the right elements in the right place at the right time for the formation and maintenance of body tissues. However, human growth and development involves far more than the physiologic process alone. It encompasses social and psychologic influences and relationships—the whole of the environment and culture that nurtures individual growth potential. As you have learned, food and feeding practices, food behavior, and food habits do not develop in a vacuum but

are intimately related to the total growth and development process—both physical maturation and psychosocial development. Therefore this framework will be used for study. Age group nutritional needs and the food that supplies them will be adapted to the general psychosocial as well as physical maturation normally achieved at each age. The following questions may be helpful guides for your study:

1. What is the normal physical growth pattern for children?
2. What are some ways to measure adequate growth?
3. What psychosocial problems face the growing child? What related developmental tasks are learned in each age period? How are these related to food and feeding?
4. What are the basic nutritional needs for normal growth and development of children?
5. How may these combined physical and psychosocial needs in the age group be met in food choices and feeding practices?

Throughout your study, remember that,

although the discussion is in terms of general needs at a given age level, wide individual variations exist within normal ranges. Thus in the care of children never lose sight of the *individual* child and his own unique needs and growth potential.

NORMAL LIFE CYCLE GROWTH PATTERN

The normal human life cycle follows four general phases of overall growth: infancy, the latent period of childhood, adolescence, and adulthood.

Infancy

During the first year of life the infant grows rapidly, with the rate tapering off somewhat in the latter half of the first year. At age 6 months birth weight will probably have doubled, and at 1 year it may have tripled. Thus a baby weighing 7 pounds at birth will weigh approximately 14 pounds at 6 months and about 21 pounds at 1 year of age. This rapid growth rate during the first year of life closely parallels the rapid growth that occurred during the fetal period preceding.

Latent period of childhood

During the years between infancy and adolescence, however, the rate of growth slows and becomes erratic and irregular. At some periods there are plateaus; at other times small spurts of growth occur. The overall rate, therefore, affects appetite accordingly. At times, a child will have little or no appetite and at other times will eat voraciously.

Adolescence

With the beginning of puberty the second rapid growth spurt occurs. Because of the hormonal influences involved, multiple body changes occur, including growth of long bones, development of sex characteristics, and fat and muscle mass development.

Adulthood

In the final phase of a normal life cycle, growth levels off on the adult plateau and then gradually declines during old age.

WAYS OF MEASURING ADEQUATE GROWTH

The important consideration in the growth of children and the wisest counsel that can be given to parents is that children are *individuals*. Thus physical growth occurs with wide variance. Parents should avoid comparing one child with another and assuming that inadequate growth is taking place when the rate does not parallel that of another child. General measures of growth in children, however, relate to physical, mental, emotional, and social and cultural growth.

Physical growth

Weight and height. These common general measures of physical growth form a crude index without giving finer details with individual variations. Generally as the child grows, his weight and height are compared to average grids of weight and height for that age.

Body measurements. Body measurements may be helpful indications of growth. These include the length of the infant while lying flat as compared to the standing height as he grows older; head circumference; measures of chest, abdomen, and leg at the calf; pelvic breadth; skin fold thicknesses; and similar measures.

Clinical signs. A general observation of vitality; a sense of well-being; posture; condition of gums and teeth, skin, hair, and eyes; muscle development; and nervous control all contribute measures of the state of health, well-being, and optimum growth. Compare the signs of nutritional status as given in Table 1-1 (p. 7).

Laboratory tests. In addition, finer measures are obtained by various laboratory tests. These may include studies of blood and urine to determine levels of hemoglobin and vitamins. Roentgenograms of the bones in the hand and wrist may also be taken to indicate degree of bone development.

Nutritional analysis. A measure of the growth of a child may be based on a nutritional analysis of his general eating habits. This will give some measure of the adequacy of the diet to meet his growth needs. The guides given in Chapter 12 (pp. 134 to 136) may be used for such a diet history and analysis. Results of the analysis may then be used as a basis for diet counseling with the parents.

Mental growth

Measures of mental growth usually involve the testing of abilities in talking and other forms of communication and the development of ability to handle abstract and symbolic material in thinking. The child originally thinks literally. As he develops in mental capacity, he increasingly can handle more than single ideas and develop constructive concepts.

Emotional growth

Emotional growth is measured in the capacity for love and affection and the ability to handle frustration and its anxieties, to control aggressive impulses, and to channel hostility from destructive to constructive activities.

Social and cultural growth

Social development of a child is measured in terms of his ability to relate to others and to participate in group living in his culture. These social and cultural behaviors are first learned through his relationships with his parents and his family. As his horizon broadens, he develops relationships with others outside the family, with friends, and with those in the community. For this reason, a child's play in the early years is a highly purposeful activity.

RELATIONSHIP OF BASIC NUTRIENTS TO THE GROWTH PROCESS

A review of the nutritional requirements for growth and development reveals their vital relationship to the overall growth process.

Calories

During childhood the demand for calories is relatively large. For example, 55% of the 5-year-old's calories are involved in the metabolic activity of basal metabolism and food digestion. Physical activity requires 25% of calories, growth needs consume 12%, and 8% is represented in fecal loss. Of these calories, carbohydrate is the main energy source and is also important as a protein-sparer to ensure that protein vital for growth will not be diverted for energy needs. Fat calories are important to ensure certain fatty acids that are essential, especially linoleic acid, although an excess of fat, especially from animal sources, should be avoided.

Protein

Protein is the *growth element* of the body. The eight essential amino acids that are necessary for formation and maintenance of muscle and nerve tissue and of bone matrix are supplied from protein sources. Protein also serves as an integral part of other body fluids and secretions such as enzymes, hormones, lymph, and plasma. It is essential to remember that these key amino acids have to be supplied in proper amounts, proportion, and timing for tissue protein to be synthesized; hence the necessity for a diet containing a variety of protein food sources is evident. By and large, the healthy, active, growing child will consume the needed amount of protein in the variety of food provided.

Water

Water is essential to life, second only to oxygen. The infant's need for water is even greater than that of an adult for two reasons: (1) a greater percentage of his total body weight is made up of water, and (2) a larger proportion of total body water is outside the cells and hence is more easily lost. Generally an infant consumes daily an amount of water equivalent to 10% to 15% of his body weight, as compared with the adult daily consumption of water equivalent to only 2% to 4% of body weight.

Minerals

A number of minerals relate to special body functions and are essential in growth and development. Two important minerals involved in growth are calcium and iron.

Calcium. Calcium is a necessary mineral for bone-building, which takes place rapidly during growth. Calcium is also needed for the developing teeth, for muscle contraction, nerve irritability, blood coagulation, and the action of the heart muscle.

Iron. Iron is necessary for the formation of hemoglobin. To avoid anemia additional food must be added to the milk diet of the infant before fetal stores of iron are depleted. Several key vitamins are associated with iron in the formation of hemoglobin and hence are partners in this important function. Also zinc and copper are two additional minerals associated with iron in growth processes.

Vitamins

A large number of vitamins are essential for growth and maintenance.

Vitamin A. Vitamin A is a necessary constituent in the eye for the maintenance of the vision cycle. It is also essential for bone and tooth development and in the formation and maturation of epithelial tissue throughout the body.

B-complex vitamins. These vitamins have many functions associated with growth. Thiamine is directly related to energy production and many tissue-building activities, which demand energy. Niacin is important in protein metabolism and tissue synthesis. Riboflavin acts as a coenzyme and is particularly involved with increasing size and change in muscle mass and body weight. Several B vitamins are associated with the proper formation of red blood cells and are therefore important during growth. These include cobalamin (vitamin B_{12}), pyridoxine (vitamin B_6), and folic acid.

Vitamin C. This key vitamin plays a number of important roles during the growth period, particularly in association with tissue synthesis. It deposits an intercellular cement substance in all tissues.

Vitamin D. Vitamin D is essential during growth for the absorption and utilization of the calcium and phosphorus demanded for rapid bone development.

Vitamin K. Vitamin K is essential for the formation of prothrombin by the liver, an initial element in the blood-clotting mechanism.

Vitamin E. Although the precise function of vitamin E is not clearly understood, it has many associations with growth in tissue synthesis, muscle metabolism, and red blood cell integrity. Apparently its function is related to the antioxidant role of maintaining the strength and integrity of the cell wall by protecting the cell lipids from oxidative breakdown.

Hypervitaminoses A and D. Hypervitaminoses A and D (pp. 42 and 45) are possibilities during the growth period when for prolonged periods excess amounts of the vitamins are given because of misunderstanding, ignorance, or carelessness. Parents should be counseled to use only the amount directed and no more. Symptoms of toxicity from excess vitamin A include loss of appetite, slow growth, drying and cracking of the skin, enlargement of the liver and spleen, swelling and pain of long bones, and bone fragility. Symptoms of toxicity from excess vitamin D include nausea; diarrhea; weight loss; excess or night urination; and eventually calcification of soft tissues, including those of the kidneys, blood vessels, bronchi, stomach, and heart.

For review and reference a summary of the nutritional requirements for growth is given in Table 13-1.

AGE GROUP NEEDS

Throughout the human life cycle food and feeding not only serve to meet nutritional requirements for growth and maintenance but also relate intimately to personal psychosocial development. The nutritional age group needs of children cannot be understood apart from the child's overall maturation as a *person*.

The eight stages of human growth as developed by Erikson provide a helpful framework for study. At each one of the stages, the child struggles between a positive and a

Table 13-1. Recommended daily dietary allowances for growth (National Research Council, 1973 revision)

| | AGE (YR.) | WT. (LB.) | CALORIES | PROTEIN (GM.) | CALCIUM (MG.) | IRON (MG.) | VITAMIN A (I.U.) | VITAMIN B COMPLEX | | | VITAMIN C (MG.) | VITAMIN D (I.U.) |
								THIAMINE (MG.)	RIBOFLAVIN (MG.)	NIACIN (MG.)		
Infants	0 to ½	14	702	13.2	360	10	1,400	0.3	0.4	5	35	400
	½ to 1	20	908	18	540	15	2,000	0.5	0.6	8	35	400
Children	1 to 3	28	1,300	23	800	15	2,000	0.7	0.8	9	40	400
	4 to 6	44	1,800	30	800	10	2,500	0.9	1.1	12	40	400
	7 to 10	66	2,400	36	800	10	3,300	1.2	1.2	16	40	400
Boys	11 to 14	97	2,800	44	1,200	18	5,000	1.4	1.5	18	45	400
	15 to 18	134	3,000	54	1,200	18	5,000	1.5	1.8	20	45	400
Girls	11 to 14	97	2,400	44	1,200	18	4,000	1.2	1.3	16	45	400
	15 to 18	119	2,100	48	1,200	18	4,000	1.1	1.4	14	45	400

conflicting negative ego value. Given favorable circumstances, a growing child develops the positive aspect of the developmental problem at each life stage and therefore builds increasing strength to meet the next life crisis. These eight stages of growth and development include the following:

Infant—trust vs. distrust
Toddler—autonomy vs. shame and doubt
Preschooler—initiative vs. guilt
Young school-age child—industry vs. inferiority
Adolescent—identity vs. role confusion
Young adult—intimacy vs. isolation
Adult—generativity vs. stagnation
Aged—ego integrity vs. despair

The struggle at any one age, however, is not forever resolved at that point. A residue of the negative remains and in periods of stress, such as illness, regression in some degree usually occurs. However, as the child gains mastery at each stage of development assisted by significant relationships of a positive nature, integration of self-controls takes place. In each of these stages of childhood food choices and feeding practices are related to the general age group characteristics.

INFANT (BIRTH TO 1 YEAR)
The premature infant

Physical characteristics. Although premature infants vary in weight and development, a child is usually considered premature if he is born before completion of 270 days of prenatal life or if he weighs less than 5½ pounds at birth. The premature infant lacks the nutritional and developmental resources provided in the final weeks of normal prenatal life. Thus he faces survival hazards. He is a fragile, unfinished product. This infant has much more water and less protein and minerals per pound of body weight than the full-term baby. Little subcutaneous fat is present, and his bones are poorly calcified. The neuromuscular system is incompletely developed, making normal sucking reflexes weak or absent. The digestive ability and kidney function may be limited. The immature liver lacks adequate iron stores and developed metabolic enzyme systems.

Food and feeding. Despite these handicaps, however, relatively simple feeding routines are usually effective, and good growth may be expected if the child is also kept warm and free from infection.

Breast milk alone is seldom adequate because it lacks sufficient protein for the rapid growth of the premature infant, and fat is poorly tolerated because of the immaturity of the digestive apparatus. Therefore the usual milk of choice is skimmed or partially skimmed, diluted cow's milk with added carbohydrate as needed, which may be supplemented by breast milk should the mother desire. Until the infant is strong enough to nurse at the mother's breast, her milk may be expressed manually or with a common hand breast pump. Initial feedings are given slowly in small amounts. Generally one needs to proceed more slowly with the smaller infants and never hurry with any of them.

Methods of feeding will vary with the infant's strength. The feedings may be given by medicine dropper, by a bottle with a soft nipple having larger than usual holes, or by gavage. Care must be taken in all methods to avoid aspiration, especially with the gavage method. For gavage feeding a tube is passed through the nose into the stomach, and the formula is fed through this tube. Careful control of amount of feeding and rate of flow is necessary.

The full-term infant

Physical characteristics. The growth rate during infancy is rapid. Consequently energy requirements are high. The full-term infant has the ability to digest and absorb protein, a moderate amount of fat, and simple carbohydrates. He has some difficulty with starch, since amylase, the starch-splitting enzyme, is not being produced at first. However, as starch is introduced, this enzyme begins to function. His renal system functions well, but he needs more water relative to his size than an adult does to manage urinary excretion. Teeth do not erupt until about the fourth month, so the initial food must be liquid or semiliquid. He has limited nutritional stores remaining from fetal development, especially in iron, so that he needs supplements of vitamins and minerals. These are first given in concentrated drops and later in solid food additions to his milk. The *newborn's rooting reflex* and somewhat recessed lower jaw are natural adaptations for feeding at the breast.

Psychosocial development. The core problem in infancy is the development of *trust vs. distrust.* Feeding is the infant's main means of establishing human relationships. The close mother-infant relationship in the feeding process fills his basic need to build trust. The need for sucking and the development of oral organs, lips and mouth, as sensory organs represent adaptations to ensure an adequate early food intake for survival. As a result, food becomes the infant's general means of exploring the environment and is one of his main early means of communication.

As muscular coordination involving the tongue and the swallowing reflex develops, he will accept solid foods beginning about the second month. Later, as physical and motor maturation develop, the infant will want to help in the feeding process. When these stages of development occur, he should be encouraged to explore his new powers. If his needs for food and love are fulfilled in this early relationship with the mother or other feeding adult and in broadening relationships with other family members, trust is developed. He shows this trust by an increasing capacity to wait for his feedings while they are being prepared.

Breast-feeding. The female breast, or mammary, glands are highly specialized secretory organs. The secreting glandular tissue is composed of from fifteen to twenty lobes, each containing many smaller units called *lobules.* The secretory cells, called *alveoli* or *acini*, that form milk are located in these lobules. They are serviced by a rich capillary system in the connective tissue to supply them with the nutrients necessary for milk production. During pregnancy the breast is prepared for this lactation process by enlarging, and the alveoli enlarge and multiply. Toward the end of the prenatal period the alveoli begin to secrete a thin, yellowish fluid, called *colostrum*. After delivery the initial breast secretion is colostrum for 2 to 4 days (10 to 40 ml. a day) until the actual milk production begins about the third day. This colostrum provides initial nutrition for the infant. It contains more protein and minerals than breast milk, but less carbohydrate and fat, and is also thought to impart healthful antibodies to the newborn.

Milk is produced under the stimulation of a hormone, *prolactin*, from the anterior pituitary gland. After the milk is formed in the mammary lobules by the clusters of secretory cells (alveoli or acini), it is carried through converging branches of the *lactiferous ducts* to reservoir spaces under the *areola*, the pigmented area of skin surrounding the nipple. These reservoir spaces under the areola are called *ampullae*. From 15 to 20 excretory lactiferous ducts carry the milk from the ampullae out to the surface of the nipple.

Two other pituitary hormones, principally *oxytocin* and to a lesser extent *vasopressin* (ADH), stimulate the ejection of the milk from the alveoli to the ducts, releasing it so that the baby can obtain it. This is commonly called the "let down" reflex. It causes a tingling sensation in the breast and the flow of milk. The initial sucking of the baby stimulates this reflex.

FEEDING TECHNIQUES. The rooting reflex of the newborn, his oral needs for sucking, and his basic hunger drive, usually make breast-feeding simple for the healthy, relaxed mother who is nutritionally sustained by an adequate diet for milk production. Several suggestions to the mother who chooses to nurse her baby may be helpful:

1. Assume the position that is most relaxing. It may be reclining in bed initially (Fig. 13-1). Later a rocker or other comfortable chair with arm support and a low footstool usually provide support.

2. Cradle the baby in the arms in a semireclining position against the breast. The warm touch of the breast on his cheek will stimulate the natural rooting reflex, causing

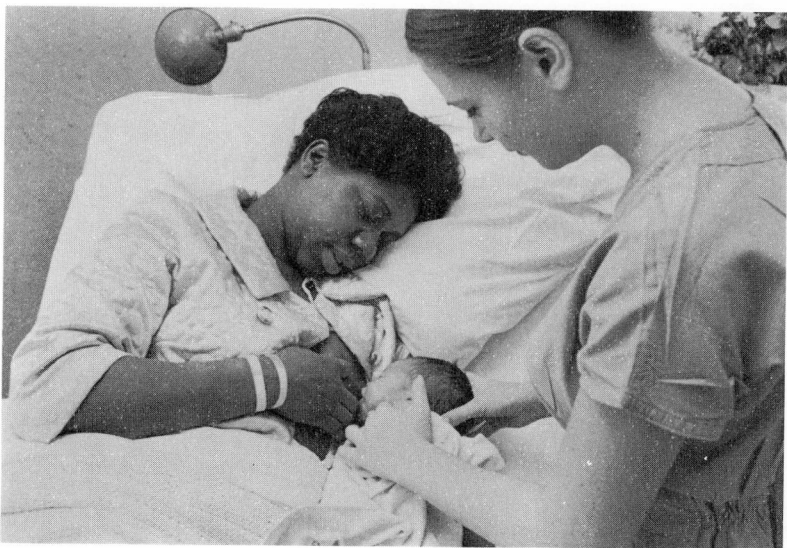

Fig. 13-1. Breast-feeding the newborn infant. Note that the nurse, in assisting the mother, avoids touching the infant's outer cheek so as not to counteract his natural rooting reflex at the touch of the breast.

him to turn his head *toward* the direction of the touch and begin sucking motions. Therefore his outer cheek away from the breast should not be touched with the hand in an effort to turn his head toward the breast. This only confuses him, because the reflex causes his head to turn away from the breast toward the touch of the hand.

3. The baby's mouth should grasp most of the areola, not merely the outer tip of the nipple. This wider grasp compresses the ampullae underneath the areola and expresses the milk. If he grasps only the tip of the nipple his mouth will clamp off the milk flow instead and may cause nipple irritation.

4. In the beginning use both breasts at one feeding if desired. After lactation is well-established, probably alternate breasts will be used for each feeding.

5. Usually a hungry infant will get his fill of milk in about the first 5 minutes of nursing, or he may continue for some 20 minutes. He has had a sufficient amount and is obviously satisfied when he stops nursing and is disinterested in obtaining more.

6. Feedings may be given according to the hunger needs of the baby. Usually these will be at closer intervals for the newborn, perhaps every 2 to 3 hours. About 3- to 4-hour intervals will suffice as development proceeds.

7. After each feeding hold the baby erect on the shoulder to allow expulsion of swallowed air. Sometimes that is necessary during the feeding also or after he has been back in his crib.

8. After lactation is established, an occasional bottle may replace the breast-feeding if the mother wishes or needs to be away.

9. No particular food per se in the mother's diet influences milk production or disturbs the infant. The mother's basic needs are for specific nutrients and fluid, as outlined in the lactation diet (p. 152).

CARE OF THE BREASTS. A properly fitting brassiere should be worn at all times to provide adequate support, with a daily change to a clean one. A folded clean white cloth, for example a large handkerchief, placed inside the brassiere will absorb any milk that may leak between feedings. Plastic brassiere liners should be avoided, since they curtail air circulation and prevent adequate drying of the nipple area.

Plain water is best for cleansing. Soap and alcohol are too drying. Boric acid should not be used. The nipple should be dried well. If difficulty with nipples (cracking or infection) should occur, the milk may be expressed with a hand breast pump and fed to the baby in bottles for a few days until the nipples heal. A nipple shield is sometimes satisfactorily used while healing occurs.

Bottle-feeding. The objective in mixing a formula for feeding an infant is to modify cow's milk to make it as nearly like breast milk as possible. A comparison of the ratio of nutrients in the two milks indicates that the protein content of cow's milk is greater than that of breast milk, and hence water dilution is required. However, the carbohydrate content of breast milk is greater than that of cow's milk, indicating a need for addition of a carbohydrate source to the formula. Thus the main ingredients are cow's milk, water dilution, and an additional source of carbohydrate, such as corn syrup or Dextri-Maltose. A basic 24-hour formula is given in Table 13-2.

Table 13-2. Basic 24-hour formula

AGE	OUNCES OF WHOLE MILK PER POUND OF BODY WEIGHT PER DAY	SUGAR*	WATER
First 2 weeks	1½ (¾ oz. evap.)	½ oz. (1 tbsp.)†	Add amount necessary
2 weeks to 2 months	1½ to 2 (1 oz. evap.)	¾ to 1 oz. (2 tbsp.)†	to bring total solution
After 2 months	2 (1 oz. evap.)	1 oz. (2 tbsp.)†	to amount required

*May be granulated, corn syrup, or maltodextrin preparation.
†2 tablespoons granulated sugar or corn syrup = 1 oz.; 4 tablespoons Dextri-Maltose = 1 oz.

Table 13-3. Suggested schedule on an approximately 4-hour basis

AGE	OUNCES PER FEEDING	NUMBER OF FEEDINGS	TIME OF FEEDINGS
First week	2 to 3	6	6, 10, 2, 6, 10, 2
2 to 4 weeks	3 to 5	6	6, 10, 2, 6, 10, 2
Second to third months	4 to 6	5	6, 10, 2, 6, 10
Fourth and fifth months	5 to 7	5	6, 10, 2, 6, 10
Sixth and seventh months	7 to 8	4	6, 10, 2, 6
Eighth to twelfth months	8*	3	7, 12, 6

*4 oz. milk may be given at midafternoon.

Table 13-4. Guideline for addition of solid foods to infant's diet during the first year*

WHEN TO START	FOODS ADDED	FEEDING
First month	Vitamins A, D, and C in multivitamin preparation (according to prescription)	Once daily at a feeding time
Second to third month	Cereal and strained cooked fruit; Egg yolk (at first hard boiled and sieved, later soft boiled or poached)	10:00 A.M. and 6:00 P.M.
Third to fourth month	Strained, cooked vegetable and meat	2:00 P.M.
Fifth to seventh month	Zwieback or hard toast	At any feeding
Seventh to ninth month	Meat: beef, lamb, or liver, (broiled or baked and finely chopped) Potato: baked, boiled and mashed, or sieved	10:00 or 6:00 P.M.

SUGGESTED MEAL PLAN FOR AGE 8 MONTHS TO 1 YEAR OR OLDER		
7:00 A.M.	Milk	8 oz.
	Cereal	2 to 3 tbsp.
	Strained fruit	2 to 3 tbsp.
	Zwieback or dry toast	
12:00 noon	Milk	8 oz.
	Vegetables	2 to 3 tbsp.
	Chopped meat or one whole egg	
	Puddings or cooked fruit	2 to 3 tbsp.
3:00 P.M.	Milk	4 oz.
	Toast, zwieback, or crackers	
6:00 P.M.	Milk	8 oz.
	Whole egg or chopped meat	
	Potato, baked or mashed	2 tbsp.
	Pudding or cooked fruit	2 to 3 tbsp.
	Zwieback or toast	

*Semisolid foods should be given immediately after breast- or bottle-feeding. One or two teaspoons should be given at first. If food is accepted and tolerated well, amount should be increased to one to two tablespoons per feeding.

Note: Banana or cottage cheese may be used as substitution for any meal.

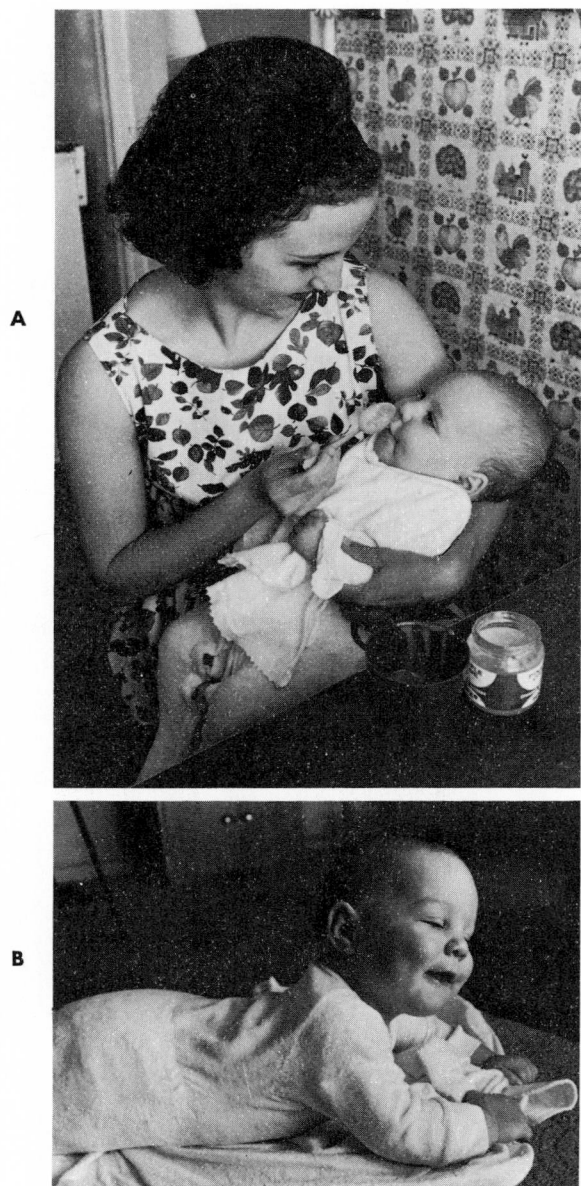

Fig. 13-2. A, This 5-month-old boy is taking a variety of solid food additions and is developing wide tastes. Here feeding has become a bond of relationship between mother and child and is not only serving as a source of physical growth, but also of psychosocial development. **B,** Optimum physical development and security are evident, the result of sound nutrition and loving care.

A simple evaporated milk formula is usually the most economical. Many special formulas are on the market but are more expensive and usually unnecessary. As the child grows older, he will take an increasing amount of formula at each feeding to meet his growth demands. The number of feedings a day will gradually lessen so that by the time he is a year old, he will have reached the general pattern of three meals a day. A suggested schedule for feedings during the first year is given in Table 13-3.

FEEDING TECHNIQUES. The child should be cradled in the arm as in breast-feeding. The close human touch and warmth are important to him. The bottle should be inclined, to keep the nipple filled with milk to minimize the swallowing of air. When obviously satisfied, the infant should not be forced to accept more milk, regardless of what is remaining in the bottle. A healthy infant will take what he needs—he should be the guide. After the infant has been fed, he should be held erect against the mother's shoulder to expel any swallowed air.

Solid food additions. There is no one set pattern for adding solid foods to the basic milk of an infant's diet during the first year. Individual needs and desires will vary. However, when the infant has developed sufficient muscular coordination involving the tongue and swallowing reflex to be ready to eat solid foods, they may be introduced about the second month. These foods may be added generally in any order. Usually the first foods given are those supplying additional iron, plus having a texture sufficiently smooth to be acceptable. Small amounts of cereal and strained cooked fruit are usually given first, followed by gradual additions of egg yolk (and later by whole egg), strained cooked vegetables and meat, toast, chopped meat, and potato. By the end of the first year, the infant usually is consuming a basic meal pattern of three meals and an intervening snack. A general guideline for addition of solid foods to the infant's diet during the first year is given in Table 13-4.

Individual practices will vary widely around this sequence of feedings. By the time a child is approximately 8 or 9 months old, he should have obtained a fairly good ability to eat simply seasoned, chopped, cooked family foods, without use of a large number of special infant foods. Throughout the first year of life, the infant's needs for physical growth and psychosocial development will be met by milk, a variety of solid food additions, and a loving, trusting relationship between mother and child (Fig. 13-2).

CHILDHOOD
Toddler (1 to 3 years)

Physical characteristics and growth. After the rapid growth of the first year, the mother may be concerned when she observes the toddler eating less food and at times having little appetite. Beginning with the second year and through the latent years of childhood, the rate of gain is less, and the pattern of growth changes. Important muscle development takes place as the child begins to walk. He needs to strengthen the big muscles of the back, buttocks, and thighs for erect posture and walking. Bones begin to lengthen, although the overall rate of the skeletal growth slows. There is more deposit of mineral for strengthening the bones to support the increasing weight than in lengthening the bones. Hence the child during this period needs fewer calories (less total quantity of food) but more protein and mineral matter for growth. The child has about six or eight teeth at the beginning of the toddler period. Most of the deciduous "baby" teeth have erupted by the end of the third year.

Psychosocial development. The key psychosocial problem with which the toddler struggles during this period is the conflict between *autonomy vs. shame and doubt.* He has an increasing sense of self or "I," of being a person, distinct and individual, apart from his mother and not just an extension of her. The very fact of beginning to walk gives him an increasing sense of his independence. He has a growing curiosity, which leads him into many areas of conflict. Often his constant use of "no" is not perverse negativism as much as it is the struggle with his ego needs in conflict with his mother's efforts to control him. He wants to do more for himself, but his attention span is fairly short because of his increasing diversion of interest to other things in the environment. Often his struggle for autonomy or selfhood takes the form of wanting to do things for himself before being able to do them completely.

Food and feeding. Calorie needs are not high during the toddler period, and they increase slowly. The greater emphasis is on key nutrients such as proteins, mineral matter, and vitamins to maintain the growth pattern. The bones are strengthening to keep pace with muscle development and increasing activity. To meet these needs, two to three cups of milk are sufficient for the child's needs. Sometimes excess milk intake, a habit carried over from infancy, may exclude some solid food from the diet. As a result, the child may be lacking iron and develop a "milk anemia" (p. 76). On the other hand, a child may dislike milk, in which case milk solids can be used in soups, custards, or puddings and dry milk can be used in cooked cereals, mashed potatoes, meat loaf, and other dishes. A variety of food should be offered the child, *avoiding an emphasis on refined sweets* (p. 199).

In summary, two principles are important for the mother to know, understand, and practice during this period:

1. The child needs fewer calories but more protein and mineral matter for growth. Hence a variety of foods should be offered in smaller amounts to provide key nutrients.

2. The child is struggling for autonomy. This struggle often takes the form of refusal of food and a desire to do things for himself before he is fully able to do them completely. Again, if the mother offers a variety of foods in small amounts, supports and encourages some degree of food choice and self-feeding in the child's own ceremonial matter, eating can be a pleasant, positive means of development. It can help fulfill the growing need for independence and his desire for ritual. The mother needs to maintain a calm, relaxed attitude of sympathetic interest to understand this struggle and to give help where needed but to avoid both overprotection and excessive rigidity.

Preschooler (3 to 6 years)

Physical characteristics and growth. Physical growth continues in spurts. On occasion the child bounds with energy; his play is hard play—running, jumping, and testing his new physical resources. At other times he will sit for increasing periods of time engrossed in passive types of activities. His mental capacities are developing. He is doing more thinking and is exploring his environment.

Specific nutrients need emphasis. Protein requirements continued to be relatively high. He continues to need calcium and iron for storage and vitamins A and C, especially for tissue growth and development.

Psychosocial development. Each age period builds on the previous one. The toddler whose physical and psychosocial needs have been fulfilled by understanding and able parents has a foundation on which the preschool period builds. The child is continuing to form life patterns in attitudes and basic eating habits as a result of his social and emotional experiences. The twofold guiding principle for parents remains the same—to provide a variety of right foods to meet physical needs and the climate to promote and support social and emotional growth.

The core problem with which the preschool child struggles during these ages is essentially that of *initiative vs. guilt.* He is beginning to develop his superego (conscience). As his powers of locomotion increase, so do imagination and curiosity. This very capacity often leads to troubled feelings about his changing attitudes, especially toward his parents. This is a period of increasing imitation and of sex identification. The little boy will imitate the father. The little girl will imitate the mother. In their play, much of this becomes evident in the use of grown-up clothes and role playing in domestic situations. Eating therefore assumes greater social significance. The family mealtime is an important means of socialization and sex identification. The children imitate their parents and others at the table. Depending on the example of the parents and other family members, this may be negative rather than positive training.

Food and feeding. Because of his developing social and emotional needs, the preschool child frequently follows food jags that may last for several days. However, this is usually short lived and of no major concern. Again variety is a keynote in offering foods. He usually prefers single foods to combination dishes such as casseroles or stews. With mental development and the learning of language the child prefers a single food that he can identify and name because it has retained its characteristic texture, color, and form. He likes foods that he can eat with his fingers. Often raw fruit and raw vegetables cut in finger-sized pieces and offered to a child for his own selection help to meet these needs.

The child should set his own goals in quantity of food. His portions need to be relatively small. Often if he can pour his own milk from a small pitcher into a little glass he consumes a greater amount. The quantity of milk consumed usually declines during the preschool years. The child will consume two to three but rarely four cups of milk during the day. Smaller children like their milk more lukewarm, not icy cold. Also they prefer it in a small glass that will hold about a half to three fourths of a cup, rather than a large adult-size glass.

As the child begins to eat increasingly away from home, group eating becomes significant as a means of socialization. He may be involved in nursery or playschool situations in which he eats with other children. Here he learns a widening variety of food habits and forms new social relationships.

Young school-age child (6 to 12 years)

Physical characteristics and growth. The elementary school–age period has been called the *latent period of growth* because the growth rate slows and body changes occur gradually. Resources, however, are being laid down for the growth demands to come in the adolescent period. By now the body type is established, and growth rates vary widely. Girls usually outdistance boys by the latter part of the period.

Psychosocial development. The core problem with which the child struggles during these years is the tension between *industry vs. inferiority.* With the stimulus of school and a variety of learning activities comes increasing mental development, ability to work out problems, and competitive activities. The child begins moving from a dependence on parental standards to the standards of his peers, in preparation for his own coming maturity. Pressures are generated for self-control of his growing body. There is a temporary disorganization of previous learning and developed personality, a kind of loosening up of the personality pattern for the inevitable changes ahead in adolescence. It is a diffuse period of gangs, cliques, hero worship, pensive daydreaming, emotional stresses, and learning to get along with other children.

Food and feeding. The slowed rate of growth during this latent period results in a general decline in the food requirement per unit of body weight. This decline continues up until the latter part of the period just prior to the adolescent period. Likes and dislikes are a product of earlier years. As horizons widen and interests are increased in many things, there is a competition from mealtime, and often family conflict ensues. Meals may be hurried or skipped, and the maturing child is left increasingly alone and prepares food for himself. In some situations meals are makeshift or nonexistent. The School Lunch Program provides a nourishing noon meal for many children who would not otherwise have one. Midafternoon snacking is common, but it is often sweets or empty calories.

Adolescent (12 to 18 years)

Physical characteristics and growth. During the adolescent period with the onset of puberty, the final growth spurt of childhood occurs. Maturation during this period varies so widely that chronologic age as a reference point for discussing growth ceases to be useful if indeed it ever was. *Physiologic age* becomes more important in dealing with individual boys and girls. It accounts for wide fluctuations in metabolic rates, in food requirements, in scholastic capacity, and even in illness.

The body changes in the adolescent period result from hormonal influences regulating the development of the sex characteristics. The rate at which these changes occur varies widely and is particularly distinct in emerging growth pattern differences between the sexes. A 13-year-old girl, for example, who is past puberty is about 2 years ahead of a boy the same age in development—sometimes she feels as if it were 5.

Other physical growth differences between the sexes emerge. In the girl there is an increasing amount of subcutaneous fat, particularly in the abdominal area. The hip breadth increases, and the bony pelvis widens in preparation for reproduction. A pelvic girdle of subcutaneous fat results. This is often a source of anxiety to many figure-conscious young girls. In the boy, physical growth is manifested more in increased muscle mass and long bone growth. His growth spurt is slower than that of a girl, but he soon passes her in weight and height, and at the age of 18 years weighs about 140 pounds. In both sexes increased activity of sweat glands and lack of good skin care make acne of face and back a common and vexing problem.

Psychosocial development. Adolescence is an ambivalent period full of stresses and strains. On the one hand, the child looks back to the securities of earlier childhood and, on the other, reaches for the maturity of adulthood. As a result, the core problem with which the adolescent struggles is that of *identity vs. role confusion.* The profound changes in body image associated with sexual development cause resulting tensions in maturing boys and girls. During this period the identity crisis, resulting largely from sexual development in preparation for an adult role

in a complex society, produces many psychologic emotional and social tensions. The period of rapid physical growth is relatively short—only 2 to 3 years—but the attendant psychosocial development and its problems continue over a longer period. The pressure for peer group acceptance is strong, and fads in dress and food habits are common. These conflicts may have nutritional consequences as the teen-ager eats away from home more often and develops a snacking pattern of his own food choices.

Food and feeding. To support the rapid physical growth of this period, caloric needs increase to meet the metabolic demands, although individual needs vary and girls consume fewer calories than boys. There is an increased appetite characteristic of this period that leads the adolescent to satisfy hunger with carbohydrate foods and to slight essential protein ones. Protein demands for adolescent growth are large, especially for the development of muscle mass in boys. Minerals particularly needed are calcium and iron. Long bone growth demands calcium. Menstrual iron losses in the adolescent girl predispose her to simple iron-deficiency anemia. Iodine may be another concern in areas where iodized salt use does not ensure sufficient iodine for the increased thyroid activity associated with growth. Vitamins are necessary regulators of these increased metabolic activities. The B vitamins are needed in increased amounts, especially by boys, to meet the extra demands of energy metabolism and muscle tissue development. Intakes of needed vitamin C and vitamin A may be low because of erratic food intake. Peer group pressure often leads to greater snacking habits and dependence on only a few foods rather than a variety.

Most United States surveys show the adolescent girl to be the most vulnerable person nutritionally. Two factors combine to help produce this result: (1) because of her physiologic sex differences associated with fat deposits during this period and her comparative lack of physical activity, she gains weight

Table 13-5. Food intake for good nutrition according to food groups and the average size of servings at different age levels *

FOOD GROUP	SERVINGS PER DAY	AVERAGE SIZE OF SERVINGS AT EACH AGE LEVEL					
		1 YEAR	2 TO 3 YEARS	4 TO 5 YEARS	6 TO 9 YEARS	10 TO 12 YEARS	13 TO 15 YEARS
Milk and cheese (1.5 oz. cheese = 1 cup milk)	4	½ cup	½ to ¾ cups	¾ cup	¾ to 1 cup	1 cup	1 cup
Meat group (protein foods)	At least 3						
Egg		1 egg	1 egg	1 egg	1 egg	1 egg	1 or more
Lean meat, fish, poultry (liver once a week)		2 tbsp.	2 tbsp.	4 tbsp.	2 to 3 oz. (4 to 6 tbsp.)	3 to 4 oz.	4 oz. or more
Peanut butter			1 tbsp.	2 tbsp.	2 to 3 tbsp.	3 tbsp.	3 tbsp.
Fruits and vegetables	At least 4, including:						
Vitamin C source (citrus fruit, berries, tomato, cabbage, cantaloupe)	1 or more (twice as much tomato as citrus)	⅓ cup citrus	½ cup	½ cup	1 med. orange	1 med. orange	1 med orange
Vitamin A source (green or yellow fruits and vegetables)	1 or more	2 tbsp.	3 tbsp.	4 tbsp. (¼ cup)	¼ cup	⅓ cup	¾ cup
Other vegetables (potato, legumes)	2 or more	2 tbsp.	3 tbsp.	4 tbsp. (¼ cup)	⅓ cup	½ cup	¾ cup
or							
Other fruits (apple, banana)		¼ cup	⅓ cup	½ cup	1 medium	1 medium	1 medium
Cereals (whole grain or enriched)	At least 4						
Bread		½ slice	1 slice	1½ slices	1 or 2 slices	2 slices	2 slices
Ready-to-eat cereals		½ oz.	¾ oz.	1 oz.	1 oz.	1 oz.	1 oz.
Cooked cereal (including pastes, rice, etc.)		¼ cup	⅓ cup	½ cup	½ cup	¾ cup	1 cup or more
Fats and carbohydrates	To meet caloric needs						
Butter, margarine, mayonnaise, oils: 1 tbsp. = 100 calories		1 tbsp.	1 tbsp.	1 tbsp.	2 tbsp.	2 tbsp.	2 to 4 tbsp.
Desserts and sweets 100 calorie portions: ⅓ cup pudding or ice cream, 2-3 in. cookies, 1 oz. cake, 1⅓ oz. pie, 2 tbsp. jelly, jam, honey, sugar		1 portion	1½ portions	1½ portions	3 portions	3 portions	3 to 6 portions

*From Bennett, M., and Hansen, A.: Nutritional requirements. In Nelson, W., editor: Textbook of pediatrics, ed. 8, Philadelphia, 1964, W. B. Saunders Co., p. 123.

easily and (2) social pressures and personal tensions concerning figure control will sometimes cause her to follow unwise self-imposed crash diets for weight loss. As a result she may be malnourished at the very time in her life when her body is laying down reserves for possible coming reproduction. The hazards of such eating habits to her future course during potential pregnancies is clear.

SUMMARY OF NEEDS FOR GROWTH AND DEVELOPMENT

Throughout human growth, therefore, it is apparent that nutritional resources to meet physical growth are conditioned by the food habits and feeding practices that are psychosocially and culturally derived. Large numbers of growing children have these resources and arrive at adulthood vigorous and happy. Unfortunately, many others do not.

A helpful tool for reviewing these developmental needs and the foods that approximately supply nutritional needs is given in Table 13-5 for review and reference. As a result of your study you should have a more realistic, sound, *working knowledge* of normal growth and development needs. This will enable you to help young children who are struggling to grow up and their parents who are trying to guide them.

CHAPTER 14 NUTRITION FOR THE AGING AND THE AGED

In the previous chapters the human life cycle has been reviewed from the point of conception through the prenatal period to birth and continuing through the growth and development years of childhood to maturity. In the care of individuals at each of these stages of growth, these basic human developmental needs have been related to optimum nutritional care. This chapter views the adult years of the life-span in the same way—as part of the whole growth pattern. Each phase of development along the way has meaning only in relation to the whole.

As you study the developmental needs of individuals in these adult years, the following questions may be useful guidelines:

1. What stages of psychosocial development continue during the adult years?
2. What social and economic problems does the aging person face in American society?
3. What is the biologic nature of the aging process? Is it the same in all aging persons?
4. What is the role of nutrition in the aging process? Are needs for specific nutrients changed in any way?
5. What clinical problems may aging individuals encounter? How is nutrition related to these problems?
6. What practical daily living problems might the aged patient have related to eating?

7. Are community resources available to help meet the aged person's needs?

Two important concepts should develop, therefore, as a result of study: (1) aging is an *individual* process and (2) aging is a part of a *total life* process. These two basic concepts will govern all other aspects of need during these years—biologic, nutritional, socioeconomic, psychosocial, and spiritual.

AGING AND THE AGED

The two terms *aging* and *aged* have comparable yet distinct meanings.

The aging process

Aging is a life process. The age of a person or an object is from the point of its beginning existence to the present time. Thus human aging is the total life process. It begins at conception and ends at death. It may be somewhat startling to think that even now all persons are aging and have been aging since the moment of conception—this is a biologic truth.

The aged

Aged refers to one who is old. He has arrived near the end of the aging process and bears visible physical signs of a gradual process of decline. Sometimes people are spoken of as young-old (those between the ages of 60 and 75 years) and as old-old (those over 75 years of age) because marked distinctions may exist between persons in these two age brackets.

Senescence and senility

The word "senescence" comes from a Latin verb, *senescere*, which means to grow old. It refers to the process of growing old or more specifically to the latter period of life, old age. It is similar to the Latin root for adolescence, for example, which means to grow up or the latter period of attaining physical maturity. The word "senile" is from the Latin word *senilis*, which simply means old. However, common usage has given it a negative clinical connotation. This negative meaning should not be attached to *normal* old age.

Thus the pattern of a *life continuum* emerges. Aging is a positive concept. It encompasses the whole of life, and each period has its own unique potentials and fulfillments. The period of adulthood—young, middle, and older—is no exception. Its own particular capacities can be lived to the fullest.

PSYCHOSOCIAL DEVELOPMENT STAGES OF ADULTHOOD

After the tumultuous adolescent period from 13 to 18 years, when youth in American society is struggling with the core problem of identity vs. identity diffusion, of learning who they are and where they are going, individuals finally emerge into adulthood. Three more basic stages in the human life-span, as identified by Erikson (p. 162), complete development.

Young adulthood (18 to 40 years)

In the years of young adulthood the individual is now launched on his own for better or worse. Each one must resolve the core problem of *intimacy vs. isolation.* If a person achieves the goal of intimacy, he is able to build an intimate relationship leading to marriage or self-fulfillment in other personal relationships, but in failing to do so he becomes increasingly isolated from others. These are years of many stresses and fulfillments. They are the years of career beginnings, of establishing one's own home, of

parenthood, of starting young children on their way through the same life stages. These are the years of early struggles to make one's way in the world with its attendant joys and heartaches.

Middle adulthood (40 to 60 years)

In the years of middle adulthood, the core problem the individual faces is *generativity vs. self-absorption.* The children have now grown and gone to make their own lives in turn. These are the years of the "empty nest." Each person must come to terms with what life has offered. He must find some kind of expression for stored learning in passing on life's teachings. It is a regeneration of one life in the lives of young persons following the same way. To the degree that these inner struggles are not won, there is increasing self-absorption, a turning in on oneself, and a withering rather than a regenerating.

Older adulthood (60 to 80 plus years)

In the last stage of life—old age, or senescence—the final core problem is resolved either in *ego intregrity vs. despair.* At this point, depending on one's individual resources, which are the outcome of all one's life before, there is either a predominant sense of wholeness and completeness or a sense of distaste, of bitterness, of revulsion, and of wondering what life was all about. If the outcome of life's basic experiences and problems has been positive, the individual arrives at old age a rich person—rich in wisdom of the years. Building on each previous level, psychosocial growth has reached its positive human resolution.

Not all the older adult patients with whom one deals, however, will be able to feel this richness. In the United States values are placed on youth, activity, and productivity. These characteristics cannot be expressed by the elderly person; hence less value is generally placed on older people in our society, and they are often made to feel unwanted and unneeded. Moreover, some of them will not have resolved the core psychosocial conflicts and struggles with which they wrestled in previous stages of life. They arrive at middle and later years poorly equipped to deal with the adjustments and health problems that may face them. Many others, however, will have been enriched by life's experiences in their maturing process. They in turn bring enrichment to others, and the resulting relationship is mutually rewarding.

SOCIOECONOMIC AND PSYCHOLOGIC FACTORS

The increasing industrialization and urbanization of American society, the complexity of the culture that it is building, and the changes in age distribution in the population have all brought about changes in the life of the aging person in the United States today.

Population changes

Not only has the general population been increasing rapidly, but significant shifts have also occurred in the age distribution. More persons are living longer. By 1975, 12%, or over 22 million, of the American population will be 65 years of age or over. In general, this increased length of life is influenced by two factors, medical care and improving living standards.

Medical care. The great progress in care of infants and children has reduced infant mortality, controlled communicable diseases, and improved child care. The increased availability and quality of medical care during adult years is also a factor in health during maturing years. However, there has been relatively little progress in control of chronic disease in old age or relating general medical care practices to the needs of the aged.

Improved general living standards. With increasing national affluence, general United States living standards are high. For many this factor has led to increased education, better housing, and improved nutrition during the growth and early adult years. In older age, however, socioeconomic problems increase for many.

Social and economic factors

America's increasing industrialization and subsequent changing social attitudes have affected the position of the older person in American society. Economic insecurity often creates pressures. An increasing policy of early retirement in industry and employment difficulties with advancing age create financial pressures. Changing social attitudes toward the elderly person and his capacities have increased institutional care and segregation in living situations. The older person is often removed from the necessary stimulus of involvement in the activities of society.

Psychologic factors

Financial pressures and a decreasing sense of acceptance and accomplishment have caused many older persons to feel anxieties and a loss of personal value. Many feel inadequate. They do not have a sense of belonging, of self-esteem, or of achievement. They are often lonely, restless, unhappy, and uncertain. The experience of health workers has demonstrated several basic needs common to older persons:

1. *Economic security.* An income through some socially useful and personally satisfying means is needed.

2. *Personal effectiveness.* There is a need for a sense of maximum self-worth, of being able to contribute something worthwhile.

3. *Housing.* A suitable place in which to live is a basic necessity.

4. *Leisure-time activities.* Some type of constructive activity to fill leisure time is needed.

5. *Social relationships.* A sense of positive and well-integrated social relationships must be found within the family and community.

6. *Spiritual values.* As life draws nearer its close, there is an increasing sense of need to achieve and maintain some satisfying spiritual values and personal goals.

BIOLOGIC CHANGES IN THE AGING PROCESS
General physiologic changes

From a biologic standpoint there is limited knowledge of the process of aging. The general biologic process extends over the entire life-span and is conditioned by experiences that have gone on before. In the later ages, however, there is a cell loss and reduced cell metabolism. During the 30- to 90-year age period there is a gradual reduction in the performance capacity of most organ systems. For example, the speed of conducting a nerve impulse diminishes by 15%. The rate of blood flow through the kidneys is reduced 65%, and the resting cardiac output is reduced by 30%. The pulmonary function (maximum voluntary ventilatory capacity) is reduced 60%. There is a reduced recovery rate after a displacing stimulus. For example, in a glucose tolerance test, the blood sugar level takes longer to return to normal. After exercise the pulse rate and respiration take longer to return to normal. Overall there seems to be a gradual reduction in the body's reserve capacities, an important cause of which is the gradual reduction of cellular units. For example, nephron units are lost from the kidney as functional tissue. Some resulting physiologic factors may also affect food patterns. For example, there may be a diminished secretion of digestive juices, a decreased motility of the gastrointestinal tract, and a decreased absorption and utilization of nutrients.

Possible role of vitamin E

The gradual diminishing of cells in the aging process may be in part caused by the gradual breakdown observed in the cell wall as part of this process, a result of the deterioration of the lipids that comprise a large part of the cell wall structure. It is in this context that vitamin E has been discussed in relation to the aging process. Its antioxidant capacities protect the lipids that construct the cell wall and therefore help to maintain its strength and integrity (p. 46).

Individuality of the process

The biologic changes are general. However, persons in the advancing years of life will display a wide variety of individual reactions. Each person bears the imprint of individual trauma and accumulation of dis-

ease experience, which has a direct effect on his individual aging process. Therefore specific needs of individuals must always be remembered and considered when caring for general aging and nutritional needs. It seems, therefore, that the greatest influence of nutrition on the aging process takes place in earlier years. Nutrition's most effective role is in the growth and middle years, which prepare the individual to meet the gradually declining metabolic processes of old age.

NUTRITIONAL REQUIREMENTS
Calories

Standard allowances. In adulthood the basal energy requirement is reduced by gradual losses in functioning protoplasm. This factor, together with the usual reduced physical activity of the adult, creates less demand for calories as age advances. In general, the reduction in the need for calories is approximately 7.5% for each decade past 25 years of age. The standard allowances of the NRC are based on estimates of a decrease in metabolic activity of about 5%. The average estimate is an approximate caloric requirement of about 1,800 calories for the adult. Men may require somewhat more—about 2,000 to 2,200 calories. These calorie requirements are highly individual according to personal activity and need. Primary consideration must also be given to the living status of the individual and the degree of physical activity. Perhaps the simplest criterion for judging adequacy of caloric intake is the maintenance of *normal* weight.

Carbohydrates. At least 70% to 75% of the total calories should be provided in the form of nonprotein calories—carbohydrate or fat. Otherwise part of the protein will be diverted for use as energy rather than tissue maintenance. The actual optimum amount of carbohydrate intake is unknown, but it is usually recommended that about 50% of the calories come from carbohydrate foods. A fairly free choice from a wide variety of carbohydrate foods according to individual digestive or metabolic situations is usually best.

Fats. Fats usually contribute about 20% of the total calories. They provide a source of energy, important fat-soluble vitamins, and essential fatty acids. A reasonable objective is the avoidance of large quantities of fat with more emphasis on the quality of the fat consumed. Wise conusel seems to center around the use of more unsaturated fats from plant sources and less saturated fat from animal ones (pp. 19 and 250).

Proteins

Standard allowances. Age itself does not alter adult protein needs. The NRC recommends a continuation of the daily protein intake for the aging individual at the same adult allowance given for age 25—0.8 gm. per kilogram of body weight. Even this amount provides an allowance for wide variation in individual needs. The need for protein may be increased during illness or convalescence or after a wasting disease, but not under normal circumstances.

Protein value. Protein needs are influenced by two basic factors: (1) the biologic value of the protein (the quantity and ratio of its amino acids) and (2) adequate caloric value of the diet. It is estimated that one fourth to one half the protein intake should come from animal sources with the remainder from plant sources. If animal and plant protein foods are eaten at the same meal, there is better use of the incomplete plant protein for tissue synthesis, since the lacking amino acids may be supplied by the animal proteins. Protein should supply from 15% to 20% of the day's total calories. Supplemental amino acid preparations are not needed as some faddists may claim. They are expensive, unpalatable, irritating, impractical, and an inefficient source of available nitrogen.

Vitamins

The sale of so-called geriatric vitamin preparations, especially of the B complex, implies that the requirement for these vitamins increases with age, which is not necessarily true. There may be gradually decreasing tissue stores with normal aging, but long-term studies show no difference in requirement from that for normal adults. The problem in some individual cases may stem from inadequate normal intake rather than from increased need. A well-selected mixed diet with a wide variety of foods should supply all the essential vitamins in normally needed quantities. Increased therapeutic needs in illness should be evaluated on an individual basis.

Minerals

There is also no need for increased minerals in normal aging. The same adult allowances are sufficient on a continuing basis and are supplied by a well-balanced diet. Two essential minerals that may be lacking in poor diets, however, are iron and calcium. Encouragement may have to be given to some individuals to ensure adequate dietary sources of these minerals among their daily food choices.

Water

The need for water varies with the environment. A liberal intake should be assured, with thirst as the general guide.

CLINICAL PROBLEMS

Although physiologic needs for nutrients do not increase with age, other environmental factors may contribute to illness and produce special clinical problems.

Malnutrition

By and large, poor dietary habits in young adulthood, like any other personal habits, tend to be set and accentuated in older age. Surveys usually show average adequate caloric intake but frequent evidence of inadequate nutrient consumption. For example, there may be fewer animal proteins, more use of grains and other starches, fewer vegetables and fruits, and more sweets and desserts. Also older persons are frequent victims of food faddists' claims concerning restorative food products, tonics, and regulators.

Causes. Numerous factors may contribute to the developing of malnutrition in an aging person.

ORAL PROBLEMS. Poor teeth or poorly fitting dentures may make chewing difficult. However, a denture can only be as successful as the health of the tissue on which it rests. Also an analysis of the three stages of eating food—biting, chewing, and swallowing—will provide a basis for helping the new denture wearer adjust to his dentures. Poor appetite and limited financial means for adequate dental care may discourage efforts to seek improvement of the situation. Also mucosal changes in the mouth and a decrease or change in quality of salivary secretions may cause additional difficulty in eating.

GASTROINTESTINAL PROBLEMS. Numerous gastrointestinal complaints vary from vague indigestion or "irritable colon" to specific diseases such as peptic ulcer or diverticulitis. Such problems generally reduce appetite and food intake; thus the needed nutrients are not taken in. A variety of acute or chronic illnesses may limit food intake or utilization.

PERSONAL FACTORS. Financial resources may be limited, with little money available to purchase needed food. A knowledge of the food needed for a well-balanced diet may be lacking. Furthermore boredom, loneliness, anxiety, insecurity, and apathy may compound the problem. Especially if an older person lives alone, the social value of eating is gone. Adequate cooking, refrigeration, or storage facilities may be lacking. He may have no means of transportation to obtain food and bring it back home. Often a vicious cycle ensues: funds are low, he hesitates to spend, goes without, and feels increasing weakness and lethargy, which leads to still less interest and incentive. Finally he is ill.

Obesity

In a different sense, obesity may be considered a form of malnutrition. It is a potential health hazard, as indicated in its being a factor in a number of degenerative diseases. It seems clearly evident at this point that a pre-

vention of obesity in earlier growth years may be the major nutritional measure one may take in preparation for old age.

Causes. Many of the same living situations and emotional factors may also contribute to obesity. They may lead to overeating as a compensation, and poor food choices result. Also physical activity is usually decreased, and the caloric requirement is lessened, but the food habits continue.

Chronic disease

Chronic illness such as heart disease often creates additional problems for adults, especially the aging. Food needs may be modified by the presence of the disease, which may require fat modification or sodium restriction and create problems in procuring and preparing foods. Diabetes may also create problems in developing a more balanced, consistent pattern of food habits.

Solutions to clinical problems

Each situation has to be approached in its own context. In all cases, there is much need for understanding care and realistic support to build improved eating habits (Fig. 14-1).

In any event, helpful attitudes and actions by the health worker must always be based on an understanding and realistic approach.

Food habits must be analyzed carefully. Whatever the setting for care may be, whether in the medical or dental office, in the health center's medical or dental clinic, in the hospital, or at home, the health worker must listen well to learn the patient's attitudes, precise situation, and limiting factors. Nutritional needs can be met with a variety of foods. Many suggestions can be adapted to fit the particular needs and situation, as well as personal desires. Suggestions should be administered on the basis of knowledge of the practical reality of the living situation.

The health worker should never moralize. There is no one food per se that anyone should eat. The statement "Eat this because

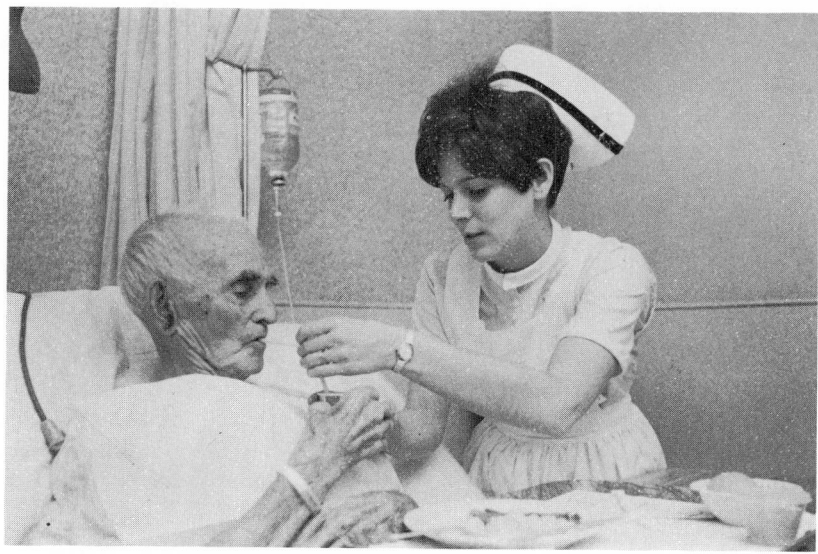

Fig. 14-1. Care and support in feeding an elderly patient. Assistance is given by the student nurse as needed to ensure optimum nutrition.

it's good for you" should be struck from everyone's vocabulary. It has little value for anyone, much less a person who is struggling to maintain personal integrity and self-esteem in a culture that largely rejects and alienates its aged.

Interest should be encouraged in food variety and seasonings. An unattractive bland diet is presumed by many to be necessary for all elderly persons. *It is not.* A variety of food and adventures with new foods, tastes, and seasonings often prove to be the needed stimuli for poor appetite and lack of interest in eating. Sometimes smaller amounts of these foods and more frequent meals are helpful.

All problems require an individual approach. A problem such as weight reduction for the older person should have reasonable approaches. Certainly no drastic measures or diets are indicated. The plan should be one for slow, gradual loss as it is needed. Because individual caloric requirements vary widely and individual personalities and problems are unique, personal and realistic planning *with* the individual patient, followed by sup-

portive guidance and encouragement, usually pays the greatest dividends.

Available resources should be explored and used. Consultation with the social worker or other resource persons on the health team, especially the nutrition specialist, is needed to determine sources of assistance. Channels of aid for the socioeconomic problems surrounding income and housing may be investigated. Also counseling with the family members or "significant others" in the older person's life may help to sensitize them to the needs of the person, which they may not have been aware of before. Beyond these more immediate means, other outside community resources are available and should be explored. Some of these possibilities are given here.

COMMUNITY RESOURCES

A number of community resources may be available for consultation and aid in meeting the needs of aging persons, including professional and volunteer organizations, government agencies, and industry-related groups.

Professional organizations

Local community groups representing health professions such as medical societies, nursing organizations, and dietetic associations sponsor a variety of programs to help meet the needs of the aged people in their respective communities. For example, the Dial-a-Dietitian program of dietetic associations may provide sound information concerning nutritional needs. Also, the Meals-on-Wheels program in various communities may provide food for homebound older persons.

Government agencies

The impact in the United States of recent federal legislation covering aid to elderly persons for medical care under the Social Security Act can hardly be minimized. The so-called Medicare bill (Title XIX) has increased the demand for high-quality medical care and its availability to elderly persons. The pressure on community nursing homes, hospitals, and related medical care resources is already being felt. Additional medical assistance programs in a number of states augment community resources on the state and local level. Some elderly persons may not be aware of these resources for health care that are provided for them under this bill.

The Department of Health, Education, and Welfare also conducts activities at a national level to coordinate care for the aged. The Federal Council on Aging conducts conferences, publishes a newsletter, *Aging*, and provides other resource materials for community workers. It also administers the Food Stamp Program, which recently has been broadened to provide for meals to elderly persons in their homes. Also the Department of Agriculture, through its extension services, state universities, and county home advisors on the local level, provide much practical aid for elderly persons and community work-

ers. Skilled professionals in public health departments work in the community through local and state agencies. They provide health guidance for elderly persons and operate chronic disease programs.

Volunteer organizations

Other volunteer organizations are available as a resource. These include the Heart Association and the Diabetes Association, both of which conduct activities related to the needs of older persons. Two national organizations in particular sponsor local community groups—Senior Citizens of America and American Society for the Aged, Inc. Often these groups provide programs in larger urban centers to involve elderly people in a variety of group activities. These programs include productive volunteer work, as well as leisure-time recreational activities. Through such channels of communication as these, social needs are met. Also nutritional support to meet physical needs is promoted through educational programs and other activities.

Industry

A number of industry-related groups, such as the Dairy Council and pharmaceutical firms, provide educational materials and sponsor research and workshops.

Special health care centers

Certain specialized needs may exist in adult patients. These include mental health and rehabilitation problems. In some communities special health care centers with specialized programs to meet these needs have been established. Often there is a team of specialists in these centers trained in the positive concepts of preventive and restorative techniques to assist the adult patient in meeting rehabilitation or mental health needs.

THREE

AN INTRODUCTION TO DIET THERAPY

CHAPTER **15** **THE HOSPITALIZED PATIENT**

NUTRITION IN CLINICAL CARE

Up to this point in your study of nutrition and its role in health care, you have considered the important basic principles of nutritional science and their role in human life. Then you have looked at people in their communities and applied these basic principles in practical everyday living and learning situations to help meet life's needs. You have looked at the whole of man's life-span and his needs throughout for normal growth and development. Now you have come to the final section of your study to complete the whole of man's nutritional needs—his modified needs in illness. Like the iceberg whose cap is seen above the water, therapeutic nutrition is but a small portion of the whole structure of basic nutrition that sustains it. A therapeutic diet is but a modification of an individual's normal nutritional needs only insofar as is necessary to meet a specific disease requirement. An understanding of diet therapy lies, therefore, in an understanding of normal human nutrition and metabolism. This has been the emphasis and order of study in this book.

Therefore this final part applying basic nutritional principles in clinical care will form a brief introduction to diet therapy. It will present modifications of normal nutrition that may be required in a particular disease condition. Because the patient is always the center of care, the first consideration will be the patient and his needs. The discussion of the disease will focus on its basis for planning nutritional care and the rationale for nutritional modification.

THE HOSPITALIZED PATIENT

The basis of care given hospital patients—children or adults—is the need each individual presents in the course of his illness and its medical treatment. Thus to give good patient care all health workers need to understand the factors at work in three basic areas: (1) in the patient himself and his personal needs and goals; (2) in the hospital setting with its strengths and impingements; and (3) in the personnel, those health team members providing care, and their various functions and relationships. On this basis and with this background, one may help to identify personal health needs and plan relevant individual care to meet these needs.

The patient

From his perspective the patient often faces a formidable environment. His illness and anxieties create psychologic tensions. He may or may not be able to cope with these tensions well. Also he brings with him his personal and social background and molding and, in whatever nature and degree they may have been developed, his spiritual resources. He is a whole person. He has physical, psychologic, social, and cultural needs, which are a part of him and must be considered in his total care.

185

Physical needs. The basic needs of ill children and adults begin with their physical needs. They are hospitalized because they have a basic illness or health problem. In relation to his specific illness a patient requires high-quality medical care. He also requires basic physical needs such as water, food, comfort, and safety. If relevant and valid nutritional care is to be planned, the health worker's first task is to gain knowledge of physical details such as age, sex, general physical condition, and presence and degree of symptoms of illness. Much may be learned through alert observation during general care. For example, skin conditions, either injuries or irritations, disabilities, and general nutritional status may be determined. A major aspect in the care of a child, for example, is the close observation of the child's food attitudes and food and fluid intake and keeping the physician and dietitian informed of these attitudes and needs (Fig. 15-1).

Psychologic factors. The hospitalization experience itself is psychologic stress for the patient. It causes the patient to use various coping, or defense, mechanisms developed over his growing years in his attempt to relieve these tensions. He may become depressed or withdrawn. He may repress his feelings. He may attempt to compensate for his loss of self-esteem with boasting or constant demands for attention. He may rationalize as a protective function to give comfort. He may substitute another goal to combat his frustration when his desired goal is not attainable in his situation. He may transfer his anxiety concerning his illness, for example, to his food service or his special diet

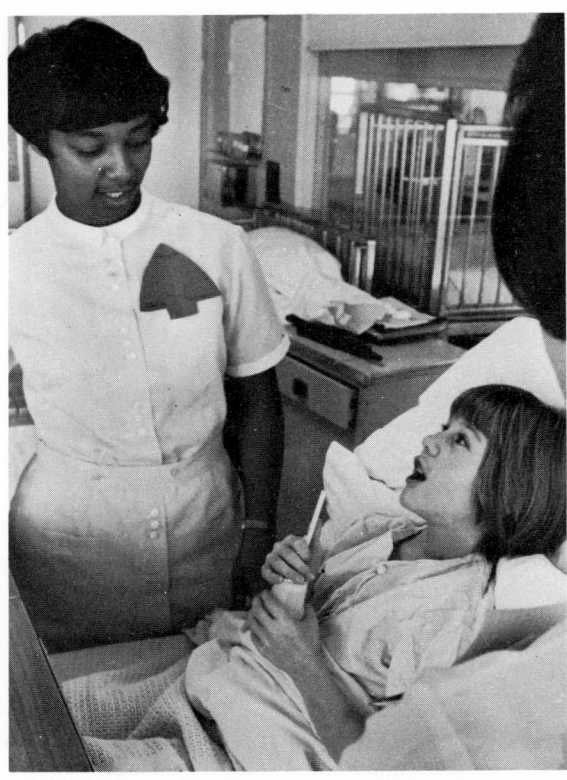

Fig. 15-1. Adequate fluid intake is essential for children, especially during illness. Here student nurses encourage a child to drink some orange juice.

restrictions. The hospitalized child especially has need for emotional support. Usually his anxieties and fears stem from separation from his family, especially his mother, and from his fears concerning his illness and its treatment. A number of factors influence his adjustment to hospitalization, including his age, how ill he is, and the kind of care that he receives. The kind of inner personal resources that he may have developed thus far from all his past experiences may or may not enable him to cope with his present situation. An additional problem is added, especially in the very young child, by his inability to communicate adequately his fears or his pains to the health workers taking care of him.

Social and cultural factors. A number of factors in the living situation of the patient play a large part in his reaction to hospitalization.

FAMILY. Persons live in families, whether they be near or far or no longer present. These family relationships directly influence the patient's development in his present situation.

GROUP MEMBERSHIPS. Memberships in various community group situations outside the family also influence a patient's responses or provide supportive group resources for him. These may be business or professional, volunteer service, social, civic, or religious groups. In the case of children, especially teen-agers, friends in their peer group may provide particular support.

OCCUPATION. Occupational roles in society develop related behavior patterns. Occupation also helps to determine a person's social class status and thus, in many instances, his reaction to illness.

FINANCIAL RESOURCES. Direct pressures may result from anxieties concerning the high cost of medical care and limited personal financial resources to pay the bills. Often help may be worked out for some source of financial assistance through consultation with the social workers on the hospital staff.

HOUSING. The patient's living situation may still offer problems in planning his continuing care.

CULTURAL FACTORS. A person is a direct product of his culture, ethnic and religious, and bears the imprint of its values, attitudes, and behaviors. Within the broad culture are also significant influential food habits and the reaction to illness and medical treatment.

Hospital setting

The hospital setting provides strengths and healing resources but, at the same time, also places restrictions on the patient. Often he is no longer a person: he is a case. No matter what his illness, for example, he is immediately bedbound and stripped of clothing, other personal identification, and all rights of decision making or independent action. Even such a homely and necessary task as going to the toilet is listed on his chart as a "privilege." He is punctured, plumbed, and palpated with innumerable fearsome-looking gadgets and machines with little explanation of what is happening. He is repeatedly given lectures as if he had no knowledge at all.

Therefore the complicated structure of the modern community hospital or extended-care facility, especially in larger cities, often bewilders and confuses many patients. It is both a medical complex devoting its energies and resources to healing and at the same time a large social community with many overt and subtle networks of relationships.

Complex medical center. Many departments contribute specialized medical and allied services. Numerous medical specialty personnel work with laboratory, x-ray, nursing service, dietary, social service, pharmacy, publications, medical records, library, and other groups. Also necessary departments to carry on the day-to-day business of the hospital include accounting, reception, maintenance, central supply, purchasing, housekeeping, and many others. A representative procession of these persons files in and out of the patient's room daily with a confusing and often conflicting array of requests and a denial of privacy. Through a labyrinth of corridors, doorways, and elevators he may be wheeled or escorted by or to

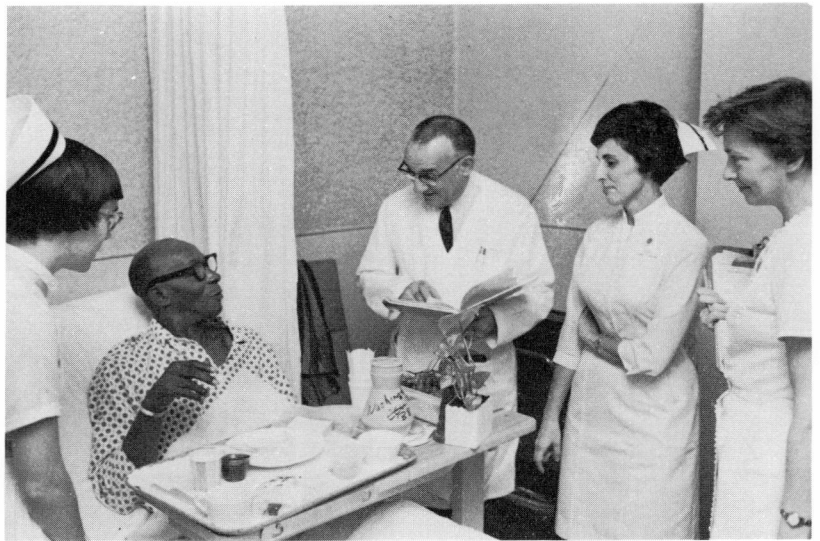

Fig. 15-2. The health team on ward rounds. Here the physician, nurse, dietitian, and student nurse confer with a patient recovering from a coronary occlusion.

these various hospital staff members. Often the purpose for these movements is vague and undefined to the patient.

Health team personnel. Among the many groups of persons comprising the hospital staff and personnel there are numerous interrelationships. Sometimes the patient may find himself caught in the middle of conflicts or overlapping interests among these groups so that his interests suffer.

However, as change takes place, the use of the health team in the various aspects of the patient's care increases. This team approach recognizes the unique contribution of special skills and knowledge and the value to the patient and health workers of such a team effort. In the care of the hospitalized patient, key persons related to his day-to-day welfare include the physician and assistant medical house staff, medical officers, the nurse and assistants such as the practical and the licensed vocational nurse, the dietitian and diet technician, the social worker, and other specialists as needed. In many places the hospital chaplain, who is especially trained in pastoral counseling, is also included. Group work of the health team includes such activities as ward rounds (Fig. 15-2) and case conferences.

PLANNING NUTRITIONAL CARE
The patient's health needs: nutritional diagnosis

In the setting provided by the individual hospital with its strengths and despite its shortcomings the members of the health team must care for the patient. The diagnosis of the patient's nutritional care needs is a prime responsibility. Under the guidance and direction of the physician and the nutrition specialist—usually a dietitian or nutritionist with advanced education in medical dietetics—the needs of the patient will be determined and a plan of care outlined. Useful and necessary background knowledge may come from several sources. These sources include the patient, the patient's chart, the family or other relatives, oral or written communication with other hospital personnel, and related research. In determining present patient care it will be helpful for the health worker to think of the patient's needs in three areas—past, present, and future. The following outline may be used as a guide:

I. Influence of past experience on present needs (here the needed skill is history taking to obtain needed information relevant to the patient's care)
   A. Social history—general socioeconomic and cultural background (family, living situation, occupations, and other important individual information)
   B. Medical history—previous illnesses, surgery, and reactions—(drug and food sensitivities, hospitalizations, and treatments)
   C. Nutrition history and analysis—general dietary habits, marketing and cooking methods, food behavior, likes, dislikes, food meanings, typical day's food intake, and analysis of nutritional status (see discussion in Chapter 11 to provide background material for nutrition history and analysis)
II. Present nutritional needs
   A. General nutritional needs of hospitalized patients
      1. Physical needs—food safety and food tolerance needs
      2. Basic physiologic needs
         a. Nutrition—including water and electrolytes
         b. Hygiene—cleanliness and elimination
         c. Rest and sleep
         d. Exercise, body mechanics, and physical energy requirements
      3. Basic psychosocial needs
         a. Minimal stress—nonthreatening environment and familiar foods
         b. Effective communication and meaning
         c. Integrity and fulfillment of desires and goals
   B. Nutritional needs of present illness (classic picture of disease and individual patient response and experience with it)
      1. Nature of the illness, its effect on the body, and clinical signs and symptoms
      2. Treatments and medications; patient responses and food interactions
      3. Diet therapy—specific order, rationale for each principle, and foods affected; meals planned (selected menu), mode of food service, and any needs for eating aids; patient response
III. Future nutritional needs for continuing care
   A. The physician's plan for continuing medical care
   B. Care facilities—home, relatives, nursing home
   C. If indicated, discussion of the patient's care plans with the person responsible for care—family member, visiting nurse, home health aide

The patient's health care: nutritional care plan

Communication skills. On the basis of background information—knowledge of specific nutritional care relative to present illness and general needs—the health team under the direction of the nutrition specialist will construct a nutritional care plan for the patient. All members of the health team, especially those working closely with the patient, such as the licensed vocational nurse or diet technician, will contribute to the plan. It will have to be flexible. Results must be checked from day to day or even hour to hour and the plan reevaluated according to need. Involvement of the patient in the plan is essential. Thus communication skills in interviewing and alert observation are vital parts of planning good nutritional care.

Points to consider. Generally, in the plan of care these points will be considered:
   1. Identified needs
   2. Goals related to specific needs
   3. Relevant background knowledge
   4. Related plan of action
   5. Results

Identified nutritional needs will be related to the personal goals of the patient. These needs may be related to present meals being served or to instruction concerning special diet needs. Related background knowledge of the nutrients and food therapies will apply. The related plan of action will involve getting a diet history, analyzing the patient's food intake, planning instructional needs, and following through with him to determine future care needs. In clinical conferences with the dietitian or the clinical nutrition specialist various members of the health team, including the nursing assistants and the diet technician, will clarify and enlarge their various activities.

BASIC CONCEPTS OF DIET THERAPY
Normal nutrition base

The primary concept of diet therapy is that such treatment is based on normal nutritional requirements of the patient. This is an important initial fact to grasp and to impart to the patient. For example, it is a great source of encouragement to the mother of a newly diagnosed diabetic child that his diet plan will be based on his normal growth and development needs and will use regular foods. Again a therapeutic diet is but a modification of normal nutritional needs, modified only insofar as the specific disease in the specific individual necessitates.

Disease application

The principles of a specific therapeutic diet will be based on modifications of the nutritional component of the normal diet. These changes may include one or more of the following types of modification:
1. *Nutrients*—modifications in one or more of the basic nutrients such as protein, carbohydrates, fat, minerals, and vitamins
2. *Energy*—modification in energy value as expressed in calories
3. *Texture*—modification in texture or seasoning, such as liquid, bland, or low residue

Background information needed

Three areas of knowledge are needed to plan and carry out valid nutritional care in therapeutic diets:
1. *Disease.* How does this disease affect the body and its normal metabolic function?
2. *Diet therapy.* How and why does the diet need to be modified in terms of its nutritional components to meet the needs created by this particular disease?
3. *Diet guidelines.* How do these necessary nutritional modifications affect daily food choices?

Individual patient adaptation

A workable plan for a specific person must be based on his food habits in his personal life situation. This can only be achieved through careful planning *with the patient* based on an initial interview to obtain a diet history and knowledge of his food habits,

living conditions, and related factors. Thus the diet principles may be understood and motivation secured to follow through. Whatever the problem, nutritional care is valid only to the extent that it involves these knowledges, skills, and insights. Individual adaptations of the diet to meet individual needs is imperative for successful therapy.

HOSPITAL FOOD SERVICE
Dietary department

The hospital dietary department is responsible for providing nourishing food for all the patients. The department may provide meals for the staff also. According to each patient's nutritional needs as related to his illness, his diet is usually ordered by his physician. In some settings the nutrition specialist, dietitian or nutritionist may outline the dietary prescription and plan of care. The dietary staff must then interpret this order in terms of specific foods required. They must see that these foods are purchased, prepared, and served correctly. A number of staff personnel, different types of food service, and various relations with other hospital departments, especially nursing, are involved in carrying out this important responsibility.

Personnel. The personnel of the dietary department includes a number of persons. The chief administrative dietitian or food service manager is responsible for the smooth running of the food service. This food service administrator must supervise the planning of all meals and other forms of food service, the purchase of all necessary food required by the plan, and the preparation and service of this food to all the patients and staff. Other staff dietitians include various ward or therapeutic dietitians, who are responsible for patient care. They work more directly with the patient and the ward staff to see that the patient gets the proper diet and to provide whatever learning experiences are needed to help the patient understand his diet needs. Other staff persons include diet technicians and clerks, who assist the dietitian in administrative food service and patient care responsibilities. They may help with tray service, distribute and collect menus, help tally food orders, and keep various records. They may assist in taking diet histories and in teaching. Other dietary aides include cooks, maids, porters, and others who assist in food preparation and service.

Types of food service. A variety of types of food service may be found in different hospitals. The service may be centralized so that all trays are served from one central kitchen or decentralized so that food is conveyed to ward areas and trays are assembled and served from the ward kitchen. Some hospitals have a type of automated food service in which food is purchased already prepared and portioned, usually in frozen form, and final preparation for service to patients is managed with the use of electronic ovens. This provides a food service similar to that used on airlines.

Menus used in various hospitals may be of a cyclic nature, being repeated by season or month. They may be standard ones served to all patients according to the type of diet ordered. In other instances the hospital may provide a selective menu from which patients may choose among different entrées and accompaniments.

Relations with nursing service department. Successful food service in any hospital requires close cooperation between the dietary and nursing service departments. Of all the persons on the health team, perhaps the nursing assistants (licensed vocational and practical nurses) and the dietary assistants (diet technicians) are closest to the patient. They can provide day-to-day help to dietitians concerning individual needs of the patients. In many instances they convey diet orders to the dietary department and aid patients in marking their menus. Often they are responsible for or participate in tray service.

Routine hospital diets

A schedule of routine "house" diets is followed in most hospitals for those patients who do not require a special diet. According to the patient's general need and tolerance, the diet ordered for him may be either a clear or full liquid one if he cannot tolerate solid food. The only difference between a clear and a full liquid diet is that milk and items made with milk may be used on the full liquid diet but not on the clear liquid one. The diet may be soft, including no raw food and being generally bland in seasoning. It may be a regular diet, including a full normal diet for age. Occasionally an interval step between soft and regular will be used—the light diet. A summary of routine hospital diets is given in Table 15-1. It indicates the usual progression and food choices at each stage.

Serving food to patients

Objective. It is well to remember that *all* diets are therapy, whether they are regular hospital diets or special ones. Each diet provides the nutritional base for healing or convalescence from illness and regaining strength and is hence an integral part of total treatment and care.

Without proper nourishment to build sound body tissue and provide needed energy no other treatment given the patient can succeed. However, beyond meeting these vital physical needs, food also helps to meet other personal, emotional, and social needs of the patient.

Acceptance of food. No matter how well planned his diet may be, unless the patient accepts and eats the food, it cannot help him. Here the health team has a prime responsibility for helping the patient obtain and enjoy the right foods. Various members of the health care team may do this in several ways: by preparing the patient, serving the tray, and assisting the patient.

PREPARING THE PATIENT. Prepare the patient for meals by helping to make him as comfortable as possible. Nurses may offer bedpans and urinals ahead of time. Wash the patient's face and hands. Try to have him in a calm, relaxed frame of mind, free from pain and discomfort. Make his environment as

Table 15-1. Routine hospital diets

FOOD GROUPS	CLEAR LIQUID	FULL LIQUID	SOFT	LIGHT	GENERAL
Soup	Broth, bouillon	Same, plus strained soups	Same, plus unstrained soups	All	All
Cereal			Refined cooked cereals, cornflakes, rice, noodles, macaroni, spaghetti	Same	All
Bread			White bread, crackers, melba toast, zwieback	Same plus graham and rye bread	All
Protein foods		Milk, cream, milk drinks	Same, plus eggs (except fried), mild cheese, fowl, fish, sweetbreads, tender beef, veal, lamb, liver, bacon, gravy	Same	All
Vegetables			Potatoes—baked, mashed, creamed, steamed, escalloped; tender cooked, whole bland vegetables (may be strained or pureed)	Same—cooked whole, bland	All
Fruit and fruit juices	Apple juice	All fruit juices	Same, plus bland cooked fruit; peaches, pears, applesauce, peeled apricots, white cherries, bananas, orange and grapefruit sections without membrane	All	All
Desserts	Plain gelatin, water ice	Same, plus sherbet, ice cream, puddings, custard	Same, plus plain cakes—sponge and other types—cookies, simple puddings	Same	All
Miscellaneous	Ginger ale, carbonated water, coffee, tea	Same	Same, plus butter, salt, pepper	Same	All

pleasant as possible by avoiding unpleasant treatment and dressings at this time. If necessary, open the windows to rid the ward of unpleasant odors. Raise the head of the bed if permissible, to put the patient in a physically comfortable position in which eating is easier. Clear the bedside stand and have the extension table over the bed in position and cleared for the tray.

SERVING THE TRAY. Provide food for the patient in as attractive a manner as possible. Place the food and dishes so that the patient can reach everything. See that the tray and everything on it are as neat, clean, and attractive as possible. Give moderate-sized servings unless otherwise ordered. Servings that are too large may discourage the patient to the point of not eating at all. Often some items may be reserved and offered between meals to encourage the patient's appetite. Serve hot foods hot and cold foods cold. Remember that the object is to entice the patient to eat a well-balanced meal in spite of a sometimes poor appetite. Check the name and diet for each patient and tray to see that the right diet gets to the right patient. If the patient does not eat, try to determine the cause and seek to remedy it. Discuss any unsolved dietary problems that come up with the team leader or the nurse or dietitian in charge.

ASSISTING THE PATIENT. According to the patient's ability to feed himself, he may need assistance. Patients usually like to help themselves as much as possible and should be encouraged to do so. If necessary, have the meat cut up and the bread buttered before bringing it to the bedside. If the patient is unable to use his right hand, place the utensils and food convenient to his left. Try to learn each patient's needs and limitations so that little things can be done without making the patient feel inadequate. When complete assistance is needed, have the tray within the patient's vision; then relax, sit down beside the bed if this is more comfortable, and make simple conversation or remain silent as the patient's condition indicates. Offer

small amounts. Do not rush the feeding. Give ample time for the patient to chew and swallow or rest between mouthfuls. Offer liquids between the solids, using a drinking tube if necessary, Wipe the patient's mouth with a napkin as needed during and after the meal. Let the patient hold the bread if he is able.

When feeding a blind patient or one with eye dressings, give a description of the food on the tray so that the patient will have a mental image that will make him want to eat. Sometimes it is helpful to use the face of a clock to help him visualize the position of certain foods on the plate, such as indicating that the meat is at 12 o'clock and the potatoes are at 3 o'clock. Warn him that the soup feels particularly hot when it is taken through a glass straw and tell him if he is being fed which foods are being served before giving them to him.

Observations. During service of meals and assistance of the patient, opportunities arise for making important observations. The nurse or dietitian and team members can observe the patient's physical appearance closely, his response to the food served, the meaning of food to him, and his appetite and tolerance for certain foods. These observations can help in adapting the patient's diet to meet his particular needs.

Reasons for food rejection by children. A number of factors may contribute to a child's poor appetite and refusal of food.

ILLNESS. The child may be too ill or weak to eat. He may have some physical intolerance for food. He may require liquid or soft food, food substitutions, or gentle help in feeding (Fig. 15-3).

ANXIETY. The child may be tense and frightened because he is separated from his family, especially his mother. The strange and unfamiliar surroundings may frighten him. He may be concerned about his illness and its outcome. Involving his parents in planning for his care or helping to make arrangements for his mother to be with him usually provides needed security and support. Also help-

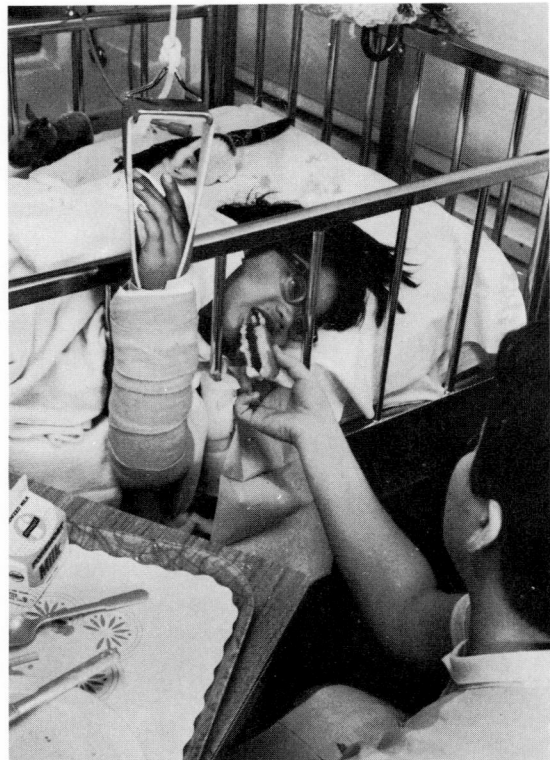

Fig. 15-3. Child with fractured arm is assisted in eating by student nurse.

ing him to talk about his fears, understanding and accepting him and his fears, or providing simple, brief explanations of his care and treatment as needed all help to reduce his anxiety, to gain his confidence, and to give him added resources with which to cope.

PRESENTATION OF FOOD. Often the child rejects food because of the way in which it is presented to him. For example, an ill 2-year-old is confronted with a tray filled with one food and adult-sized utensils unceremoniously planted before him by a large, forbidding, strange adult with the command "Now eat!" and is overwhelmed. Worse yet, force-feeding a child who has inner conflicts only adds more trauma. Some children are already wearing battle scars of home combat with an adult over food.

Ways of achieving food acceptance by children. Nurses, dietitians, and their assistants experienced in caring for children have devised numerous ways of presenting food. Basically these ways of helping a child to eat revolve around two related factors: (1) self-selection and (2) warm mealtime atmosphere.

SELF-SELECTION. Allowing a child to have some degree of choice in his food is helpful. Although a variety of meal services may not be possible in all hospitals, a selective menu from which the child, with guidance, may help choose his own food is a step in that direction. Some consideration of a child's likes and dislikes, with encouragement in convalescence to try out new tastes in food, also helps achieve warm acceptance.

WARM MEALTIME ATMOSPHERE. The manner in which the food is served and a warm atmosphere at mealtime are major influences on the child's reaction. The following may help to create this atmosphere: personnel, group eating, festive days, familiar food, and family involvement.

Personnel. The warm, supportive manner of the personnel serving the food is of inestimable value. They must know the children and have a feeling for them. Food is served attractively in proper-sized small portions and in correct child-sized utensils. Bedbound patients are made as comfortable as possible and assisted as needed.

Group eating. Often ambulatory patients may eat at small tables in family style. Interest is heightened if the children are involved in the preparation. For example, they may help set the tables, serve as host or hostess, pass the food, and refill serving dishes as needed. Various staff persons may eat with the children occasionally and find in sharing food not only a means of observing and learning more about their patients but also an important vehicle of establishing feeling relationships with them.

Festive days. Observance of holidays and birthdays with special food decorations will help to interest children and give support.

Familiar food. Consideration should be given to ethnic food habits. Sometimes a familiar food or dish from home that is not contraindicated by the child's illness will stimulate appetite and interest in eating, thus securing needed nourishment for him. Preparing food and ethnic dishes to which the child is accustomed or flavoring food according to familiar tastes is helpful to a child, especially one confined to bed for an extended period.

Family involvement. Explorations with his mother of the child's home eating habits and of the ways that she prepares and serves his food will often give helpful background for planning the child's nutritional care while he is in the hospital. Also such discussions provide opportunity for parents to express their anxieties about the child and lead to mutual learning about the normal growth and development needs of children. If the child requires any special diet modifications, these needs may also be discussed with the parents, helping them to explore ways that the child's needs may be fitted in with the family eating habits.

NUTRITION EDUCATION OPPORTUNITIES

Helping the patient to learn more about his diet and nutritional needs is an important part of his total care. If he understands the role that his food plays in his health and in helping him to regain his strength and recover from his illness, he is more likely to accept his diet. He is also encouraged to continue to follow through with these sound eating habits when he is discharged from the hospital.

The nursing and dietetics assistants, as well as other team members, can work with the dietitian or nutritionist and the nurse to provide important nutrition and diet teaching in several informal ways.

Planned conversations

While giving general nursing care, for example, the nurse can have "planned conversations" with the patient. The health worker can talk with him about general observations of his needs. Together they can explore ways that the patient's needs can be met and why certain foods are particularly important to his health. Likewise the diet technician can make informal visits to patients' rooms on ward rounds to discuss general diet needs or the nutritional bases for food selections. Often the selective menu is an excellent vehicle for such conversations. The health worker can make suggestions for food items that the patient may need more than others and can discuss with him the comparative food values.

Food service

Food service itself presents opportunities for teaching. When serving his meal tray or assisting him with eating, the nurse or other team members can point out certain food items on the tray as examples of foods that supply specific nutrients to the body. For example, if he has had surgery and particularly needs protein for tissue healing, the nurse can point out the protein foods on the tray and suggest that he eat these foods first while his appetite may be better.

The patient's family

Sometimes the health worker can plan to talk with the patient's family about his diet needs or get additional information from them about his food habits. It may be possible to help the person who will be preparing the patient's food to know what his diet needs are and to learn some practical ways of meeting these needs.

Resources

Many nutrition education resources exist in the hospital and community to assist the patient in learning about his diet needs or to help the health worker in this part of patient care. The hospital dietitian, for example, can provide information and some simple teaching tools and reference materials. The nurse and the health team members may also consult with the dietitian or the diet technician concerning the patient's needs. In the community other persons are available to help the patient after he goes home. If there is an outpatient department, the dietitian in the clinic section of the hospital can continue the patient's nutrition education. The nurse may refer the patient to this dietitian. Other general community resources include nutritionists with the public health department, school nurses, agricultural extension service home advisors, nutrition teachers in local schools, school lunch program supervisors, dietitians in health agencies such as the Heart Association or with industry-related groups such as the Dairy Council. Sometimes an organized interagency nutrition council exists in the community. These groups develop and sponsor a number of nutrition education programs and provide a variety of resource materials.

CHAPTER 16

GASTROINTESTINAL PROBLEMS

GASTROINTESTINAL TRACT AND ACCESSORY ORGANS
Physiologic functions

The digestion and absorption of the food a person eats is accomplished in the gastrointestinal tract through a series of intimately related secretory and neuromuscular mechanisms. In Chapter 8 this normal network of functions was summarized. This background now forms the basis for a study of problems related to the gastrointestinal tract. Any disease state can best be understood in terms of the specific interference it brings to the normal function involved at that point. Thus the general dietary modifications used in disease states relate specifically to the normal physiologic operation of the organs involved.

Psychologic influences

The individual's particular emotional make-up and manner of dealing with life's day-to-day problems and challenges will often be reflected in the functions of his digestive tract. The gastrointestinal tract is indeed a sensitive mirror of the individual human condition. Its physiologic functioning reflects both physical and psychologic conditioning. In helping to adapt diet therapy for patients with gastrointestinal problems, the health worker will be dealing not so much with a specific food item per se as with the state of the body that receives it. Far more truth than mere humor exists in the statement "Surrounding every stomach there is a person."

Factors involved in diet therapy

Diet therapy for various gastrointestinal problems, therefore, will be determined by a consideration of four basic factors involved:
1. *Chemical secretions*—the secretory functions that provide the necessary environment and agents for chemical digestion
2. *Muscle activity and structural integrity* —the neuromuscular functions and their structures that provide the necessary motility and mechanical action for digestion and move the food mass along
3. *Absorbing mucosa*—the absorptive functions, which enable the end products of digestion (the nutrients) to enter the body's circulation and nourish the cells
4. *Psychologic factors*—the person himself and his coping mechanisms

Now these factors involved in diet therapy will be considered in relation to each successive section of the gastrointestinal tract: (1) mouth and esophagus, (2) stomach and duodenum, and (3) intestines. Also involved are two additional concerns: (1) food intolerances and allergies and (2) the accessory organs— liver, gallbladder, and pancreas.

MOUTH AND ESOPHAGUS
Cleft palate

Feeding difficulties in infants and young children may result from abnormalities in the structure of the mouth. When the parts of the upper jaw and of the palate separating the mouth and the nasal cavity do not fuse properly during fetal development, the anatomic abnormality creates difficult feeding problems. If this fusion of the parts of the upper jaw and mouth fails to occur, cleft lip (harelip) or cleft palate or both result. Since the infant is unable to suck adequately with this abnormality, early feedings are tiring and lengthy. A softened nipple with enlarged openings through which the infant can obtain milk by chewing motion is helpful. In some instances a medicine dropper or gavage feedings (p. 164) may be used initially. The infant should be held in an upright position and fed slowly in small amounts to avoid aspiration. There should be brief rest periods and frequent burping to expel the large amount of air swallowed. If acid foods such as orange juice are irritating, ascorbic acid supplement is usually prescribed. As solid foods are added, they may be mixed with milk in the bottle and given in gruel or thickened form through a large nipple opening.

Surgical repair of a cleft palate is usually carried out over the growth years, depending on the extent of the deformity and the growth of the child. During this period the child may be cared for by a group of specialists to handle his overall development. This group may be found in larger medical centers and is called the Cleft Palate Team. Preparation for surgery demands good nutritional status. After surgery good nursing and nutritional care are essential. The infant or child is usually fed a fluid or semifluid diet using a medicine dropper or spoon. Great care must be exercised to protect the suture line and avoid any strain.

Dental caries

Incidence. Of all the problems affecting the teeth, dental decay is the most prevalent among young children. Almost no one escapes it. According to surveys, over 99% of the children in the United States are affected by it at one time or another, and its incidence seems to have little pattern. It is found both in well-fed and in undernourished children. It may have small effect and cause little difficulty, or it may be rampant and cause considerable destruction of teeth and thus influence eating ability. Perhaps because it is so common and does not usually cause grave problems, it is often dismissed with indifference or ignored. Yet it remains and continues to disfigure, cause pain, create nutritional problems, and cost money.

Causes. Three factors contribute to tooth decay and work together to sustain the problem: a susceptible host, various oral bacteria, and the child's diet.

SUSCEPTIBLE HOST. Differences in susceptibility to dental caries vary widely among individual children. Some of these differences are hereditary, in that the anatomic characteristics and shape of the tooth are at fault. However, the ultimate cause is basic interrelationships between the shape of the tooth and the environment of the mouth that sustains tooth development during formative periods of growth. Since teeth once formed are stable structures, a positive nutritional influence can have effect only during growth and development of the enamel-forming organ in the gums and tooth bud. Certain vitamins and minerals, especially vitamins A and D, calcium, and phosphorus, play a part during this period of tooth formation (p. 43). Studies also indicate that fluoride ingestion during this period may have a direct influence on tooth formation.

ORAL BACTERIA. Dental plaque is the gelatinous coating of a tooth. These plaques contain a number of bacteria. In humans streptococci are the bacteria in greatest number in these dental plaques. These bacteria seem to have a particular affinity for carbohydrates and act on them rapidly. Controlled tests show that only 13 minutes after carbohydrate is present in the mouth, streptococci alone can increase the acidity of the dental plaque a great deal. However, the oral flora is complex, and bacterial effects vary among several microorganisms. Whatever the microorganism involved, the necessary material for them to feed on is the caries-producing base. This material is carbohydrate.

THE CHILD'S DIET. As carbohydrate food accumulates in the mouth, therefore, it provides the necessary media for the normal growth of these acid-producing microorganisms, which cause tooth decay. In sites on the tooth where the shape contributes to retention of food particles, especially of sticky, gummy foods, which adhere and remain more readily on these tooth surfaces, this bacterial activity is greatest. Persistent and continuous snacking of such sticky carbohydrates, therefore, is a prime factor in tooth decay. A number of studies have indicated this fact. When concentrated carbohydrate snacks such as candy have been consumed at numerous times throughout the day, the incidence of caries is greatly increased, especially when candy is of a sticky nature such as carmels. During periods when the candy has been withdrawn, the caries rate has decreased.

The other dietary element that has a large influence on dental caries is *fluoride*. Repeated studies consistently confirm about 60% reduction in the incidence of dental caries in children with both prenatal and postnatal exposure to fluoridated water. Extensive research on the dental caries activity in children from eleven areas in five western states (Oregon, Idaho, Montana, Utah, and Washington) found that the one most significant factor was the presence of fluorides in the water supplies.

Dietary implications. Although the problem of dental caries is by no means solved, recent advances in the knowledge of nutrition and its relationship to caries provide helpful steps in that direction. In summary, therefore, two nutritional factors seem to be involved: sweets and fluoride.

SWEETS. Adhesive carbohydrates such as candy bars, caramels, and other sweets consumed at frequent intervals increase dental caries. Carbohydrates in liquid form may be somewhat less cariogenic than those in solid form.

FLUORIDE. Fluoridated public water supplies decrease dental caries rates. Public health authorities have advocated the fluoridation of public drinking water in the amount of 1 part per million in areas where the drinking water is low in fluoride content.

Dentures

In some older persons, ill-fitting dentures may cause problems with chewing and hence digestion of foods. The health of the gums on which the dentures rest is imperative for successful fit and use of dentures. Vitamins A and C are particularly related to the integrity of gum tissue and hence may need special attention in the diet when healing or strengthening may be necessary. When dental problems exist or when dentures are not present, a *mechanical soft* diet may be used. In this diet all foods are soft cooked foods, and meats are ground and sometimes mixed with sauces or gravies, thus requiring less chewing to make eating easier.

Fractured jaw

A fractured jaw poses obvious problems in chewing food. After the initial injury has

Table 16-1. High-protein, high-calorie formula for milk shakes

INGREDIENTS	AMOUNT	APPROXIMATE FOOD VALUE	
Milk	1 cup	Protein	40 gm.
Eggs	2	Fat	30 gm.
Skimmed milk powder or	6 to 8 tbsp.	Carbohydrate	70 gm.
Casec	2 tbsp.	Calories	710
Sugar	2 tbsp.		
Ice cream	1 in. slice or 1 scoop		
Cocoa or other flavoring	2 tbsp.		
Vanilla	Few drops, as desired		

been corrected with surgical wiring together of the jaws, the resulting immobility prevents the normal taking in of food. A high-protein, high-calorie liquid diet is needed to provide healing nutrients in a texture that can be taken in without movement of the jaw. A straw is used to drink the liquid formula. A typical high-protein, high-calorie formula for milkshakes to use in such situations is given in Table 16-1. As healing occurs and chewing gradually can be resumed, soft foods, which require little effort in chewing, are introduced at first.

Hiatus hernia

Problems of the lower esophagus may be caused by hiatus hernia. This is a condition caused by a protrusion of a part of the upper stomach into the thorax because of an opening created by a weak spot in the diaphragm. This outpouching at the juncture of the esophagus and the stomach allows food to be held in this pouch and thus hinders normal food passage at this point. Since the food is held near the bottom of the esophagus and begins some mixing with the stomach acids, it may be pushed back up into the lower esophagus and cause heartburn as a result of this regurgitation.

Depending on the degree of the problem, much discomfort after eating may be involved. Usually the problem can be controlled by eating more frequent small meals, so that less volume is introduced into the stomach at one time. The patient is more comfortable if he does not lie down immediately after eating, since gravity would tend to pull the food more readily back up into the esophagus and cause discomfort. There may be a need for sleeping in an elevated position using a triangular support under the pillow. This prevents gastric secretions from getting back up into the esophagus and causing difficulty. In situations of greater involvement surgical repair may be the treatment of choice.

STOMACH AND DUODENUM

The most common clinical problem affecting the upper gastrointestinal tract is peptic ulcer—the general term given to an eroded mucosal lesion in the stomach or duodenum. Occasionally the lesion may be located in the lower esophagus. Gastric ulcers are less common. The majority occur in the duodenal bulb, where the gastric contents emptying into the duodenum through the pyloric valve are most concentrated in acid.

Peptic ulcer

Causes. The fundamental cause of peptic ulcer is not clear. However, two main factors seem to be involved: (1) the amount of gastric acid and pepsin secreted and (2) the degree of tissue resistance to the digestive action of these secretions. In the development of gastric ulcers, although the presence of acid is essential, the degree of tissue sensitivity seems to be the paramount factor. In the development of duodenal ulcers excessive production of acid and pepsin is the primary factor. In either case hydrochloric acid in the gastric juice is generally acknowledged to be the essential factor in the development, perpetuation, and recurrence of peptic ulcer.

The psychologic factor in peptic ulcer is variable. The so-called ulcer personality has been described in many tests. Although overdrawn perhaps in some sources, the ulcer-prone individual does tend to be anxious or tense, aggressive, and competitive. Peptic ulcer usually occurs in men between the ages of 20 and 50 years. This is a time of life when career and personal strivings are likely to be at a peak.

Clinical symptoms. Increased gastric contractions that are especially painful when the stomach is empty are cardinal symptoms of peptic ulcer. The amount and concentration of hydrochloric acid is increased in duodenal ulcer but may be normal in gastric ulcer. Nutritional deficiencies may be seen in low plasma protein levels, anemia, and loss of weight. Hemorrhage may be the first sign of the ulcer in some patients. Confirmation of the diagnosis comes from clinical findings, x-ray tests, or visualization by gastroscopy.

General medical management. Three factors form the basis of treatment: (1) *drug* *therapy and antacids* to counteract the hypermotility and hypersecretions, (2) *rest,* both physical and mental, aided as necessary by sedatives, and (3) *diet therapy* to provide maximum healing and prevent further tissue damage.

Diet therapy. The general term *bland* has been used to describe the various ulcer diets found in common practice. The word comes from the Latin word *blandus* meaning a smooth tongue or soothing and has taken on the meaning of something insipid, dull, uninteresting, and unattractive. Such meanings are all too often conveyed by the usual ulcer diets in many hospitals. These diets are often nutritionally inadequate, esthetically unappealing, scientifically unsound, and emotionally disturbing. That such a state is not necessary is increasingly made evident by research that indicates that the usual rigid and restrictive approach is based more on tradition and assumption than on scientific fact. Perhaps a better perspective may be gained by seeing the background development of diet therapy for peptic ulcer, which forms the rationale given for the two basic approaches to treatment: (1) the traditional conservative management and (2) the liberal individual approach.

TRADITIONAL, CONSERVATIVE DIETARY MANAGEMENT. In the latter part of the nineteenth century the prevailing belief concerning treatment for peptic ulcer was that food was harmful to the ulcer and that only complete rest, meaning an empty stomach, would permit healing. Therefore semistarvation regimens became the accepted practice among European physicians and were soon introduced to the United States.

In 1915 an American physician, Bertram Sippy, began the principles of continuous control of gastric acidity through diet and alkaline medication. His rather rigidly outlined program of milk and cream feedings with slow additions of single soft food items over a prolonged period of time allowed little variation for individual need or nutritional adequacy. Some increase in the diet was made in 1935 by a Danish physician, Meulengracht,

who introduced a somewhat more liberal approach in feeding peptic ulcer patients, especially as a treatment for hemorrhage. In the main, however, Sippy's regimen, although clearly establishing the important acid-neutralizing principle of frequent feedings, continued to place rigid restrictions on the traditional dietary programs followed in common practice.

Although many changes in the details of management have occurred since Sippy's day, his general restrictive pattern has been the mold for much of the traditional conservative management still used by some clinicians today. This traditional diet therapy is based on several principles. The food must be both acid neutralizing and nonirritating.

Acid-neutralizing food. Assumptions underlying this rigid form of therapy are unfounded and have not been supported by recent research. The therapy usually begins with milk and cream feedings every hour or so, allegedly to neutralize free acid with the milk protein, suppress gastric secretion with the cream, and generally "soothe" the ulcer by "coating" the stomach. However, after the food has been mixed with stomach acids, its physical nature changes. No coating of the stomach results.

Afterward, soft, bland foods are added gradually, and some food is kept in the stomach at all times to mix with the acid to prevent its corrosive action on the ulcer. These bland foods are usually limited to choices of white toast or crackers, refined cereals, egg, mild cheeses, a few cooked pureed fruits and vegetables, and later ground meat.

Nonirritating food. This therapy is concerned with eliminating chemical, mechanical, and thermal irritation:

1. *Chemical irritation.* Any food believed to stimulate gastric secretions is prohibited. These would include any highly seasoned, fried, or spiced foods.

2. *Mechanical irritation.* Any foods believed to be abrasive in their effect on the ulcer are prohibited, including all raw food, plant fibers, whole grains, and gas formers.

Graduated bland diet for peptic ulcer

GENERAL DESCRIPTION

1. Avoid overeating at any one meal. It is better to eat smaller amounts more often.
2. Eat slowly and chew thoroughly. Sip liquids slowly, especially hot or cold ones.
3. Avoid worry, tension, argument, hurry, and fatigue, particularly at mealtime.
4. Avoid monotony in diet by varying the foods used as much as the diet allows.
5. Use no spices or seasonings except salt. Avoid concentrated sweets. Small amounts of sugar may be used.
6. Do not drink more than a glass of liquid with each meal, but drink as much as desired between meals.
7. Take medications regularly as directed.
8. Follow all directions carefully, and include only that part of the following diet list that is prescribed. Make the additions to the diet only when the physician advises it.
9. Maintain regular hours for eating, and take meals regularly.

STAGE I

FOOD	ALLOWED	NOT ALLOWED
Milk	Regular or homogenized, buttermilk	
Cream	Plain or mixed with milk	
Fats	Fresh butter or fortified margarine	Any other
Eggs	Boiled, poached, coddled, scrambled in double boiler; plain omelet; eggnog with vanilla only	Fried eggs
Cereals	Cooked, refined or strained; oatmeal, Cream of Wheat, farina, Wheatena, precooked infant cereals; also plain buttered noodles, macaroni, spaghetti, or white rice Dry cereals such as cornflakes, puffed rice, Rice Krispies, without bran	Whole grain cereals and those containing bran or shredded wheat
Desserts	Plain custard, Jell-O, rennet, plain cornstarch, tapioca, or rice puddings; plain vanilla ice cream (if allowed to melt in mouth)	Any other
Bread	Enriched white; fine rye or fine whole wheat bread at least one day old (may be plain or toasted); soda crackers, zwieback, melba toast, hard rolls	Whole wheat and other whole grain bread; graham or coarse crackers; hot or fresh bread
Cheese	Cream, cottage cheese, mild processed American, and Swiss	Any other
Sweets	Jelly (clear, plain), honey, sugar (in moderation), strained cranberry sauce	Any other
Potato	or baked sweet potatoes or yams in moderate amounts	
Cream soups	Cream soups homemade from the following pureed vegetables: asparagus spinach peas potatoes green beans tomatoes	Canned cream soups; soups from any other vegetables; dehydrated and chicken soups, broths, meat stock, bouillon

STAGE II

FOOD	ALLOWED	NOT ALLOWED
Fruit juices	Strained orange juice, beginning with ¼ cup, diluted with water and taken at end of meal Later can be undiluted; prune juice if necessary for bowel regulation; grapefruit juice may be added later if tolerated	Any other

Graduated bland diet for peptic ulcer—cont'd

FOOD	STAGE II ALLOWED	NOT ALLOWED
Plain cake	Angel food, sponge, pound, butter cake (without frosting)	Any cakes made with nuts, dates, spices, frostings
Vegetables (Group 1)	Winter, banana, or acorn squash; tomato juice if tolerated. The following cooked and strained or strained vegetables for infants: asparagus, peas, carrots, green beans, beets, spinach	Any other, also raw or coarse vegetables
Fruits (Group 1)	The following stewed fruits, which have been strained (or fruits strained for infants): pears, peaches, prunes, apricots, applesauce	All other

	STAGE III	
Fowl	Tender white or dark meat boiled, broiled, roasted, or baked, of turkey, chicken, squab, or pheasant	Fried, braised, or in any other form; skin, gristle or fat
Fish	Fresh or frozen; boiled, broiled or baked; scalded canned tuna or salmon, oysters, fresh or canned	Other fish canned or prepared in any other manner; smoked, pickled, preserved fish, crab, lobster, sardines
Meats	At first only finely ground plain beef; later tender cuts of beef, veal, lamb; also liver, sweetbreads, brains (boiled, broiled, creamed, roasted)	Fried, smoked, pickled, cured; skin, gristle, fat, meats with tough fiber; delicatessen pork, ham, bacon, salami, wieners

	STAGE IV	
Desserts	Prune or apricot whip, plain vanilla, chocolate, or sugar cookies or wafers; plain sherbet, ices, ice cream if eaten slowly; fine graham crackers	Rich pastries or pies, nuts, raisins, coconut, gingerbread, spice cake, candy
Vegetables (Group 2)	Tender whole cooked vegetables: asparagus, squash, carrots, spinach, peas, string beans, beets, mushrooms, tomatoes, peeled	Onions, celery, sauerkraut, cucumbers, peppers, turnips, radishes, cabbage, cauliflower, broccoli, brussel sprouts; any coarse vegetables; hulls or fibers of green vegetables; coleslaw or other salads
Fruits (Group 2)	Canned or cooked without skins or seeds: pears, apricots, peaches, persimmons. Nectar from pears, peaches or apricots; juice of apples, grapefruits, or oranges	
Beverages	Weak tea, weak cocoa, Sanka, Postum; plain milk shakes	Coffee, strong tea, iced drinks, soft drinks, alcoholic beverages of any kind
Miscellaneous	Homemade mayonnaise without spices; duck; crisp bacon; vegetable oils or shortening; less tender cuts of meat (properly prepared) such as beef round, cutlet; sour cream, yogurt; brown sugar, powdered sugar; mint jelly	Spices or condiments, pepper, horseradish, meat sauces, catsup, mustard, vinegar, pickles, relishes, olives; spicy foods, fried foods; gravies; hot cakes and other hot breads; chewing gum

3. *Thermal irritation.* Any hot or cold foods believed to irritate the lesion by their effect on surface blood vessels are prohibited, including hot beverages and soups, frozen desserts, or iced beverages.

After the initial hourly milk and cream, the diet is gradually increased as the ulcer heals. Such a traditional conservative routine usually follows a progressive four-stage pattern similar to that shown in the graduated bland diet (pp. 202 and 203).

LIBERAL INDIVIDUAL APPROACH. Accumulating experience and research, however, has begun to challenge the validity of some of these beliefs. In contrast to the traditional, conservative management stands the increasingly accepted liberal individual approach. Numerous studies have found that healing is related not so much to restrictive diet and medications as to the personal care and concern of the health team. In all instances results have indicated that the current concept of rigid dietary treatment is not verified as superior or even sound therapy. Bland foods do not increase the rate of healing, and no particular benefit accrues from avoidance of all foods thought to be commonly irritating.

Traditional practices questioned. Current studies have refuted several traditional practices:

1. *Gastric irritation.* A number of spices and herbs and other such substances have been tested to determine their effect on gastric acidity. No significant change in gastric pH was noted with any of these items with four basic exceptions. These exceptions are black pepper, meat extracts, caffeine, and alcohol. No food (such as orange juice) was found sufficiently acid of itself to cause a significant pH change or direct irritation of an ulcer.

2. *Buffering foods.* Protein foods are effective buffering agents because of their amphoteric nature (p. 31). Milk has some buffering effect, but other protein foods seem to be as effective or more so. All proteins influence acid secretion, however, more than do carbohydrates and fat. Any form of fat tends to suppress gastric secretion and motility. A volume of any food sufficient to exert pressure on the stomach wall stimulates gastric secretion.

3. *Fiber or residue.* The routine omission of any fiber in the diet also seems to have no basis in fact. Individual modes of eating, improper chewing, and rapid consumption of meals are more involved as sources of irritation. So-called coarse or rough foods, such as lettuce, raw fruits, celery, cabbage, and nuts, do not necessarily hurt a peptic ulcer when they are properly chewed and mixed with saliva. Grinding or straining of food is needed only when teeth are poor or absent.

4. *Gas formers.* Foods labeled "gas formers" also are questionable routine omissions for all persons with peptic ulcer. Tests have shown little consistency in the responses of hospitalized patients to a variety of foods such as onions, fried foods, cabbage, baked beans, orange juice, milk, nuts, and spiced foods. Because of the wide variance in symptoms and responses among patients tested, individual tolerances seem to be the basic factor. It is entirely a matter of individual response.

Basic principles of liberal dietary management. In the light of such findings and the cumulative experiences of many physicians and nutritionists in daily practice, what reasonable principles of diet therapy for peptic ulcers may be deduced? That sound dietary management does play an important part in total therapy is clear, but it seems equally clear that the individual must be the focus of treatment. It is not *an* ulcer; it is *his* ulcer. It is conditioned by his unique makeup and life situation, and the presence of the ulcer in turn affects the patient's life. Therefore two basic principles guide the more liberal approach:

1. *The individual must be treated as such.* A careful initial history will give information about daily living situations, attitudes, and food reactions and tolerances. On the basis of such a history a reasonable and adequate dietary program *that the patient can follow* may be worked out.

2. *The activity of the patient's ulcer will influence dietary management.* During acute

periods of active ulceration more vigorous treatment is necessary to control acidity and initiate healing. However, when pain disappears, feedings should be liberalized according to individual tolerance and desire using a *variety* of foods. Optimum nutrition and emotional outlook are essential for recovery. Both these are more likely to be supported by such a liberal program. During quiet periods and for long-term prophylaxis when the patient does not have symptoms, he fares better from judicious choice of a wide range of foods and regular, unhurried eating habits.

SUMMARY OF GENERAL DIET THERAPY. The following is a summary of the diet therapy principles for patients with peptic ulcer:

1. *Optimum total nutrition* based on individual needs and food tolerances is necessary to support recovery and maintenance of health.

2. *Protein* must be adequate for tissue healing needs and for buffering.

3. *Fat* should be used in moderate amounts for suppression of gastric secretion and motility. When cardiovascular disease is a concern, reduction of saturated fat may be desirable and substitution made of polyunsaturated fats (p. 250).

4. *Meal intervals and size* should be adequate to maintain individual control of gastric secretions. Frequent small feedings may be required during more active stress periods. Regular meals, moderate in size and sufficient in number for individual need, should be an established habit.

5. *Positive individual needs on a flexible program* rather than negative blanket restrictions on a rigid regimen should be the guide. In any event treatment based on the elimination of prejudiced ideas and the use of wise individual counseling instead forms the keystone of therapy.

General gastric disturbances in young infants

Infantile colic. Infantile colic is the name given to intermittent periods of loud, continuous crying. It is not uncommon in newborns and lasts no longer than the third month. It is usually seen only in firstborn infants and seldom in their subsequent brothers and sisters. Because it occurs rather routinely in the evening hours between 5 or 6 P.M. and midnight, medical, nursing, and nutritional care are usually better directed toward the ragged nerves of the new, inexperienced parents than to the infant himself. It is a self-limiting difficulty, ending spontaneously during the first 3 months. However, to young, tense parents this brief interval of time may seem an eternity.

Treatment usually involves careful history taking to discover attitudes and feeding practices. The child may be underfed and simply screaming because of hunger or he may be overfed by a zealous young mother and have abdominal discomforts. In other cases an experimenting mother may be rapidly changing his formula from day to day.

The common pacifier is much more in current vogue than formerly with the blessing of most pediatricians. At least the pacifier has the value of closing the opening from which the noise emanates. Mostly, however, treatment involves explanation and moral support to the parents with reassurance that their child is growing normally. They may take courage from the knowledge that such an active, energetic child with high neuromotor functions often develops faster than his more passive peers. He may hold up his head, walk, sit, and talk sooner. He has excellent energy potential for becoming a vigorous and vocal adult.

Simple functional vomiting. Regurgitation, or spitting up, is common in most young infants. Its cause is usually gastric distention from overfeeding or from swallowing air during feeding or crying. Other related factors may be ineffective burping or leaving the baby in a supine (on his back) position rather than a prone (on his stomach) position after feeding. Also overactivity and semiacrobatics at the hands of doting fathers and grandparents soon after he has been fed may stimulate regurgitation. Temperature of the feeding may be a factor, since feedings that are too hot may induce vomiting. Milk at room temperature is better tolerated. Even cold feedings have evoked no difficulty in a number of infants. Again simple attention to possible causative factors and reassurance to the young mother will provide adequate care.

INTESTINES
General functional disorders

Irritable colon. The term *irritable colon* is given to the condition of general discomfort in the lower abdomen because of excessive motility or hyperactivity of the colon or a decrease in muscle tone. It is manifested in general changes in bowel habits, either frequent stools of a soft, segmented nature or larger, hard stools, which are difficult to pass. It is best treated by attending to the underlying causes and giving symptomatic care. Adjunct therapy with diet will usually involve fluid intake, modification of fiber content, and adjustment of specific foods according to individual tolerances.

Constipation. Dietary manipulation for constipation is often not a fundamental cure, but simply a helpful adjunct. In children psychogenic constipation may occur during the ages of 1 to 2 years, while the child is being toilet trained. Sometimes a compulsive, anally fixated mother who believes in an arbitrary timetable of elimination ("a daily bowel movement is absolutely essential to health") imposes stringent toilet disciplines on the child and scolds him for failures or rewards him for perfect performance. The child soon learns that he can suppress the natural impulse to defecate, and he uses this power as a weapon in his conflict with his mother. In time the habit weakens normal peristalsis, and stools become dry and difficult to pass. Correction of the problem involves adjustment of the parent-child relationship and a resultant easing of the conflict and tensions. The mother needs to learn two simple physiologic facts: toxins are not absorbed from fecal material, and therefore a *daily* stool is not essential to the child's health.

Occasionally in children there occurs simple physiologic constipation, which is usually short in duration. It is aided by moderately reducing the milk intake, increasing the carbohydrate intake (for example, increasing the sugar somewhat in an infant formula), and increasing fruits, vegetables, and water intake. Similar diet adjustments are helpful to adults: increased water intake; increased fiber (bran), as in whole grains; more raw or lightly cooked fruits and vegetables; and more naturally laxative fruits such as dried prunes (or juice) and figs.

Diarrhea. Diarrhea in infants is a serious problem, especially if it is prolonged and associated with infection. Because of his relatively high water content and his large area of intestinal mucosa in proportion to body surface area, the infant's fluid and electrolyte reserves may be rapidly depleted. The sequence of steps leading to dehydration may be reviewed in the discussion of water balance (p. 80).

Common mild diarrhea usually responds to simple treatment. This consists of reducing the food intake, especially carbohydrate and fat in the formula, and increasing the water intake, sometimes including in it oral electrolyte replacements. More serious forms involving infection and producing marked dehydration and acidosis are medical emergencies calling for immediate intravenous fluid and electrolyte therapy. The loss of potassium can be dangerous, since lowered blood levels of potassium affect action of the heart muscle.

After initial essential replacement of fluid and electrolytes and when the infant is able to take oral feedings more readily, they are resumed. Water, glucose, and balanced salt solutions may be used. These are followed by milk mixtures, breast milk, or substitutes such as Probana (a high-protein formula with banana powder) or Nutramigen (a casein hydrolysate free of galactose) as the stool volume decreases. Calories are increased to normal requirements as soon as possible.

Such agents as pectin and kaolin may thicken the stools, but most authorities agree that they have little or no therapeutic usefulness in severe infant diarrhea. Although views differ, pediatricians generally discount the previous practice of starving patients with acute diarrhea. This was a practice based on the erroneous belief that avoidance of oral intake puts the bowels at rest. Also tea should not be given to the child. The xanthines in tea stimulate and excite children and in some cases cause excessive urination, which in turn only aggravates the fluid imbalance.

Organic diseases

Organic diseases of the intestine may be classified into three general groups: (1) those involving anatomic changes, as in diverticulosis; (2) those relating to malabsorption difficulties, as in sprue and celiac disease; and (3) inflammatory and infectious mucosal changes, as in ulcerative colitis.

Diverticulosis and diverticulitis. Diverticula are small protrusions from the intestinal lumen, usually the colon, and produce the condition *diverticulosis.* More often diverticulosis occurs in older people and develops at points of weakened musculature in the bowel wall. The condition is usually without symptoms unless the diverticula become inflamed, a state called *diverticulitis.* In such conditions, fecal residue may cause increased irritation. There are pain and tenderness, usually localized in the lower left side of the abdomen, nausea, vomiting, distention, intestinal spasms, and fever.

DIET THERAPY. During acute periods oral feedings may be limited to clear liquids with gradual progression to full liquids (p. 192). Follow-up diet therapy is based on texture modification—at first a residue-free diet if necessary and then maintenance according to individual need on a low-residue dietary program. An outline of such a low-residue diet plan is given on p. 208.

In contrast, more recently there are indications that a high-residue diet may be better therapy for diverticular disease. Patients tend to develop pockets of high pressure in the colon because of segmental contractions of the bowel. Some clinicians suggest that these segmental contractions may occur more commonly in patients on a low-residue diet because of the ability of the colon when empty to contract completely, thus producing pressure and pain. Therefore a high-residue diet is used to prevent such contractions of the bowel. Advocates of this therapy recommend including 2 to 3 tablespoons of bran with each meal, mixed with the various foods used.

Malabsorption syndrome (sprue and celiac disease). Adult nontropical sprue is similar in nature to childhood celiac disease. In fact, most adults with sprue give a history of having had episodes of celiac disease as children.

CLINICAL SYMPTOMS. The characteristic diarrhea in sprue consists of multiple foamy, malodorous, bulky, greasy stools. Poor absorption of fat is evident in the large amounts appearing in the stools as soaps (fatty acids saponified with calcium salts) and fatty acids. Poor absorption of iron produces anemia. In other persons a lack of folic acid will produce another specific type of anemia. Poor absorption of vitamin K may lead to hemorrhagic tendencies. Poor calcium absorption may produce the disturbed serum calcium:phosphorus ratio with resulting tetany (p. 67).

The condition varies widely among individuals, but four basic types of symptoms of intestinal malabsorption are general: (1) malnutrition, (2) multiple foul, bulky, foamy, greasy stools, (3) distended abdomen because of accumulation of improperly digested and absorbed material and gas accumulation, and (4) secondary vitamin and mineral deficiencies.

DIET THERAPY. Since the discovery that *gluten* is an important factor in the cause of nontropical sprue or celiac disease, the gluten-free or low-gluten diet has been widely used with great effect. Gluten is a protein found mainly in wheat, with additional amounts in rye, oats, and barley. Therefore these four grains (wheat, rye, oats, and barley) are eliminated from the diet. Corn and rice are the substitute grains used. The offending

Low-residue diet

	ALLOWED	NOT ALLOWED
Beverages	Only 2 glasses of milk, if allowed, boiled or evaporated; fruit juices, coffee, tea, carbonated beverages	Alcohol
Eggs	Prepared in any manner except fried	Fried eggs
Cheese	Cottage, cream, mild American, Tillamook (use in small amounts)	Highly flavored cheeses
Meat or poultry	Roasted, baked, or broiled tender beef, bacon, ham, lamb, liver, veal, fish, chicken, or turkey	Tough meats, pork; no meats fried or highly spiced
Soup	Bouillon, broth, strained cream soups from foods allowed	Any others
Fats	Butter, margarine, oils, 1 oz. cream daily	None
Vegetables	Canned or cooked, strained vegetable such as asparagus, beets, carrots, peas, pumpkin, squash, spinach, young string beans, tomato juice	Raw or whole cooked vegetables
Fruits	Strained fruit juice, cooked or canned apples, apricots, white cherries, peaches, pears, dried fruit puree; ripe bananas and avocados; all without skins or seeds	All other raw and cooked fruits
Breads and crackers	Refined bread, toast, rolls, crackers	Pancakes, waffles, whole grain bread or rolls
Cereals	Cooked cereal, such as Cream of Wheat, Malt-O-Meal, strained oatmeal, cornmeal; cornflakes, puffed rice, Rice Krispies, puffed wheat	Whole grain cereals; other prepared cereals
Potatoes and substitutes	Potatoes, white rice, macaroni, noodles, spaghetti	Fried potatos, potato chips, brown rice
Desserts	Gelatin, tapioca, angel food or sponge cake, plain custards, ices or ice cream without fruit or nuts, rennet or simple puddings	Rich pastries, pies, anything with nuts or dried fruits
Sweets	Sugar, jelly, honey, syrups, gumdrops, hard candy, plain creams, milk chocolate	Other candy; jam, marmalade
Miscellaneous	Cream sauce, plain gravy, salt	Nuts, olives, popcorn, rich gravies, pepper, spices, vinegar

grains are obvious in cereal form, but they are also used as ingredients such as thickeners or fillers in many commercial products. Therefore close attention should be given to label reading and food preparation. The gliadin fraction of the gluten proteins seems to be the offending agent in sensitive individuals. A gluten-free diet for nontropical sprue or celiac disease is given on p. 209. In addition, the basic principles of therapy for

patients with celiac disease, especially in the early stages, are as follows:

1. Calories—high, usually about 20% above normal requirement to compensate for fecal loss
2. Protein—high, usually 6 to 8 gm./kg. body weight
3. Fat—low, but not fat free because of impaired absorption
4. Carbohydrate—simple, easily digested

Gluten-free diet for nontropical sprue

CHARACTERISTICS

1. All forms of *wheat, rye, oat, buckwheat,* and *barley* are omitted except gluten-free wheat starch (Cellu Products Co.).
2. All other foods are permitted freely unless otherwise specified by the physician.
3. The diet should be high in protein, calories, vitamins, and minerals.

FOODS	ALLOWED	NOT ALLOWED
Milk (2 glasses or more)	As desired	
Cheese	Any as desired	
Eggs (1 or 2 daily)	As desired	
Meat, fish fowl (1 or 2 servings)	Any plain meat	Breaded, creamed, or with thickened gravey; no bread dressings
Soups	All clear and vegetable soups; cream soups thickened with cream, cornstarch, or potato flour only	No wheat flour–thickened soup; no canned soup except clear broth
Vegetables (2 servings of green or yellow daily at least)	As desired except creamed	No cream sauce or breading
Fruits (at least 2 or 3 daily, including 1 citrus)	As desired	
Bread	Only that made from rice, corn, or soybean flour or gluten-free wheat starch	All bread, rolls, crackers, cake, and cookies made from wheat and rye, Ry-Krisp, muffins, biscuits, waffles, pancake flour and other prepared mixes, rusks, zwieback, pretzels; any product containing oatmeal, barley, or buckwheat; no breaded food or bread crumbs
Cereals	Cornflakes, cornmeal, hominy, rice Rice Krispies, Puffed Rice, precooked rice cereals	No wheat or rye cereals, wheat germ, barley, buckwheat, kasha
Pastes		No macaroni, spaghetti, noodles, dumplings
Desserts	Jell-O, fruited Jell-O, ices or sherbets, homemade ice cream, custard, junket, rice pudding, cornstarch pudding (homemade)	Cakes, cookies, pastry; commercial ice cream and ice cream cones; prepared mixes, puddings; homemade puddings thickened with wheat flour
Beverages	Milk, fruit juices, ginger ale, cocoa (read label to see that no wheat flour has been added to cocoa or cocoa syrup); coffee (ground), tea, carbonated beverages	Postum, malted milk, Ovaltine (read labels on instant coffees to see that no wheat flour has been added)
Condiments and sweets	Salt; sugar, white or brown; molasses; jellies, jams; honey, corn syrup	Commercial candies containing cereal products (read labels)
Fats	Butter, margarine, oils	Commercial salad dressings except pure mayonnaise (read labels)

Caution: Read labels on all packaged and prepared foods.

sugars (fruits, vegetables) should provide about one half the calories
5. Feedings—small, frequent feedings during ill periods; afternoon snack for older children
6. Texture—smooth, soft, avoiding irritating roughage initially, using strained foods longer than usual for age, adding whole foods as tolerated and according to age of child
7. Vitamins—supplements of vitamins A and B in water-miscible forms, and vitamin C
8. Minerals—iron supplements if anemia present

Ulcerative colitis. The cause of ulcerative colitis is unknown, and no specific cure has been devised. However, treatment today is far more effective, based on new drug therapy with more potent antibiotics and endocrine agents. This treatment has improved the condition of many patients. Ulcerative colitis usually occurs in young adulthood. It sometimes occurs in patients having various degrees of anxiety and insecurity. However, this is by no means true in all cases.

CLINICAL SYMPTOMS. The common clinical symptom is a chronic bloody diarrhea, which occurs at night as well as during the day. Ulceration of the mucous membrane of the intestine leads to various associated nutritional problems, such as loss of appetite, nutritional edema, anemia, avitaminosis, protein losses, negative nitrogen balance, dehydration, and electrolyte disturbances. Weight loss, often general malnutrition, fever, skin lesions, and arthritic joint involvement occur.

PRINCIPLES OF TREATMENT. The management of patients with active but uncomplicated chronic ulcerative colitis involves the three important factors of rest, nutritional therapy, and sulfonamides. There must be physical gastrointestinal rest and emotional rest. Vigorous nutritional therapy must be instituted. Indeed, nutrition is the key to successful treatment.

DIET THERAPY. Nutritional therapy for ulcerative colitis is based on restoration of nutrient deficits and prevention of local trauma to the inflamed area.

High-protein diet. The raw surface of the inflamed colon may be regarded as equivalent to an extensive wound or burn of the skin. There are massive losses of protein from the colon tissue. There are losses associated with impaired intestinal absorption of protein. Only if adequate protein is provided for tissue synthesis can healing take place. The diet should supply from 120 to 150 gm. of protein per day. Protein supplements, such as between-meal feedings using nonfat dry milk, Sustagen, Gevral, Protenum, or Meritene, are helpful to achieve the necessary intake. Tasteful ways of including protein foods of high biologic value (egg, meat, and cheese) must be devised. Milk causes some difficulty with many patients, so it is usually omitted at first and then only gradually added in cooked form, such as in creamed soups or puddings.

High-calorie diet. At least 3,000 calories a day are needed to restore nutritional deficits from daily losses in the stool and consequent weight loss. Also only if sufficient nonprotein calories are present to support and protect the main function of protein—rebuilding of tissue—will healing take place and the negative nitrogen balance be overcome.

Increased minerals and vitamins. When anemia is present, iron supplements may be ordered. However, many patients do not tolerate such iron preparations, and blood transfusions may be used instead. Extra vitamins to aid in the healing process and the metabolism of the increased calories and protein are especially needed. These are vitamin C and B vitamins—thiamine, riboflavin, and niacin. Usually additional supplements of these vitamins are ordered. Potassium therapy may also be indicated because of losses of potassium from diarrhea and tissue destruction.

Low-residue diet. To avoid irritation to the colon the diet at first is fairly low in residue. In acute stages it may be almost residue free

Graduated low-residue diet for ulcerative colitis

GENERAL DIRECTIONS

1. Monotony in diet should be avoided by varying foods as much as diet prescription allows.
2. There is an individual variation in the tolerance to certain foods. If any of the foods in this diet disagrees with the patient, it may require some change in the diet schedule.

FOODS	ALLOWED	NOT ALLOWED
Beverages	Carbonated drinks (not iced) in small amounts; coffee or substitutes, tea, special mixtures as prescribed	Milk in any form; fruit juices
Bread	Enriched white or fine rye bread, plain or or toasted; plain or salted crackers, zwieback, melba toast, plain muffins	Whole wheat, dark rye, pumpernickel, or any hot breads
Cereal	Cooked, refined or strained—oatmeal, Cream of Wheat, Cream of Rice, farina, Wheatena; precooked cereals; Pablum, Pabena, Cerevim Dry cereals without bran or shredded wheat, noodles, spaghetti, macaroni, plain rice	Cereals containing bran or shredded wheat; unrefined rice, hominy
Meat	Ground or tender beef, lamb, pork, veal; sweetbreads, brains, liver; may be baked, boiled, broiled or roasted; crisp bacon	Fried, smoked, pickled, or cured meats, meat with long fibers, gristle, skin, delicatessen rare meats
Fish	Fresh fish, boiled, broiled, or baked; canned, scalded tuna or salmon; crab meat, oysters	Fried fish, lobster, other canned, smoked, pickled, preserved, or gefilte fish
Fowl	Any boiled, broiled, baked, or roasted	Gristle, skin, or fat; fried fowl
Egg	Soft or hard, boiled, poached, coddled, plain omelet, scrambled, creamed	Fried
Cheese	Cream, cottage, mild cheddar, or American	All other cheeses
Milk	None	
Fat	Butter or margarine in limited amounts, cream for beverage or cereal; crisp bacon; plain gravies in small amounts	Any other
Soup	Bouillon, broth, meat, or poultry; may add strained vegetable juices	Cream soup, vegetable soup
Vegetables	Potatoes without skins	All others
Fruit	None	All
Dessert	Plain angel food, butter, sponge, or pound cakes, plain cookies, plain sherbet or ices, plain ice cream, plain smooth puddings (rice, tapioca, bread, starch, custard), plain Jell-O in small quantities; gelatin flavored with coffee, strained fruit juices	Nuts, coconut, raisins

Continued.

Graduated low-residue diet for ulcerative colitis—cont'd

FOODS	ALLOWED	NOT ALLOWED
Sweets	Plain jelly, sugar, honey, syrup, plain hard candies, in *limited* amounts	Large amounts of any sweets, jam or marmalade, candy with nuts or fruit, concentrated sweets, rich pastry, or candy
Miscellaneous	Spices and seasonings in moderation	Nuts, olives, pickles, popcorn, horseradish, relishes

Additions:

The following foods may be added in order only when prescribed. Add each food in small amounts at first until tolerance is assured.

1. Banana, ripe
2. Orange juice—strained and diluted at first—beginning with ¼ glass at end of a main meal and gradually increasing to full glass
3. Vegetable juice, including tomato—canned, or vegetable juices prepared in a blender and strained
4. Other fruit juices—as with orange juice
5. Vegetables—cooked and strained or prepared strained baby vegetables
6. Fruits—cooked or stewed and strained or prepared strained baby fruits; canned pears; strained applesauce; baked apple without skin or seeds; no dates, figs, or other raw fruits
7. Milk—boiled for 3 minutes; served hot or cold; ½ glass once daily at first; used in creamed soups, cream sauce, milk toast, or plain pancakes; increasing slowly to ½ glass three times daily and finally to one glass at a time as prescribed; used possibly with flavoring nutrient powders or cream
8. Vegetables—tender, whole cooked or canned, not strained; gradually introducing asparagus tips, carrots, beets, spinach, squash, string beans, peas, and pumpkin; avoiding skin and seeds; no cabbage, cauliflower, onions, radishes, or turnips
9. Crisp raw lettuce (finely shredded); raw tomato; no other raw vegetables
10. Unboiled milk

(based mainly on lean meat, rice, white bread, Italian pasta, strained cereal, cooked eggs, sugar, butter, and cream). The graduated low-residue diet may be used initially with additional protein, calories, vitamins, and minerals in interval feedings.

As the patient improves, however, a full diet with high-protein feedings should be used. Only heavy roughage needs to be avoided, since the primary concern is to supply necessary nutrition in as appetizing a manner as possible.

Perhaps no other condition better illustrates the need for a close working relationship among all members of the health team and the patient than does chronic ulcerative colitis. The appetite is poor, but the nutritional intake is *imperative.* In many individually creative ways the fundamental therapeutic needs *must* be met through attractive, nourishing food given with supportive warmth and encouragement.

FOOD INTOLERANCES AND ALLERGIES

A number of conditions may cause certain food intolerances or allergies. These conditions may be of specific genetic origin or due to a less well-defined sensitivity. The resulting difficulty in handling certain foods may lie at the digestion point in the intestine or at the metabolic level in the cell.

GENETIC DISEASE
Phenylketonuria (PKU)

Metabolic defect. Phenylketonuria results from a missing enzyme, which oxidizes *phenylalanine,* an essential amino acid, to tyrosine, another amino acid. Phenylalanine therefore accumulates in the blood, and its alternate metabolites, the phenyl acids, are excreted in the urine.

Clinical symptoms. The most profound effect that may occur in untreated phenylketonuria is mental retardation. The IQ is usually below 50 and most frequently under 20. The damage to the central nervous system probably occurs within the first 2 years. The patient may learn to walk, but few learn to talk. There is increased motor irritability, hyperactivity, convulsive seizures, and bizarre behavior.

Dietary management. Treatment of phenylketonuria is totally dietary. A low-phenylalanine diet is used to reduce the serum phenylalanine levels that cause the clinical symptoms, especially the central nervous system damage.* Since phenylalanine is an essential amino acid necessary for growth, it cannot be totally removed from the diet. Thus a small amount is allowed in the formula with blood levels being constantly monitored to control this amount.

MILK SUBSTITUTE FORMULA. Milk has a relatively high phenylalanine content, so the first need for the infant is a milk substitute. The formula is usually made from Lofenalac, a special casein product balanced with fats, carbohydrates, vitamins, and minerals. It is usually well accepted by the infant.

LOW-PHENYLALANINE DIET. As the child grows, solid foods are added to the diet according to their phenylalanine content. In the diet listings foods are grouped according to their content of phenylalanine. The diet is prescribed by the physician according to the child's blood phenylalanine test and then calculated by the nutritionist in terms of numbers of food choices allowed daily from each of the food groups. Then a meal pattern of feedings is made out for the mother to follow in feeding the child.

Family counseling. The parents charged

---

*The detailed dietary management of PKU may be found in Williams, S. R.: Nutrition and diet therapy, ed. 2, St. Louis, 1973, The C. V. Mosby Co., pp. 419-425.

with the care of a phenylketonuric child face physical, emotional, and financial tensions. They must understand and accept the absolute necessity of following the diet carefully; so patient and understanding teaching must be done. Frequent home visits by the public health nurse or nutritionist and their assistants may be a source of guidance and support as the child grows older. Other family members and any subsequent brothers or sisters should be tested for phenylketonuria also. With careful control the phenylketonuric child will grow and develop normally. Such a child diagnosed at birth by widespread screening programs in many states, may expect a healthy and happy adulthood, instead of the profound disease consequences that he would probably have experienced so few years ago. Screening tests of newborn for phenylketonuria are mandatory now in most of the states.

Galactosemia

Metabolic defect. Galactosemia is also a genetic disease caused by a missing enzyme, which controls a step in the conversion of galactose to glucose. Milk, the infant's first food, contains a large amount of the disaccharide lactose (milk sugar), which is acted on by the intestinal digestive enzyme lactase to produce the monosaccharides glucose and galactose (p. 90). When the subsequent conversion of galactose to glucose cannot be made because of the absence of the specific cell enzyme necessary for this conversion, galactose rapidly accumulates in the blood and in various body tissues.

Clinical symptoms. The rapid accumulation of galactose in tissues causes damage to the untreated infant. The child fails to thrive, and clinical evidences are apparent soon after birth. Liver damage brings jaundice, cirrhosis, enlargement of the spleen, and ascites —accumulation of fluid in the abdominal cavity. Death usually results from liver failure. If the infant survives, the continuing tissue damage in the optic lens and the brain cause cataracts and mental retardation.

Foods that may be included or should be excluded in a galactose-free diet*

FOOD CATEGORIES	FOODS INCLUDED	FOODS EXCLUDED†
Milks and milk products	None; Nutramigen and soybean milks used as milk substitutes	All milk of any species and all products containing milk, as skim, dried, evaporated, condensed, yogurt, cheese, ice cream, sherbet, malted milk
Legumes	All may be included if facilities are available for monitoring erythrocyte galactose-1-phosphate	
Meat, fish, and fowl	Plain beef, chicken, fish, turkey, lamb, veal, pork, and ham	Creamed or breaded meat, fish, or fowl; sausage products, such as wieners, liver sausage, cold cuts containing milk, organ meat, such as liver, pancreas, and brain
Eggs	All	None
Vegetables	Artichokes, asparagus, beets, broccoli, cabbage, carrots, cauliflower, celery, chard, corn, cucumbers, eggplant, green beans, kale, lettuce, mustard, okra, onions, parsley, parsnips, pumpkin, rutabaga, spinach, squash, tomatoes	Sugar beets, peas, lima beans; creamed, breaded or buttered vegetables; canned or frozen vegetables; corn curls (if lactose is added during processing)
Potatoes and substitutes	White and sweet potatoes, yams, macaroni, noodles, spaghetti, rice	Any creamed, breaded, or buttered; French fried or instant potatoes if lactose is added during processing
Breads and cereals	Any that do not contain milk or milk products‡	Prepared mixes, such as muffins, biscuits, waffles, pancakes; some dry cereals; Instant Cream of Wheat (*Read labels carefully*)
Fats	Margarines and dressings that do not contain milk or milk products; oils, shortenings; bacon	Margarines and dressings containing milk or milk products; butter; cream; cream cheese
Soups	Clear soups; vegetable soups that do not contain peas or lima beans; consommés	Cream soups, chowders, commercially prepared soups containing lactose
Desserts	Water and fruit ices; gelatin; angel food cake; homemade cakes, pies, cookies made from acceptable ingredients	Commercial cakes and cookies and mixes; custard, puddings, ice cream made with milk; any containing chocolate
Fruits	All fresh; canned or frozen that are not processed with lactose	Any canned or frozen processed with lactose
Miscellaneous	Nuts and nut butters, unsalted popcorn, olives, pure sugar candy, jelly or marmalade, sugar, corn syrup	Gravy, white sauce; chocolate, cocoa, toffee, peppermints, butterscotch, caramels, molasses; instant coffee, powdered soft drinks, monosodium glutamate, some spice blends, chewing gum

*From Koch, R., Acosta, P., Ragsdale, N., and Donnell, G. N.: Nutrition in the treatment of galactosemia, J. Am. Diet. Assoc. **43:**216, 1963.
†In all instances labels should be read carefully, and any product that contains milk, lactose, casein, whey, dry milk solids, or curds should be omitted.
‡In each area bakeries should be contacted and a list of acceptable products made available.

Table 16-2. Typical uses of lactose*

Ascorbic and citric acid mixtures	Party dips
Buttermilk	Penicillin and other antibiotics
Cakes and sweet rolls	Pharmaceutical bulking agents,
Canned and frozen fruits and vegetables	fillers, and excipients
Caramels, fudge, and tableted candies	Pie crusts and fillings
Cheese foods and spreads	Powdered coffee cream
Cookies and sandwich cookie fillings	Powdered soft drinks
Cordials and liqueurs	Puddings
Cottage cheese and cottage cheese dressings	Salad dressings
Dietetic preparations	Sherbets, frozen desserts, and ices
Dried soups	Simulated mother's milk; infant
Easter egg dyes and dye carrier	food formulas
Fireworks, flares, and pyrotechnics	Sour cream
French fries and corn curls	Spice blends
Frozen cultures	Starter cultures
Health and geriatric foods	Sweetened, condensed milk
High-solids ice cream	Sweetness reducers in icings, candies,
Instant coffee	preserves, and fruit pie fillings
Instant potatoes	Tablets (food and pharmaceutical)
Meat products	Tinctures
Modified skimmed milk	Vitamin and mineral mixtures
Monosodium glutamate extender	

*From Koch, R., Acosta, R., Ragsdale, N., and Donnell, G. N.: Nutrition in the treatment of galactosemia, J. Am. Diet. Assoc. 43:216, 1963.

Dietary management. The main indirect source of dietary galactose is milk. Therefore *all* forms of milk and lactose must be removed from the diet. A galactose-free diet is used, such as that given on p. 214. The milk substitute usually used for infant feeding is Nutramigen, a complete protein compound that is free of galactose. Careful attention must be given to avoid lactose from other food sources as solid foods are added to the infant's diet. Parents must be carefully instructed to check labels on all commercial products. Table 16-2 gives products that normally contain lactose. Even drugs contain lactose occasionally as an ingredient.

Lactose intolerance

A deficiency of any of the enzymes that act on the disaccharides in the intestine—lactase, sucrase, maltase, or isomaltase—may produce a wide range of gastrointestinal problems and abdominal pain. The missing enzyme results in the inability to digest the specific sugar involved. Of these clinical problems, lactose intolerance is perhaps the most common. It is often seen in adults of certain racial backgrounds and may also occur in childhood. A diet similar to that used for galactosemia is required. Milk and all products containing lactose are carefully avoided. For children a milk substitute is used—Nutramigen, soy milk, or a meat-based formula.

The characteristic symptoms of lactose intolerance include a severe watery diarrhea after drinking milk, which results in an excessive loss of fluid from the intestine. If not treated, dehydration and serious illness may result.

In the United States population roughly 100% of Orientals past the teens, 60% to 80% of American blacks, about 100% of American Indians have lactose intolerance. Northern European Caucasians and their descendents, who comprise a large majority of the American population, maintain lactase enzyme activity until late in life. Many persons with lactose intolerance can still drink some milk. They may get intestinal gas and softening of the stools with a large intake but can usually handle from ½ to 1 cup of milk at a time, or they can tolerate cooked products containing milk.

The second most common disaccharide intolerance is that of sucrose. This condition should show up the first time that a young child is given any fruit containing sucrose— canned fruits and puddings, for example. Most mothers do not sweeten cereals. However, if sugar is used, such as in an evaporated milk formula, it is likely to show up at the time that the formula is first used. This is not too common a disorder. A good history could pinpoint exactly what food causes the symptoms, and then it can be verified with dietary measures. Most persons can tolerate a small amount of the sugars to which they are intolerant—about 5 or 6 gm. of the sugar at a time. These small amounts will not precipitate an acute case of diarrhea. There may be minor softening of stools or a slightly bulkier stool, but the gastrointestinal result will not be sufficient to eliminate a great number of nutrients with the stools.

FOOD ALLERGIES

The care of the allergic child is often frustrating. A wide variety of environmental, emotional, and physical factors influence the child's reaction, and a suitable diet is sometimes difficult to find. Since sensitivity to protein substances is a common basis of the allergies, the early foods of infants and children are frequent offenders. Children tend to become less allergic to food sources as they grow older, however. The allergies manifested mainly in gastrointestinal problems tend to occur in younger children. The allergies manifested more in respiratory problems such as asthma tend to occur more often in older children.

Milk allergy

Cow's milk has long been and continues to be the most common cause of allergic reactions in young infants. The allergy to milk usually causes gastrointestinal difficulties, such as vomiting, diarrhea, and colic. The problem is generally identified by the clinical symptoms, family history, and a trial on a milk-free diet, using a substitute formula such as a soybean preparation (Sobee or Mull-Soy) or a meat formula.

Egg, wheat, and other foods

The albumin in egg white is a potential allergen and hence is usually added to the infant's diet after earlier use of egg yolk. Wheat is also a fairly common food allergen among allergic children. The specific biochemical sensitivity to gluten, a protein found in wheat, in the child with gluten-induced celiac disease (p. 207) is an example of such an allergy.

Dietary management

In an allergic child's diet, foods are usually added slowly, common offenders being excluded in early feedings. In some cases a series of diagnostic diets, such as the Rowe elimination diets, may be used to identify the offending food. These four diets may be compared on p. 217.

Each of the four basic diets is used for a trial period. If no change occurs in the allergic condition, the patient is given the next diet. If the patient's symptoms improve on a given diet, it is assumed that the offending food is not in that diet list. Then foods are added one at a time to test the patient's response. If a given food causes return of the allergy, the food can then be identified as an offending allergen and eliminated from use. Guidance in the substitution of special food products and in the use of special recipes should be provided for the mother in feeding the child.

Food additives

As food processing expands and the use of a wide variety of food additives increases, a greater number of allergic reactions to these chemicals are being encountered. The full scope of the problem for the allergist is indeed great. The Food Protection Committee of the National Research Council lists thirteen

Rowe elimination diets (rules enclose foods in the cereal-free elimination diets 1 and 2 and 3, a commonly used combination)*

DIET 1	DIET 2	DIET 3	DIET 4
Rice	Corn	Tapioca	Milk †
Tapioca	Rye	White potatoes	Tapioca
Rice biscuit	Corn pone	Breads made of any	Cane sugar
Rice bread	Corn-rye muffin	combination of soy,	
	Rye bread	lima, potato, and	
	Ry-Krisp	tapioca flours	
Lettuce	Beets	Tomatoes	
Chard	Squash	Carrots	
Spinach	Artichokes	Lima beans	
Carrots	Asparagus	String beans	
Sweet potatoes or yams			
		Peas	
Lamb	Chicken (no hens)	Beef	
	Bacon	Bacon	
Lemons	Pineapple	Lemons	
Grapefruit	Peaches	Grapefruit	
Pears	Apricots	Peaches	
	Prunes	Apricots	
Cane sugar	Cane or beet sugar	Cane sugar	
Sesame oil	Mazola oil	Sesame oil	
Olive oil ‡	Sesame oil	Soybean oil	
Salt	Salt	Salt	
Gelatin, plain or flavored with lime or lemon	Gelatin, plain or flavored with pineapple	Gelatin, plain or flavored with lime or lemon	
Maple syrup or syrup made with cane sugar flavored with maple	Karo corn syrup White vinegar	Maple syrup or syrup made with cane sugar flavored with maple	
Royal baking powder	Royal baking powder	Royal baking powder	
Baking soda	Baking soda	Baking soda	
Cream of tartar	Cream of tartar	Cream of tartar	
Vanilla extract	Vanilla extract	Vanilla extract	
Lemon extract		Lemon extract	

*From Rowe, A. H.: Elimination diets and the patient's allergies, ed. 2, Philadelphia, 1944, Lea & Febiger.
† Milk should be taken up to 2 or 3 quarts a day. Plain cottage cheese and cream may be used. Tapioca cooked with milk and milk sugar may be taken.
‡ Allergy to it may occur with or without allergy to olive pollen. Mazola oil may be used if corn allergy is not present.

classes of additives, which include over 2,700 individual items. Particular offenders among the food additives include food-coloring agents, sweeteners, and flavorings.

ACCESSORY ORGANS

Three major accessory organs lie adjacent to the gastrointestinal tract and produce important digestive agents that enter the intestine and aid in the handling of food substances. Specific enzymes are produced for each of the major nutrients, and bile is added to assist in the digestion of fats. These three organs are the liver, gallbladder, and pancreas. Diseases in each of these organs, therefore, can easily affect gastrointestinal function and cause problems of interference with the normal handling of specific types of food.

Diseases of the liver

Hepatitis. The exact organism responsible for hepatitis is not clearly defined. It is probably one of a group of related viruses. In infectious hepatitis the viral agent is transmitted by the oral-fecal route, a common one in many epidemic diseases. Thus the usual entry is through contaminated food or water. In serum hepatitis the organism is usually transmitted in infected blood by transfusions or by contaminated instruments such as syringes and needles.

CLINICAL SYMPTOMS. The viral agents of hepatitis produce diffuse injury to liver cells. In milder cases the tissue injury is largely reversible, but with increasing severity more extensive damage occurs. Massive damage in some cases may lead to liver failure and death. Thus varying clinical symptoms appear, depending on the degree of liver injury. *Jaundice* is a common symptom and the most obvious one. Other symptoms include general malaise, loss of appetite, diarrhea, headache, fever, enlarged and tender liver, and enlarged spleen.

TREATMENT. The importance of bed *rest* in the treatment of acute hepatitis has been clearly demonstrated. Physical exercise increases both severity and duration of the disease. A daily intake of 3,000 to 3,500 ml. of *fluids* guards against dehydration and gives a general sense of well-being and improved appetite. *Optimum nutrition* provides the foundation for recovery of the injured liver cells and overall return of strength. It is the major therapy. The principles of diet therapy relate to the liver's function in the matabolism of each of the major nutrients.

PRINCIPLES OF DIET THERAPY

High protein. Protein is essential for liver cell regeneration. It also provides lipotropic agents (p. 21) for the conversion of fats to lipoproteins and their removal from the liver, thus preventing fatty infiltration. The diet should supply from 75 to 100 gm. of protein daily.

High carbohydrate. Sufficient available glucose must be provided to restore protective glycogen reserves in the liver and meet the energy demands resulting from the disease process. Also an adequate amount of glucose ensures the use of protein for vital tissue building. This is an application of the protein-sparing action of carbohydrate (p. 31). The diet should supply from 300 to 400 gm. of carbohydrate daily.

Moderate fat. An adequate amount of fat in the diet makes the food more palatable, and hence the patient with poor appetite will be encouraged to eat. Former liver disease diets limited the fat on the rationale of preventing fat accumulations in the diseased liver. However, values of better overall nutrition for improved food intake outweigh these concerns, and a moderate amount of easily utilized fat, such as that in whole milk, cream, butter, margarine, and vegetable oil, is beneficial. The diet should incorporate from 100 to 150 gm. of such fat daily.

High calorie. From 2,500 to 3,000 calories are needed daily to fulfill energy demands of the tissue-building process, to compensate for losses because of fever and general debilitation, and to renew strength and recuperative powers.

Meals and interval feedings. The problem of supplying a diet adequate to meet the increasing nutritive demands of a patient whose illness makes food seem almost repellant to him is a delicate one. It calls for creative ideas and supportive encouragement. The food may have to be in liquid form at first, using concentrated formulas such as the one in Table 16-1 (p. 199) for frequent feedings. As the patient can better tolerate solid food, every effort should be made to prepare and serve it in an appetizing and attractive manner. Nutritional therapy is the key to recovery. Therefore a major responsibility is the devising of ways to encourage optimal food intake. The diet should include approximately the amounts given on p. 219.

High-protein, moderate-fat, high-carbohydrate diet

DAILY FOOD PLAN
  1 quart milk
  1 or 2 eggs
  8 oz. lean meat, fish, poultry
  4 servings vegetables:
    2 servings potato or substitute
    1 serving green leafy or yellow vegetable
    1 to 2 servings of other vegetables, including 1 raw
  3 to 4 servings fruit (include juices often)
    1 or 2 citrus fruits (or other good source of ascorbic acid)
    2 servings other fruit
  6 to 8 servings bread and cereal (whole grain or enriched)
    1 serving cereal
    5 to 6 slices bread, crackers
  2 to 4 tbsp. butter or fortified margarine
  Additional jam, jelly, honey, and other carbohydrate foods as patient desires and is able to
    eat them. Sweetened fruit juices increase both carbohydrate and fluid.

Cirrhosis. Liver disease may advance to the chronic state of cirrhosis. The French physician Laennec first named the disease from the Greek work *kirrhos*, meaning orange, because the cirrhotic liver was a firm, fibrous mass with orange-colored nodules projecting from its surface. Another name given to such a cirrhotic liver is a "hobnail" liver, referring to its rough, nodular surface, similar to that of the bottom of a boot. The nutritional or alcoholic form of cirrhosis bears his name, Laennec's cirrhosis.

The most common problem is fatty cirrhosis associated with malnutrition. The associated malnutrition may develop from other causes, but it usually is the result of a long history of alcoholism. The fatty liver and early cirrhosis may appear within 5 years of the onset of the alcoholism, but more often 10 to 15 years is required. Increasingly poor food intake as the excessive drinking continues leads to multiple nutritional deficiencies. Damage to the liver cells occurs as fatty infiltration, causing cell destruction and fibrotic tissue changes.

CLINICAL SYMPTOMS. Early signs include gastrointestinal disturbances such as nausea, vomiting, loss of appetite, distention, and epigastric pain. In time jaundice may appear.

There is increasing weakness, edema, ascites, and anemia from gastrointestinal bleeding, iron deficiency, or hemorrhage. A specific anemia from folic acid deficiency is also frequently observed.

Essentially the major symtoms are due to a basic protein deficiency and its multiple metabolic problems. As the disease progresses, fibrous scar tissue increasingly impairs blood circulation through the liver, and portal hypertension develops. Contributing further to the problem is *ascites,* an accumulation of fluid within the peritoneal cavity. The impaired portal circulation with increasing venous pressure may lead to *esophageal varices,* with the danger of rupture and fatal massive hemorrhage.

TREATMENT. Treatment is difficult when alcoholism is the underlying problem. Each patient requires individual supportive care and approach. Usually therapy is aimed at correction of fluid and electrolyte problems and nutritional support to encourage healing of the liver tissue as soon and insofar as possible.

PRINCIPLES OF DIET THERAPY

Protein according to tolerance. In the absence of impending hepatic coma the daily protein intake should be 80 to 100 gm. to correct the severe malnutrition, to regenerate functional liver tissue, and to replenish plasma proteins. However, if signs of hepatic coma appear, the protein is adjusted to individual tolerance.

Low sodium. Sodium is usually restricted to 500 to 1,000 mg. daily to reduce fluid retention. Low-sodium diet plans are given in Chapter 19.

Texture. If esophageal varices develop, it may be necessary to give soft foods that are smooth in texture to prevent the danger of rupture of these blood vessels.

Optimum general nutrition. The remaining overall diet principles outlined for hepatitis are continued for cirrhosis for the same reason. Calories, carbohydrates, and vitamins are supplied according to individual need and deficiency. Moderate fat is used. Alcohol is strictly forbidden.

Hepatic coma. As cirrhotic changes continue in the liver and portal blood circulation diminishes, collateral circulation develops bypassing the liver. The normal liver has a major function of removing ammonia from the blood by converting it to urea for excretion. In the diseased liver these normal reactions cannot take place. Therefore ammonia-laden blood, carrying the products of protein metabolism, approaches the liver but cannot follow the usual portal pathways. Therefore it is detoured around the liver through the collateral circulation. Then it reenters the systemic blood flow and produces ammonia intoxication and coma. This ammonia is formed mainly in the gastrointestinal tract as a result of protein digestion. Gastrointestinal bleeding, as well as intestinal bacteria production, may add still another source of ammonia.

CLINICAL SYMPTOMS. Typical responses of the patient involve disorders of consciousness and alterations in motor function. There are apathy, mild confusion, inappropriate behavior, and drowsiness progressing to coma. The facial expression is described as an absent stare. Speech may be slurred and monotonous. A typical motor system change is the coarse flapping tremor observed in the outstretched hands. The breath may also have a characteristic fecal odor.

TREATMENT. The fundamental principle of therapy is the removal of the sources of excess ammonia. Diet adjustments will focus on reduced intake of protein and control of fluid and electrolytes.

PRINCIPLES OF DIET THERAPY

Low protein. Protein intake is reduced as individually necessary to restrict the dietary sources of nitrogen in amino acids. The amount of restriction will vary with the circumstances. The unconscious patient will receive no protein, but the usual amounts given range from 15 to 50 gm. depending on whether symptoms are severe or mild. A simple dietary method for controlling the protein intake is given on p. 221. A basic meal pattern containing approximately 15 gm. of protein is used, adding small items of protein foods according to the level of protein desired.

Calories and vitamins. The amounts of calories and vitamins are ordered according to need. About 1,500 to 2,000 calories are sufficient to prevent tissue breakdown, which would be a source of more amino acids and available nitrogen. Carbohydrates and fat sufficient for energy needs are essential. Vitamin K is usually given by intravenous feeding, along with other vitamins that may be deficient.

Fluid intake. Fluid intake is carefully controlled in relation to output.

Diseases of the gallbladder

The main function of the gallbladder is to concentrate and store bile. Its powers of such concentration are great. The liver produces daily about 600 to 800 ml. of bile, which the gallbladder normally concentrates fivefold to tenfold, and stores in its small 40 to 70 ml. capacity. Through the cholecystokinin mechanism (p. 91), the presence of fat in the duodenum stimulates contraction of the gallbladder with the release of bile into the common duct and then into the small intestine.

Low-protein diets—15, 30, 40, and 50 gm. protein

GENERAL DESCRIPTION

1. The following diets are used when dietary protein is to be restricted.
2. The patterns limit foods containing a large percent of protein, such as milk, eggs, cheese, meat, fish, fowl, and legumes.
3. Avoid meat extractives, soups, broth, bouillon, gravies, and gelatin desserts

BASIC MEAL PATTERNS (CONTAINING APPROXIMATELY 15 GM. PROTEIN)

BREAKFAST	LUNCHEON	DINNER
½ cup fruit or fruit juice	1 small potato	1 small potato
½ cup cereal	½ cup vegetable	½ cup vegetable
1 slice toast	Salad (vegetable or fruit)	Salad (vegetable or fruit)
Butter	1 slice bread	1 slice bread
Jelly	Butter	Butter
Sugar	1 serving fruit	1 serving fruit
2 tbsp. cream	Sugar	Sugar
Coffee	Coffee or tea	Coffee or tea

FOR 30 GM. PROTEIN

Add: ½ pint milk
    1 ounce meat, 1 egg,
      or equivalent

EXAMPLES OF MEAT PORTIONS

1 oz. meat = 1 thin slice roast—2 in. × 1½ in.
           1 rounded tbsp. cottage
            cheese
           1 slice American cheese

FOR 40 GM. PROTEIN

Add: ½ pint milk
    2½ oz. meat or 1 egg and
      1½ oz. meat

2½ oz. meat = Ground beef patty (5
            from 1 lb.)
           1 slice roast

FOR 50 GM. PROTEIN

Add: ½ pint milk
    4 oz. meat or 2 eggs and
      2 oz. meat

4 oz. meat = ¼ lb. meat
           2 lamb chops
           1 average steak

Cholecystitis and cholelithiasis. *Cholecystitis* is an inflammation of the gallbladder, usually resulting from a low-grade chronic infection. Normally cholesterol in bile, which is insoluble in water, is kept in solution by the other bile ingredients. However, when the absorbing mucosal tissue of the gallbladder is inflamed or infected, changes occur in the tissue; the absorptive powers of the gallbladder may be altered, affecting the solubility of the bile ingredients. Excess water may be absorbed, or excess bile acids may be absorbed. Under these abnormal absorptive conditions, cholesterol may precipitate, causing gallstones composed of almost pure cholesterol to form. This condition is called *cholelithiasis.* Also a high dietary fat intake over a long period of time predisposes to gallstone formation because of the constant stimulus to produce more cholesterol as a necessary bile ingredient to metabolize the fat.

CLINICAL SYMPTOMS. When inflammation, stones, or both are present in the gallbladder, contraction from the cholecystokinin mechanism causes pain. Sometimes the pain is severe. There are fullness and distention after eating and difficulty particularly with fatty foods.

TREATMENT. Surgical removal of the gallbladder is usually indicated. This surgery is called a *cholecystectomy.* However, the surgeon may wish to postpone surgery until the inflammation has subsided. If the patient is obese, as many persons with gallbladder disease are, some weight loss before surgery is advisable. Thus the supportive therapy is largely dietary.

PRINCIPLES OF DIET THERAPY

Fat. Because fat is the principal cause of contraction of the diseased organ and subsequent pain, it should be greatly reduced.

Calories should come principally from carbohydrate foods, especially during acute phases. A diet plan for a low-fat regimen is given below.

Calories. If weight loss is indicated, the calories will be reduced according to need. Principles of weight-reduction diets are given in Chapter 17.

Low-fat and fat-free diets

GENERAL DESCRIPTION

1. This diet contains foods that are low in fat.
2. Foods are prepared without the addition of fat.
3. Fatty meats, gravies, oils, cream, lard, and desserts containing eggs, butter, cream, nuts, and avocados are avoided.
4. Foods should be used in amounts specified and only as tolerated.
5. The same pattern contains approximately 85 gm. protein, 50 gm. fat, 220 gm. carbohydrate, and 1,670 calories.

	ALLOWED	NOT ALLOWED
Beverages	Skimmed milk, coffee, tea, carbonated beverages, fruit juices	Whole milk, cream, evaporated and condensed milk
Bread and cereal	All kinds	Rich rolls, breads, waffles, pancakes
Desserts	Jell-O, sherbet, ices, fruit whips made without cream, angel food cake, rice and tapioca puddings made with skimmed milk	Pastries, pies, rich cakes and cookies, ice cream
Fruits	All fruits as tolerated	Avocado
Eggs	3 per week allowed, cooked any way except fried	Fried eggs
Fats	3 tsp. butter or margarine daily	Salad and cooking oils, mayonnaise
Meats	Lean meat, such as beef, veal, lamb, liver, lean fish, and fowl, baked, broiled, or roasted without added fat	Fried meats, bacon, ham, pork, goose, duck, fatty fish, fish canned in oil, cold cuts
Cheese	Dry or fat-free cottage cheese	All other cheese
Potato or substitute	Potatoes, rice, macaroni, noodles, spaghetti, all prepared without added fat	Fried potatoes, potato chips
Soups	Bouillon or broth, without fat; soups made with skimmed milk	Cream soups
Sweets	Jam, jelly, sugar, sugar candies without nuts or chocolate	Chocolate, nuts, peanut butter
Vegetables	All kinds as tolerated	The following should be omitted if they cause distress: broccoli, cauliflower, corn, cucumbers, green pepper, radishes, turnips, onions, dried peas, and beans
Miscellaneous	Salt in moderation	Pepper, spices, highly spiced food, olives, pickles, cream sauces, gravies

---

Low-fat and fat-free diets—cont'd

SUGGESTED MENU PATTERN

BREAKFAST	LUNCH AND DINNER
Fruit	Meat, broiled or baked
Cereal	Potato
Toast, jelly	Vegetable
1 tsp. butter or margarine	Salad with fat-free dressing
Egg, 3 times per week	Bread, jelly
Skimmed milk, 1 cup	1 teaspoon butter or margarine
Coffee, sugar	Fruit or dessert, as allowed
	Skimmed milk, 1 cup
	Coffee, sugar

Fat-free diet

GENERAL DESCRIPTION

The following additional restrictions are made to the low-fat diet to make it relatively fat free:

1. Meat, eggs, and butter or margarine are omitted.
2. Three oz. fat-free cottage cheese are substituted for meat at the noon and evening meals.

Cholesterol and gas formers. Two additional modifications sometimes found in traditional low-fat diets for gallbladder disease concern restriction of foods containing cholesterol and foods labeled *gas formers.* Neither modification has a valid basis. The body synthesizes daily several times more cholesterol than is present in an average diet. Thus restriction of cholesterol in food has no appreciable effect in reducing gallstone formation. Total dietary fat reduction is more to the point. Also blanket restriction on so-called gas formers seems unwarranted. Food tolerances are highly individual. Surveys of hospitalized patients fail to show any differences in food tolerances attributable to the presence of gastrointestinal disorders. Patients with gallbladder disease had no more incidence of specific food intolerances than patients without gastrointestinal disease.

Diseases of the pancreas

Pancreatitis. Acute *pancreatitis* is inflammation of the pancreas. This is caused by the digestion of the organ by the very enzymes it produces, principally trypsin. Normally enzymes remain in an inactive form until the pancreatic juice reaches the lumen of the duodenum (p. 90). However, gallbladder disease may cause a gallstone to enter the common bile duct and obstruct the flow of pancreatic juice or cause a reflux or backing up of bile from the common duct into the pancreatic duct. This mixing of digestive materials activates the powerful pancreatic enzymes within the gland. In such activated form they begin their damaging effects on the pancreatic tissue itself, causing acute pain. Sometimes infectious pancreatitis may occur as a complication of mumps or a bacterial disease. Also the excessive use of alcohol appears to be another factor in the disease. Mild or moderate pancreatitis may subside completely, but it has a tendency to recur.

TREATMENT. Care consists of measures recommended for acute disease involving shock. These measures include intravenous feeding at first, replacement therapy of fluid and electrolytes, blood transfusions, antibiotics and drugs for the relief of pain, and gastric suction.

DIET THERAPY. In initial stages oral feedings are withheld because entry of food into the intestines stimulates pancreatic secretions. As

Table 16-3. Principles of dietary management for patients with cystic fibrosis

PRINCIPLE	REASON
High calorie	Energy demands of growth and compensation for fecal losses—large appetite usually ensures acceptance of increased amounts of food
High protein	Usually tolerated in large amounts—excess above normal growth needs require to compensate for losses
Moderate carbohydrate	Starch less well tolerated; simple sugars easily assimilated
Low to moderate fat, as tolerated	Fat poorly absorbed, but tolerance varies widely
Generous salt	Food generously salted to replace seat losses; salt supplements in hot weather
Vitamins	Double doses of multivitamins in water-soluble form (vitamin E supplements sometimes used, since low blood levels of the vitamin have been observed); vitamin K supplements with prolonged antibiotic therapy.
Pancreatic enzymes	Large amounts given by mouth with each meal (may be mixed with cereal or applesauce for infants) to compensate for pancreatic deficiency—powdered pancreas containing steapsin, trypsin, and amylapsin (pancreatin or other pancreatic extracts, such as Cotazym or Viokase).

healing progresses and oral feedings are resumed, a light diet is used to avoid excessive stimulation of pancreatic secretions. Alcohol and excess use of coffee should also be avoided to decrease pancreatic stimulation.

Cystic fibrosis of the pancreas. Cystic fibrosis is a generalized hereditary disease of children that involves the exocrine glands, particularly the pancreas, and thus affects many tissues and organs. In past years its prognosis was poor. Few children with an early onset survived past 10 years of age. However, with better knowledge of the disease, improved diagnostic tests, clinical treatment, and antibiotic therapy, prognosis has improved.

CLINICAL SYMPTOMS. Cystic fibrosis usually produces characteristic clinical symptoms:

1. Pancreatic deficiency with greatly diminished digestion of food caused by the absence of pancreatic enzymes
2. Malfunction of mucus-producing glands with accumulation of thick viscid secretions and subsequent respiratory difficulties and chronic pulmonary disease
3. Abnormal secretions of the sweat glands containing high electrolyte levels
4. Possible cirrhosis of the liver arising

from biliary obstruction and increased by malnutrition or infection

TREATMENT. As a result, treatment is based on three factors: (1) control of respiratory tract infections, (2) relief from the effects of an extremely viscid bronchial secretion, and (3) the maintenance of sound nutrition. The digestive deficiency and malabsorptive character of cystic fibrosis is evident in the nature of the child's stools. They are similar to those in celiac disease (typically bulky, mushy, greasy, foul, and foamy), but they also contain more undigested food. Only about half—50% to 60%—of the child's food is absorbed. Thus the child with cystic fibrosis has a much more voracious appetite.

DIET THERAPY. The basic objective of nutritional therapy is to compensate for the large loss of nutrient material resulting from the insufficiency of pancreatic enzymes. Apparently protein hydrolysates, split fats (emulsified simple fats), and simple sugars are used more easily. There is a wide variation, however, in tolerance for fat, and the amount of fat intake is usually prescribed according to the character of the stools. Large increases of protein seem to be well tolerated and are needed for the replacement of losses and for growth. Diet guides for cystic fibrosis are similar to those outlined for celiac disease. The food used varies in form according to the age of the child. The important principles of dietary management for patients with cystic fibrosis are summarized in Table 16-3.

17 THE PROBLEM OF OBESITY AND WEIGHT CONTROL

THE PROBLEM OF OBESITY

Obesity is a problem of societies wealthy enough to afford it. It results from excess intake of food as compared with energy demands on the body for its use. Abundant statistical evidence indicts obesity as a health hazard. It increases the risk of a number of diseases, such as coronary artherosclerosis and hypertension. It complicates other diseases, such as respiratory difficulties in emphysema, chronic bronchitis, and asthma. It increases surgical risk. It disturbs growing adolescents. It reduces life expectancy.

Although rare forms of obesity caused by endocrine disorders exist, it is the so-called simple obesity seen in everyday clinical practice that concerns both patient and health worker. In the face of overwhelming and obvious evidence of its effect on health, the obesity problem continues to plague victims and health workers alike, and efforts to combat it are largely frustrating to both. It soon becomes evident, therefore, that so-called simple obesity is not so simple after all.

Reports indicate that approximately 10% of children in the United States are obese. Similar figures are given for adults. The difficulty of the problem of controlling weight stems generally from two factors—its unsure definition and its many causes.

Definitions

Ideal weight. The term *obesity* is used to indicate the presence of excess body weight of 15% or more above the ideal. The problem, however, lies in defining the word "ideal." It is generally defined in reference to average weight according to height and frame. However, persons vary widely in these health values. For example, body composition plays a part in defining obesity, since a large person may not necessarily be obese because a large percent of the body mass is muscle instead of fat. This would be true of a professional football player.

Associated definitions. Also different words associated with obesity and weight control require definition. In view of the controversy and divergent opinions concerning exact terminology, the Committee on Nutrition of the American Academy of Pediatrics recently gave these definitions for common terms used:

1. *Hunger*—a biologic phenomenon predominately unlearned and unconditioned, a basic physiologic drive
2. *Appetite*—a learned response, usually in intimate association with past food experiences
3. *Anorexia*—the absence of desire for food in circumstances in which one might ordinarily anticipate such a desire

4. *Satiety*—the lack of desire to eat that ensues after eating, predominately determined by postingestion factors
5. *Palatability*—related to preingestion factors, such as taste, aroma, texture, appearance, color, temperature, and association with past experiences

Types of obesity

Recognition of different types of obesity adds to the problem of definition. It is not merely a matter of total weight. The ratio of lean body mass or muscle to body fat is involved. The two basic types of obesity, which differ in ratio of muscle, or lean tissue, to fat tissue are developmental and reactive.

Developmental obesity. This type of obesity begins early in life and steadily continues into adult years. Studies indicate that, at birth, fat accounts for about 12% of the infant's body weight. The middle of the first year there is usually more fat in boys than in girls. By the time that the infant is 1 year old, fat accounts for about 24% of the body weight. As the child continues to grow throughout the childhood years, the percent of fat normally remains essentially constant relative to the desired weight for height and age. The peak for onset of juvenile obesity occurs during the first 4 years of the child's life, and it is established by the time that the child is 11 years old. About the twelfth year the percent of body fat increases in girls, and the development of lean body mass begins to rise sharply in boys.

Thus the developmental form of obesity begins early in life. The cells become supersaturated with fat, and additional cells are recruited from connective tissue for fat deposit. With the increasing weight, additional bone and muscle cells must also increase to help carry the load. As a result these children are usually taller, have an advanced bone age, and have been consistently obese since infancy. Their percent of lean body mass is high, and so also is the fat deposit. This type of obesity thus produces a higher ratio of lean body mass, along with the fat.

Reactive obesity. The reactive type of obesity usually results from intense and oft repeated episodes of emotional stress. As a result of the stress period the child overeats, and his weight often assumes an up-and-down type of weight pattern. His body composition is high in fat but not in the lean body mass observed in the developmental type of obesity. Thus in the reactive type of obesity associated with emotional stress of the growth years, an excess ratio of fat is produced.

CAUSES OF OBESITY

The complexity of "simple" obesity is further increased by its many causes.

Physical factors

The basic physical laws of energy exchange as described in Chapter 4 account for obesity. This means that an intake of more energy potential (calories) in food than output of energy (calories) in total energy metabolism, including basal needs and physical activity, produces obesity. Table 4-2 lists a general criteria for measuring basal energy needs, the energy required for the work of the body at rest, and additions for physical activities.

The maintenance levels of calories required by various individuals varies widely. It is also influenced by activity level. Obese persons generally consume fewer calories than nonobese ones, but their activity level is usually lower also. Obese, sedentary persons therefore simply cannot afford to eat as much as their leaner counterparts.

Physiologic factors

The normal physiology of the growth years contributes to the deposition of fat tissue. Numerous studies indicate that there are critical periods for the development of obesity. Several implications appear reasonable in considering food and feeding habits of the early growth years.

Fat content and quantity feeding of infant formulas. With the knowledge regarding the rapid growth of the first year and the normal laying down of fat during that period, questions can be raised concerning the fat content of infant diets and formulas. The attitude of mothers who insist on the infant's finishing the bottle with every feeding of formula, whether or not desired, can also be questioned.

Sex differences in early years. If the sex differences in calorie expenditure at the early age of 2 or 3 years are considered, it should be realized that all toddlers are not going to eat the same amount of food. The basic metabolic rate is higher in the boy than in the girl during the second and third years of life. Therefore parents should be prepared for early differences between young boys and girls. Food should not be pushed at children during the latent period of growth, when the normal rate of growth is slowed and the child's need is less.

Overfeeding in preschool years. Overfeeding during the years of slow growth can make a large contribution to the development of continuing obesity. The peak onset of developmental types of obesity is during these early years. Mothers of young children would be well advised to offer them the enjoyment of a wide variety of food in realistic smaller portions.

Decreased activity of elementary school years. Prior to the beginning of the school years the child engages in much strenuous physical play, testing his developing strength and motor capacity. Usually this is independent, spontaneous activity, and there is not yet a set schedule for the day. With the continuing experiences of school, however, the child becomes more sedentary in his recreational pattern, as well as his school activities. This great change in energy expenditure between the ages of 7 to 11 years calls for guidance from parents concerning habits of food intake.

Adolescent sex differences in body composition. The increasing tendency for fat deposit in the teen-age girl in comparison to the greater increase in lean body mass in the boy of the same age makes weight control a greater problem for the girl. Guidance from parents in a supportive, accepting manner, especially for young girls, is needed.

Adult adjustment problems. Other critical periods for beginning of the obesity problem occur in the adult years. For example, the woman encounters a critical period after the age of 21 because of being less active without adjusting her caloric intake accordingly. Other times are during the first pregnancy and after menopause because of the hormonal factors that are operating. For the man a critical period is between the ages of 25 and 40, generally caused by decreasing activity with no consequent change in the habit formed during adolescence of eating large amounts of food. Both men and women tend to gain weight after the age of 50 because of the lowered basal metabolic requirement and decreased activity with failure to lower caloric intake also.

Hereditary factors

There is apparently no basic genetic factor in obesity. It is true that obese children are more likely than nonobese ones to have obese parents. Surveys indicate that when one parent is obese, approximately 40% of the offspring are obese. When both parents are obese, 80% of the offspring are obese. These results are probably due to the family influence, however. It is a situational problem caused by the molding of food habits. Excessive food preparation and consumption is a family habit pattern. It tends to be perpetuated in adulthood and then passed on to successive generations.

Social and cultural factors

The class values placed on the obese state by different social groups will also influence the incidence of obesity. Generally a greater number of obese persons are found in the lower socioeconomic status groups than in the higher ones. Increasing upward mobility usually causes a decline in obesity, since a greater value is placed on weight control in upper economic groups. In the lower socioeconomic groups obesity is more common and therefore considered normal.

Many cultural factors also condition food habits. Much seasonal emphasis is placed on feasting such as at Christmas and Thanksgiving. Also meal patterns differ in different cultures. The three-meals-a-day pattern is a cultural one, not a biologic necessity. Some indication exists that less food taken more often may be a better pattern to control weight than larger meals taken less frequently. Also some consideration has to be given to the type and frequency of snacks. Too often among growing children these foods tend to be rich in carbohydrates and relatively low in the content of other nutrients and serve only to provide excess calories.

Psychologic factors

The relation of emotional factors to obesity is well established. The obese state may well be the individual's protective resolution of deeper emotional problems. In such cases, to remove it without providing an alternative and satisfying resolution may create further problems. Overeating may often result from boredom, loneliness, or a sense of being socially rejected by one's peer group.

DIET THERAPY FOR WEIGHT CONTROL
Principles and rationale

In common practice the general approach to the control of simple obesity is based on the underlying physical energy exchange cause and the patient's situational needs. In other words, the amount of energy taken in as food must be reduced below the amount of energy demanded by the patient's basal and total energy requirements. It must also be based on individual patient needs. Such a program has three main principles: (1) individual decision and support, (2) individual diet with calorie and situational adaptations, and (3) a planned follow-up program.

Motivation and support. The degree of patient motivation is a prime factor. There must be a point of decision on the part of the indi-

vidual and a determination to follow through. Initial interviews seek to determine individual needs, attitudes toward food, and the meaning of food for the patient. Recognition is given to the emotional factors involved in a reduction program, and support is provided by the health team to meet the patient's particular needs. Shame or scare tactics have no place in such a program.

Diet control. Wise and effective diet control is based on the patient's situational needs, a personal diet plan, and some type of definite follow-up program.

INITIAL INTERVIEW. On the basis of careful interviewing, the patient's food habits and situational factors can be determined. Using a guideline such as that given in Chapter 11, the health worker can gather this important background information. Then a balanced diet can be made out for the individual patient based on his normal nutritional needs. The calorie level of the the weight reduction diet is adjusted to meet his individual weight reduction requirement. One thousand fewer calories daily is the necessary adjustment to lose about 2 pounds a week; 500 fewer calories, to lose 1 pound a week. The basis of this calculation is given in Table 17-1. Usually the energy value of the adjusted diet will range between 800 and 1,500 calories.

INDIVIDUAL DIET PLAN USING EXCHANGE SYSTEM. A simple system for establishing weight control plans is the basic exchange system of dietary control. In this system foods are grouped according to approximate food value, so that choices may be made on the basis of a meal plan outlined for the individual patient. A description of this exchange system of dietary control is given on p. 230. A listing of food exchange groups is given on pp. 231 and 232.

Using the various weight-reduction diet levels from 800 to 1,500 calories given in Table 17-2, the health worker may make out a pattern for the patient according to his required adjustment in calories. Then a variety of sample menus can be developed from the food pattern, so that the patient may have

Table 17-1. Calorie adjustment required for weight loss

To lose 1 pound a week—500 fewer calories daily
Basis of estimation:

1 lb. body fat	=	454 gm.
1 gm. pure fat	=	9 calories
1 gm. body fat	=	7.7 calories (some water in fat cells)
454 gm. × 9 cal./gm.	=	4,086 calories per lb. pure fat
454 gm. × 7.7 cal./gm.	=	3,496 (or 3,500) calories per lb. body fat
500 cal. × 7 days	=	3,500 calories = 1 lb. body fat

The exchange system of dietary control

The exchange system set up by professional organizations including the American Dietetic Association is based on a simple grouping of common foods according to generally equivalent nutritional values. The system may be used for any situation requiring calorie and food value control.

The foods are divided into six basic groups called the exchange groups (pp. 231 and 232). Each food within a group contains approximately the same food value as any other food item in that same group, allowing for free exchange *within any given group*. Hence the term *food exchange* is used throughout. The total number of exchanges per day depends on individual nutritional needs, based always on normal nutritional recommendations of the Food and Nutrition Board, National Research Council.

Although some variation occurs in the composition of foods within the exchange groups, for simplicity the following values for carbohydrate, protein, and fat are used:

FOOD	APPROXIMATE MEASURE	CARBO-HYDRATE (GM.)	PROTEIN (GM.)	FAT (GM.)	CALORIES
Fruit exchange	Varies	10	—	—	40
Bread exchange	1 slice	15	2	—	70
Meat exchange	1 oz.	—	7	5	75
Vegetable (B) exchange	½ cup	7	2	—	40
Milk exchange	1 cup	12	8	10	170 (skimmed = 80)
Fat exchange	1 tsp.	—	—	5	45

much flexibility in food choice and still maintain a sufficient reduction in calories as indicated. When the meal pattern is made out with the patient, his individual living situation, desires, and cultural patterns are taken into consideration.

FOLLOW-UP PROGRAM. A follow-up schedule of appointments is then outlined with the patient, and its values are discussed with him. On subsequent clinical visits, progress records are kept. Problems are discussed and solutions to them mutually decided. Continuing support and positive reinforcement for progress achieved are given. A number of practical suggestions to dieters have evolved from much experience. These are given on p. 233. Such suggestions as these may help the patient to anticipate needs, avoid pitfalls, and sustain motivation.

Essential characteristics of a sound diet for weight control

Much experience has shown that there are no real shortcuts in weight control. In the face of many periods of discouragement the patient may be harried, vexed,

Food exchange groups

LIST 1. MILK EXCHANGES

Whole	1 cup	(Cream portion of whole milk equals
Skimmed	1 cup	two fat exchanges. One cup
Buttermilk	1 cup	whole milk equals 1 cup skimmed
Evaporated	½ cup	milk plus two fat exchanges.)
Nonfat dry	¼ cup	
Yogurt, plain	1 cup	

LIST 2. VEGETABLE EXCHANGES (AS SERVED PLAIN, WITHOUT FAT SEASONING OR DRESSING; ANY FAT USED IS TAKEN FROM FAT EXCHANGE ALLOWANCE)

Group A. (Use as desired: negligible carbohydrate, protein, and fat in amounts commonly eaten)

Asparagus	Greens	Mushrooms
Bak choi, gai choi	Beet greens	Okra
Bamboo shoots	Chard	Peppers (bell, chili, etc.)
Broccoli	Collards	Radishes
Brussels sprouts	Kale	Sauerkraut
Cabbage	Mustard	String beans
Cauliflower	Spinach	Squash, summer
Celery	Turnip greens	Tomatoes
Chicory		Watercress
Chinese cabbage	Salad greens	Parsley
Cucumbers	Lettuce	Pimientos
Escarole, endive		
Eggplant		

Group B. (½ cup equals one-serving)

Artichoke (1 medium)	Peas, green	Squash, winter
Beets	Pumpkin	Turnips
Carrots	Rutabaga	
Onions		

LIST 3. FRUIT EXCHANGES (UNSWEETENED—FRESH, FROZEN, CANNED, COOKED; ONE EXCHANGE IS PORTION INDICATED BY EACH FRUIT)

Berries		Dried fruits		Others	
Blackberries	1 cup	Apricots	4 halves	Apple	1 small
Blueberries	⅔ cup	Dates	2	Apple juice	⅓ cup
Raspberries	¾ cup	Figs	1 small	Applesauce	½ cup
Strawberries	1 cup	Prunes	2 medium	Apricots (fresh)	2 med.
		Raisins	2 tbsp.	Banana	½ small
Citrus fruits				Cherries	10 large
Grapefruit	½ small			Fig (fresh)	1
Grapefruit				Grapes	12 med.
juice	½ cup			Grape juice	¼ cup
Orange	1 small			Peach	1 med.
Orange				Pear	1 small
juice	½ cup			Pineapple	½ cup, 1 slice
Tangerine	1 large			Pineapple	
				juice	⅓ cup
Melons				Plums	2 med.
Cantaloupe	¼ med.			Prunes (fresh)	2
Honeydew	⅛ med.			Prune juice	¼ cup
Watermelon	½ 1 in. center slice				

Continued.

Food exchange groups—cont'd

LIST 4. BREAD EXCHANGES (EQUIVALENT PORTIONS INDICATED BY EACH ITEM)

Bread

Bagel	½
Biscuit, roll (2 in. diam.)	1
Bread (white or dark)	1 slice
Cornbread (1½ in. cube)	1
Frankfurter roll	1 small
Hamburger roll	½ large
Tortilla	1 med.

Crackers

Animal	8
Graham (2½ in. square)	2
Oyster	½ cup
Round, thin (½ in. diam.)	6 to 8
Saltines (2 in. square)	5
Soda (2½ in. square)	3
Matzos (6 in. diam.)	1 piece
Muffin (2 in. diam.)	1
Melba thins	4
Pretzels (22 per lb.)	1 med.
Pretzel sticks (av. thin)	14

Cereals

Cooked	½ cup
Dry (flakes, puffed)	¾ cup
Flour	2½ tbsp.
Rice, grits (cooked)	½ cup
Corn	⅓ cup
Spaghetti, macaroni, noodles (cooked)	½ cup

Vegetables, and other

Baked beans, no pork	¼ cup
Beans, peas (dried, cooked)	½ cup
Corn on the cob	½ large ear
	1 small ear
Popcorn (popped)	1 cup
Parsnips	⅔ cup
Potatoes, white	1 small
Potatoes, mashed white	½ cup
Potatoes, sweet, or yams	¼ cup
Sponge cake, plain (1½ in. cube)	1
Ice cream, vanilla (omit 2 fat exch.)	½ cup
Ice milk, vanila	½ cup

LIST 5. MEAT EXCHANGES (ALL ITEMS REFER TO COOKED WEIGHT)

Lean meat, poultry	1 oz.
Cold cuts (4½ × ⅛ in.)	1 slice
Frankfurter (8 to 9/lb.)	1
Egg	1
Cheese, cheddar type	1 ounce
Cheese, cottage	¼ cup
Sausage (3 × ½ in.)	2

Fish

Cod, halibut	1 oz.
Salmon, tuna, crab, lobster	¼ cup
Shrimp, clams, oysters, etc.	5 small
Sardines	3 med.
Scallops (12/lb.)	1 large
Peanut butter (limit 1 exch. per day)	2 tbsp.

LIST 6. FAT EXCHANGES

Avocado (4 in. diam.)	⅛
Bacon, crisp	1 slice
Butter or margarine	1 tsp.
Cream, light (20%)	2 tbsp.
Cream, heavy (40%)	1 tbsp.
Cream cheese	1 tbsp.
Cheese spreads	1 tbsp.

French dressing	1 tbsp.
Half-and-half (10% cream and milk)	4 tbsp.
Mayonnaise	1 teaspoon
Nuts	6 small
Oil or cooking fat	1 tsp.
Olives	5 small
Sour cream	2 tbsp.

MISCELLANEOUS FOODS ALLOWED AS DESIRED (NEGLIGIBLE CARBOHYDRATE, PROTEIN, FAT)

Artificial sweeteners	Gelatin, plain	Rennet tablets, plain
Bouillon, fat-free	Lemon	Rhubarb
Broth, clear	Mustard	Spices
Coffee	Pepper	Tea
Cranberries, unsweetened	Pickles, dill and sour	Vinegar
Catsup		

Table 17-2. Weight reduction diets, using the exchange system of dietary control

FOOD EXCHANGE GROUP*	APPROXIMATE MEASURE	800 CALORIES	1,000 CALORIES	1,200 CALORIES	1,500 CALORIES
		TOTAL NUMBER OF EXCHANGES PER DAY			
Milk (nonfat)	1 cup	2	2	2	2
Vegetable (A)	As desired	Free	Free	Free	Free
Vegetable (B)	½ cup	1	1	1	1
Fruit	Varies	3	3	3	4
Bread	1 slice	1	3	4	4
Meat	1 oz.	6	6	7	9
Fat	1 tsp.	1	1	2	4
		DISTRIBUTION OF FOOD EXCHANGES			
Breakfast					
Fruit		1	1	1	1
Meat		1	1	1	1
Bread		1	1	1	1
Fat		1	1	1	1
Lunch and dinner					
Meat		2 to 3	2 to 3	3	4
Vegetable (A)		Any	Any	Any	Any
Vegetable (A) (either meal)		1	1	1	1
Bread		0	1	1 to 2	1 to 2
Fat		0	0	0 to 1	1 to 2
Fruit		1	1	1	1 to 2
Milk		1	1	1	1

*See food exchange groups, pp. 231 and 232.

Practical suggestions to dieters

GOALS	Be realistic. Don't set your goals too high. Adjust your rate of loss to one to two pounds per week. If visible tools are helpful motivation techniques, use them.
CALORIES	Don't be an obsessive calorie counter. Simply become familiar with the food exchanges in your diet list, and learn the general calorie values of some of your favorite home dishes so that you may occasionally make substitutions.
PLATEAUS	Anticipate plateaus. They happen to everyone. They are related to water accumulation as fat is lost. During these periods increase your exercise to help you get started again.
BINGES	Don't be discouraged when you break over and have a dietary binge. This happens to most other people, too. Simply keep them infrequent, and, when possible, plan ahead for special occasions. Adjust the following day's diet or the remaining part of the day accordingly.
SPECIAL DIET FOODS	There is no need to purchase special low-calorie foods. Learn to read labels carefully. Most special diet foods are expensive, and many are not much lower in calories than regular foods.
HOME MEALS	Try to avoid a separate menu for yourself. Adapt your needs to the family meal, adjusting the seasoning or method of preparing family dishes to lower caloric values of added fats and starches.

Continued.

Practical suggestions to dieters—cont'd	
EATING AWAY FROM HOME	Watch portions. When a guest, limit extras such as sauces and dressings, and trim meat well. In restaurants select singly prepared items rather than combination dishes. Avoid items with heavy sauces or fat seasonings. Select fruit or sherbet as desserts rather than pastries.
APPETITE CONTROL	Avoid dependence on appetite-depressant medications. Usually they are only crutches. Beginning efforts to control the appetite may be aided by nibbling on food from the free list or by saving over meal items such as fruit for use between meals.
MEAL PATTERN	Eat three or more meals a day. If you are used to three meals, leave it at that. If you are helped by snacks between meals, then plan part of your day's allowance to account for them. The main point to remember is not to take all your calories at one sitting. Avoid the all-too-common pattern of no breakfast, little or no lunch, and a huge dinner!

and tempted to grab for pills, formulas, or fads. However, a sound dietary approach to weight control that holds hope of achieving a degree of lasting success must be based on five characterictics: realistic goals, calories lowered according to need, nutritional adequacy, cultural adaptation, and calorie readjustment to maintain weight.

Realistic goals. Goals must be realistic in terms of overall loss and rate of loss.

Calories lowered according to need. The diet must be low enough in calories in relation to individual levels of energy expenditure to effect a gradual weight loss. Usually a rate of 1 to 2 pounds a week is recommended.

Nutritional adequacy. The diet must be nutritionally adequate. Lower calorie levels may need supplementation. The nutrient ratio should supply no less than 12% to 15% of the calories as protein; no more than 35% of the calories as fat, with reduced intake of saturated fats; and the remainder of the calories as carbohydrates, using little or no sucrose and including a variety of food sources.

Cultural adaptation. The food plan must be enough like the eating pattern of the individual to form the basis for *permanent* reeducation of his eating habits. In other words, he must be able to live with it. Personal adaptation is mandatory.

Calorie readjustment to maintain weight. When the desired weight level is reached, the calories are adjusted accordingly, but the reeducation achieved in basic habits is the continuing means for weight control.

BEST APPROACH TO WEIGHT CONTROL

In the last analysis, in the approach to the problem of obesity and its control the best goal seems to be *prevention*. In the face of knowledge about the hazards of obesity, the causes of it in early developmental years and in subsequent adult life situations, and the difficulties and frustrations involved in attempting to control it in the adult years, indications are that early nutrition education and support to young parents and children before obesity occurs would be the most successful approach.

CHAPTER 18 DIABETES MELLITUS

Diabetes is an ancient disease. As far back as 1500 B.C. its symptoms were written down on an Egyptian papyrus. Later, in the first century the Greek physician Aretaeus described a malady in which the body "ate its own flesh" and gave off large quantities of urine. He named the disease *diabetes* from the Greek word meaning siphon or to pass through. Much later, in the seventeenth century, the word "mellitus" was added to distinguish it from a similar disease, *diabetes insipidus*, in which large amounts of urine were passed. The word "mellitus" comes from the Latin word for honey and indicates the sweet nature of the urine. Diabetes insipidus, on the other hand, although manifested by similar symptoms of excess urine, does not produce a sugary urine and is caused by a different disorder located in the pituitary gland. Also it is much more rare. So in common usage the single term *diabetes* usually refers to diabetes mellitus.

Many years passed, during which scientists and physicians continued to puzzle over the mystery of diabetes mellitus, but the cause remained unknown. For physicians and their patients these years could easily be called the *Diabetic Dark Ages*. Patients had short lives and were maintained on a variety of semistarvation diets. Finally in the early 1900s a beginning clue pointing to the involvement of the pancreas in the disease was discovered by a young German medical student, Paul Langerhans. He found special clusters of cells scattered about the pancreas that were different from the rest of the tissue. He called these *islands* or *islets*. Although their function was then still unknown, these cells were named for their young discoverer— the islets of Langerhans. Soon afterward in 1922, working on this lead provided by Langerhans, the two Canadian scientists F. G. Banting and his assistant C. H. Best isolated and identified the special substance produced by these islet cells in the pancreas. This substance proved to be a hormone that regulates the oxidation of blood sugar and helps convert it to heat and energy. Banting and Best called the new hormone *insulin* from the Latin word *insula*, meaning island. For his leadership in the discovery Banting received the Nobel prize and was knighted by his government.

Insulin now continues to be a main tool for the control of diabetes. The underlying metabolic problem even yet is unsolved. Recent insulin assay tests developed to measure the level of insulin activity in the blood (ILA) have found insulin-like activity in early diabetes to be two or three times the normal insulin levels. Investigators are working on the theory that the insulin is present, but bound with a protein, hence making it unavailable. Diabetes therefore results from the lack of insulin. This lack may be in the production by the pancreatic islet cells or at the level of availability in the blood.

THE NATURE OF THE DISEASE
Predisposing factors

Family history. At least one third of all diabetic patients reported the occurrence of diabetes among some of their relatives. Diabetes appears to be a hereditary disease transmitted as a recessive Mendelian trait. Inherited traits, such as sex, physical appearance, eye color, and disease probabilities, are transmitted through the chromosomes in the cell nucleus. The chromosome is a rod-shaped body in the cell nucleus that carries the genes inherited from each parent. When conception occurs, the father contributes twenty-three chromosomes in his sperm cell, and the mother contributes twenty-three in her ovum. These combine on fertilization to form forty-six chromosomes, which then align themselves in twenty-three specific pairs in the fertilized ovum. Thereafter with each successive cell division by which growth occurs in the new life, these same pairs of chromosomes are duplicated in each nucleus and govern the transmission of inherited traits. The genes on the respective pairs of chromosomes are almost identical with each other, so that they too form pairs, or so-called

links, of genes. A gene trait is *recessive* (does not manifest itself) if it does not match its partner. The recessive gene must be carried by both parents to cause a defect. A person is called a *carrier* of a trait if he carries the recessive gene but does not manifest its symptoms. Transmission of recessive traits to successive generations follows the pattern established by Mendel, as illustrated in Fig. 18-1. If two carriers marry, the risk for each birth is 25% for manifesting the trait and 50% for carrying it, with a 25% chance of neither carrying nor manifesting. If both parents of an individual are diabetic, that is, manifesting the trait of the disease, then the probability for the child developing the disease increases to 100%. Therefore blood relatives of known diabetics should maintain testing periodically to determine whether the disease is present.

Obesity. Weight is also a predisposing factor in diabetes, especially in adults. Obese persons are especially susceptible to developing the disease. Many (85%) of the adults

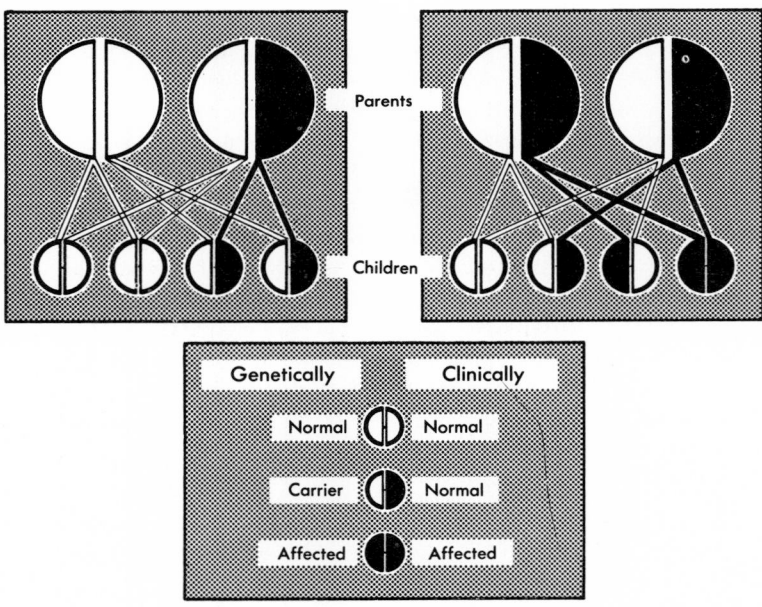

Fig. 18-1. Pattern of genetic disease. Transmission of recessive traits follows Mendel's law. If two carriers marry, one child will be normal, one child will manifest the trait, and two children will be carriers.

with diabetic onset at maturity are over-weight or have been overweight prior to the occurrence of the disease. Persons over 45 years of age appear to be more vulnerable. Diabetes may also be latent and should be watched for in mothers who have delivered large babies. All these high-risk persons should be examined regularly for evidences of diabetes.

Clinical symptoms

The symptoms of diabetes are progressive in nature. They develop from simple initial complaints to more serious complications in time if the condition continues to be un-treated and uncontrolled. These symptoms progress in the following manner:

I. Initial complaints
  A. Increased thirst (polydipsia)
  B. Increased urination (polyuria)
  C. Increased hunger (polyphagia)
  D. Weight loss (in adult maturity-onset form of diabetes the opposite is frequently true—the patient may be obese and usually is)
II. Clinical laboratory test data
  A. Sugar in the urine (glycosuria)
  B. Elevated blood sugar level (hyperglycemia)
  C. Abnormal glucose tolerance test (with a glucose load the blood sugar rises to a higher level than normal and takes a longer period to return)
III. Other possible symptoms
  A. Blurred vision
  B. Skin irritation or infections (skin irritation is particularly noticeable in the woman around the vulva because of the heavy glucose load in the urine)
IV. Results of uncontrolled diabetes
  A. Fluid and electrolyte imbalance (dehydration)
  B. Acidosis (ketosis)
  C. Loss of strength (weakness, lack of energy)
  D. Coma

Because of the symptoms of sugar in the urine and elevated blood sugar, both related to excess glucose, diabetes has been called a disease of carbohydrate metabolism. However, as more has been learned about the close relationships of carbohydrate metabolism with fat and protein metabolism, it has become evident that diabetes is a general metabolic disorder resulting from an insulin lack (absolute, partial, or caused by unavailability), which affects more or less each of the basic nutrients. The two most closely affected nutrients, however, are carbohydrate and fat because they are the main energy sources and as such are metabolized in close balance with each other (p. 21).

Types of diabetes

Juvenile-onset form. In its juvenile form diabetes develops fairly rapidly and is usually more severe and unstable. The child is usually overweight, and the family history is strongly positive for the disease. Acidosis is fairly common, and insulin therapy is required.

Maturity-onset form. In its maturity-onset form diabetes develops much more slowly. It is usually milder and more stable, and the patient is often overweight. Acidosis is infrequent. The majority of these patients are maintained on diet therapy either alone or with the aid of oral hypoglycemic drugs.

BLOOD SUGAR CONTROLS
Sources of blood glucose

Review carefully the metabolism of carbohydrate and fat in Chapters 2 and 3. A clear understanding of the controls for maintaining a normal blood sugar level is essential to understanding the diabetic imbalance in these mechanisms. The normal blood sugar level is usually maintained in a fasting state from 70 to 120 mg./100 ml. To maintain this normal range the body must have a constant source of glucose and at the same time continual controls, or uses, for that glucose.

Diet. The sources of the blood glucose are the basic nutrients in the diet—carbohydrates, proteins, and fats. Of these nutrients, the main source of blood glucose is carbohydrate. All the carbohydrate consumed is converted through digestion to glucose, and transported to the bloodstream. A small amount (10%—the glycerol portion) of fat is converted to glucose and enters the bloodstream. A fairly large proportion (58%) of protein is available for conversion to glucose, depending on the body's need. Thus these three substances in food maintain a steady supply of glucose to the blood.

Stored glycogen. Another source of supply from inside the body is the stored glycogen in the liver (p. 12). Although this is not a large storage, it is constantly being produced and hence provides a readily available source of glucose when the body requires it.

Control of blood glucose

Insulin. Insulin is the major control agent for maintaining a normal blood glucose level. As indicated, insulin is a hormone produced in special cells in the pancreas. Although its precise role is not entirely clear, insulin functions at several points to exercise this important control:

1. It facilitates the transport of glucose through the cell membrane by increasing the permeability of the cell wall. Hence it enables glucose to enter the cell, so that it can be burned for energy.

2. It aids in the conversion of glucose to glycogen and its storage in the liver (glycogenesis). Insulin also enables some glycogen to be stored in muscle tissue.

3. It stimulates the conversion of glucose to fat for storage as adipose fat tissue (lipogenesis).

Thus through these various functions insulin facilitates the use of blood sugar and prevents its rise to abnormal levels. These normal routes of entry and control of the use of blood glucose and the balance that must be maintained between the two are diagrammed in Fig. 18-2.

Glucagon. Another more recently discovered pancreatic hormone is glucagon. This hormone is also secreted by the islets of Langerhans alongside the cells that produce insulin. It is produced in different cells, however, called *alpha cells*, whereas insulin is produced by the adjacent beta cells. Thus these islets of Langerhans can be considered "glands within a gland," endocrine glands producing hormones within a larger exocrine

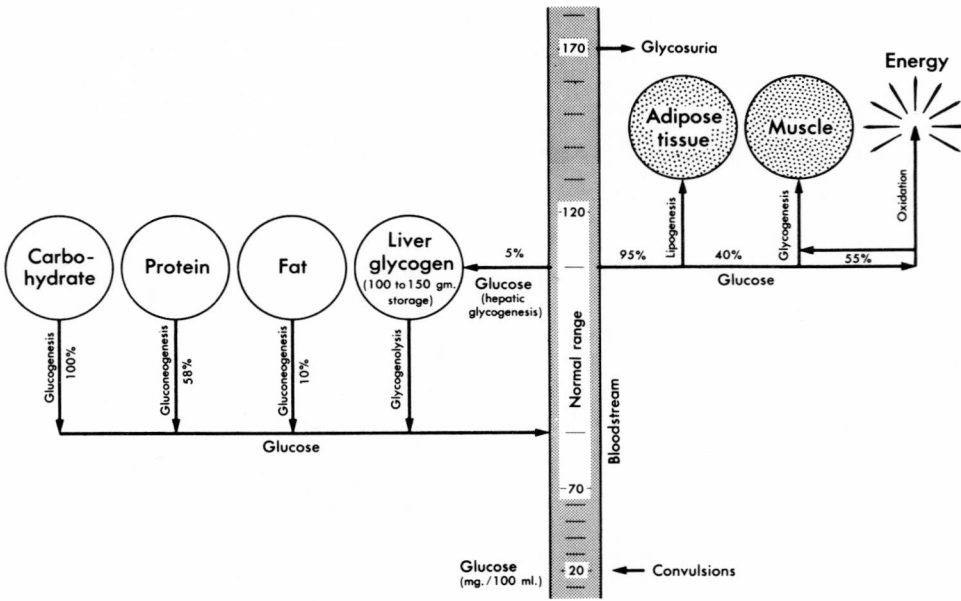

Fig. 18-2. Sources of blood glucose (food and stored glycogen) and normal routes of control.

gland that produces digestive enzymes. Glucagon gets its name from its stimulating effect on *glycogenolysis,* the conversion of glycogen to glucose. Thus it has an opposite action to insulin. It helps to break down liver glycogen and thus supply more blood glucose to bring blood glucose levels back up to normal as needed. It is sometimes used to control more brittle, or unstable diabetes. It acts as a counterbalance to excess insulin and as such is sometimes used as treatment for insulin shock or hypoglycemic reactions.

Metabolic changes in diabetes

In uncontrolled diabetes insulin is lacking to control the blood sugar level normally. Blood glucose cannot be oxidized properly in the cell to furnish energy and therefore builds up in the blood (hyperglycemia). When the blood sugar level rises to about 170 to 180 mg./100 ml., the sugar spills over in the urine (glycosuria). Some persons have a high renal threshold for glucose, and their blood sugar will rise considerably higher before appearing in the urine. Fat formation (lipogenesis) is curtailed, and fat breakdown (lipolysis) increases, leading to excess ketone formation and accumulation in the blood (ketosis) (p. 21). The appearance of one of these ketones —*acetone*—in the urine indicates the development of ketosis. Tissue protein is also broken down in an effort to secure energy, causing weight loss and nitrogen excretion in the urine.

OBJECTIVES OF NUTRITIONAL CARE IN DIABETES

The three basic objectives in the care of a diabetic patient are optimum nutrition, avoidance of symptoms, and prevention of complications.

Optimum nutrition

The patient's basic requirement is adequate nutrition for growth, development, and maintenance of an ideal weight. The lower end of the average range of weight for height is wise. Any degree of overweight should always be avoided.

Avoidance of symptoms

An effort is made to keep the patient relatively free of symptoms such as glycosuria and hyperglycemia. When the patient is receiving insulin therapy, however, it is wiser to have occasional glycosuria of small amounts as a monitoring device rather than constant negative urine tests that may indicate tendencies to low blood sugar or hypoglycemic episodes.

Prevention of complications

Complications in the eye tissue (retinopathy), in nerve tissue (neuropathy), and in renal tissue (nephropathy) occur in uncontrolled diabetes. Therefore an effort is made to prevent these complications through careful control. Coronary artery disease occurs in diabetics about four times as often as in the general population, and peripheral vascular disease occurs about forty times as often. These chronic manifestations or complications are believed to be reduced or retarded by good care and control.

Philosophies of control

Physicians vary in their approaches to controlling diabetes. Some follow a philosophy of strict *chemical control*, seeking to maintain a sugar-free urine constantly. Others follow a more moderate *clinical control* approach, seeking to maintain the patient relatively free of clinical symptoms. Still others follow a *free control* approach, placing little or no control on the patient's diet and administering insulin accordingly as necessary. Whatever the philosophy of diabetic management a particular physician may use, basic *consistency* of habit is the major need. This may be expressed as the three important R factors: *regulation, regularity,* and *routine.*

Whatever the individual physician's approach, the basic control of diabetes rests on a *balance* of three important interrelated factors: (1) diet, (2) insulin, and (3) exercise.

PRINCIPLES OF DIET THERAPY: THE BALANCE CONCEPT

The fundamental concept of diabetes control is that of *balance*. The basic principles of care then follow. The main principle may be stated simply: *individual diet therapy is always based on the normal nutritional needs of that particular person.* The necessary balance for control of diabetes, as in general health, may be viewed at three basic levels: the overall energy balance required, the nutrient balance among the necessary nutritional factors in food, and the distribution balance of these foods throughout the day.

Energy balance

The basic measure of energy balance is the maintenance of an *ideal weight*. The concept of the energy cycle has been discussed in Chapter 4. A review of these principles would be helpful at this point. The units of measure for energy are calories. Thus the diet for a diabetic patient is first outlined in terms of calorie requirements to meet his individual energy needs. These needs would be determined by ideal weight, with allowances for individual physical activity or added normal physiologic stress such as growth or pregnancy.

Thus if the patient is overweight, as is true with many adult diabetics, the diet prescription would reduce calories sufficiently to effect a gradual weight loss. Usually this would result in a diet of no more than 1,200 to 1,500 calories a day. If the patient is a fast-growing, lean adolescent boy, however, the calorie intake may need to be as high as 4,000. In any case, the number of calories prescribed will be that required for the normal nutritional needs of the individual to maintain health.

Nutrient balance

Protein. Normal age group requirements for protein govern the amount indicated for the individual patient. The optimum, or upper, range of these normal amounts is the usual guideline. For the adult man, therefore, the recommended daily average of 56 gm. indicated by the National Research Council's recommended dietary allowances is increased to give a range of 70 to 100 gm. for the diabetic. As a general rule of thumb, the protein part of the diet (as expressed in grams) should be about 5% of the number of total calories in the prescription. Thus in a 1,500-calorie diet about 75 gm. of protein would be used.

Carbohydrate. Carbohydrate should be adequate for need. It should not be restricted, as was the former rule for diabetics, but at the same time it should not be excessive. The usual daily dietary range is from 100 to 250 gm. As a general rule the carbohydrate (as expressed in grams) should be about 10% of the number of calories in the diet. Thus in a 1,500-calorie diet there would be about 150 gm. of carbohydrate. It is important to have sufficient carbohydrate to balance the metabolizing of fat, to provide sufficient energy and prevent excess fat breakdown, which leads to ketosis (p. 21). Refined, or "free," sugars should be avoided in habitual use. Sugar substitute sweeteners may be used instead.

Fat. Fat also should be adequate, but *moderation* is the guideline. Some clinicians advise substitution of vegetable fat for some of the animal fats in the diet to increase the ratio of unsaturated fatty acids. This is based on the general indication of a relationship between saturated fats and coronary artery disease and the greater risk factor of such disease in diabetes. As a general rule, the fat part of the diet prescription (as expressed in grams) is about 5% of the number of total calories. Thus in a 1,500 calorie diet there would be about 75 gm. of fat.

The general nutrient ratio. A general rule of thumb for outlining the final prescription is the determining of calorie and protein requirements first, according to known standard individual recommendations. The number of calories are established according to the amount required to maintain ideal weight and the protein according to optimum ranges of the normal recommended allowances, as indicated. Then after the protein calories have been deducted from the total, the remaining calories are divided about equally between carbohydrate and fat. Roughly, then, the carbohydrate, protein, and fat dietary ratio would be about 2:1:1. For example, an average 1,500-calorie diet may be divided into approximately 150 gm. of carbohydrate, 75 gm. of protein, and 75 gm. of fat.

Distribution balance

The third basic balance level is more important in the diabetic diet than in a normal diet for the health of nondiabetics. This is true because of the nature of the disease process involved. The factor to remember is always insulin availability in overall balance control, whether this hormone comes from the diabetic's own pancreas or is administered from the outside. The type of control of diabetes depends on the nature of the disease in a given individual. He may be controlled by diet alone in mild states of the disease. He may require oral medications to control blood sugar levels in somewhat more advanced states. He may require insulin administration in more severe forms of the disease. The distribution of food during the day therefore must be considered in relationship to the degree of insulin activity, whatever the type of control that is required.

Control by insulin. The schedule of the day's food intake pattern should be balanced with the type of insulin used and its pattern of absorption and peaks of activity.

SHORT-ACTING INSULIN. Regular crystalline insulin or Semilente Iletin are short-acting forms of insulin. These insulins cover about a 4- to 6-hour period of time and thus only the one meal following their use. Therefore these insulins are generally used in situations where short-term periods of control are indicated, such as in surgery, during labor and delivery, or in periods of illness. They may also be used in mixtures with other insulins for control of juvenile diabetes when a closer, more even control is necessary.

MEDIUM-ACTING INSULIN. NPH (neutral protamine Hagedorn), lente, and globin are intermediate insulins. NPH is the most widely used of these preparations. Medium-acting insulins are usually given in the morning, half an hour before breakfast, reach their peak of activity in 8 to 10 hours, about midafternoon, and then last in the waning period a total of 20 to 24 hours. The meal distribution pattern must account for this pattern of insulin activity. A smaller breakfast and a larger lunch and dinner pattern with allocations for a midafternoon and evening snack may be used. This would give approximately a one-fifth, two-fifths, two-fifths meal pattern. This amounts to three meals of fairly equal size with snacks from the lunch and dinner allocations for midafternoon and evening. For some, particularly adult, patients the afternoon snack may not be as important, but usually all patients require an evening snack.

LONG-ACTING INSULIN. PZI (protamine zinc insulin) and Ultralente Iletin are long-acting insulins. They are rarely used now. Long-acting insulins require a more substantial evening meal and bedtime snack to cover the prolonged period through the sleep hours. The meal distribution is about a one-seventh, two-sevenths, two-sevenths, two-sevenths pattern for each of the three meals and the bedtime snack.

MIXTURES OF INSULIN. Occasionally two types of insulin may be mixed in a syringe and given in one injection. For example, regular insulin may be mixed with NPH if more immediate morning coverage is required. In such cases a more substantial breakfast would be needed and a mid-morning snack, as well as midafternoon and bedtime snacks. The morning snack is usually more necessary for the younger child.

Control by oral hypoglycemic drugs. Several types of oral medications that are useful with some adult diabetics have been developed. These are of two basic types: (1) sulfur derivatives, the sulfonylureas, and (2) biguanides, phenformin. The first group, sulfonylureas, are believed to act on the basis of stimulation that they provide for the limited function of insulin-producing cells in the pancreas. Phenformin is believed to operate at the level of making the insulin that is produced more available for use. The sulfonylureas include tolbutamide (Orinase), chlorpropamide (Diabinese), and acetohexamide (Dymelor). The phenformin agent is marketed as DBI or Meltrol. A second form of DBI is available to avoid some of the gastrointestinal disturbances encountered as side effects by some persons. It is a slow-release preparation in modified form, DBI-TD. These various oral medications find use only in the following situations: (1) maturity-onset type of diabetes, (2) no history of ketosis or coma, and (3) the diabetes present for less than 10 years.

It is again evident that insulin activity is involved with the use of these oral hypoglycemic drugs. Therefore the meal distribution balance of the diet should be a fairly even one throughout the day to balance with this activity.

Diet control alone. Even if the diabetes requires only diet control, one still needs to consider distribution through the day in a fairly even balance of meals. Again, since by definition of the disease process a limited tolerance for handling glucose is involved, a load of this from a large meal at any one point would have to be avoided. A balance of meals throughout the day provides better overall control.

DIET MANAGEMENT
Exchange system of dietary control

Immediately after the discovery of insulin in 1922, the diabetic diet remained closely calculated. Carefully weighed-out food portions were listed for daily use. Obviously this system of diet control had many practical and psychologic drawbacks in everyday life. Thus, with recognition of the need for a more flexible and realistic approach, a new system of control was introduced in 1950. In this system foods commonly used are grouped according to like nutrient composition and designated *food exchange groups*. Six food groups are listed: milk, vegetables (A and B), fruit, bread, meat, and fat. Within any one group food items can be freely exchanged, since all foods in that group in the portion indicated have approximately the same nutrient value. These six food exchange groups are described in Table 18-1. This table gives the nutrient composition and general characteristics of each of the six food groups. The list of foods in each of the food groups that accompanies this plan is given in the previous chapter (pp. 231 and 232). This same system is also used for weight control and other conditions in which dietary management is needed. These tools, the nutrient composition of the food exchange groups and the food lists comprising each group, are the basic tools with which health workers may calculate diet needs and help patients make wise food selections and substitutions.

Steps in planning individual diet therapy

Diet prescription. The individual diet prescription is determined, as has been indicated, on the basis of the individual normal nutrition requirements and life situational needs. A careful history is taken first to determine the individual's living situation, food attitudes, and eating habits. On the basis of this information an individual prescription can be given.

Calculation of diet from prescription. Using the diet prescription, the nutritionist usually calculates the diet using the formula given in Table 18-2. In this short method of calculation the carbohydrate foods are calculated first, leaving the bread exchange group as a final control. Next in turn the protein requirement and then the fat are calculated, using the meat exchange group and the fat exchange group as controls. This then gives the total day's exchanges, allocated in terms of the number of exchanges (choices) from each of the food groups for use throughout the day. Often in common practice the specific calculation of the diet by grams of nutrients is not necessary. Working with the

Table 18-1. Food exchange groups

| FOOD GROUP | UNIT OF EXCHANGE | COMPOSITION | | | CALORIES | CHARACTERISTIC ITEMS |
		CARBOHY-DRATE (GM.)	PROTEIN (GM.)	FAT (GM.)		
Milk						
Whole	1 cup	12	8	10	170	Equivalents to 1 cup whole milk listed; 1 cup skimmed + 2 fat exchanges = whole milk
Skimmed	1 cup	12	8	—	80	
Vegetables						
A	As desired	—	—	—	—	Free use: 3% carbohydrate and below (tomatoes, green beans, leafy vegetables)
B	½ cup	7	2	—	35	Medium carbohydrate: pod and root varieties (green peas, carrots)
Fruit	Varies	10	—	—	40	Fresh or canned without sugar. Portion size varies with carbohydrate value of item; all portions equated at 10% carbohydrate
Bread	Varies; 1 slice bread	15	2	—	70	Variety of starch items, breads, cereals, vegetables; portions equal in carbohydrate value to 1 slice bread
Meat	1 oz.	—	7	5	75	Protein foods; exchange units equal to protein value of 1 oz. lean meat (cheese, egg, seafood)
Fat	1 tsp.	—	—	5	45	Fat food items equal to 1 tsp. butter or margarine (bacon, oil, mayonnaise, olives, avocados)

Table 18-2. Calculation of diabetic diet—short method using exchange system (2,200 calories)

FOOD GROUP	TOTAL DAY'S EXCHANGES	CARBO-HYDRATE (230 GM.)	PROTEIN (90 GM.)	FAT (100 GM.)	BREAKFAST	LUNCH	DINNER	SNACKS PM	HS
Milk	2	24	16	20	1				1
Vegetable A	As desired	—	—	—		As desired	As desired	As desired	
Vegetable B	1	7	2				1		
Fruit	6	60 __ 91			1	1	2	1	1
Bread	9	135 __ 226	18 __ 36		2	2	2	1	1
Meat	8		56 __ 92	40 __ 60	1	3	4		
Fat	8			40 __ 100	2	3	3		

Table 18-3. ADA meal plans for diabetics

DIET PLAN NUMBER	1	2	3	4	5*	6*	7*	8	9
Calories	1,000	1,500	1,800	2,200	1,800	2,600	3,500	2,600	3,000
Carbohydrate (gm.)	125	150	180	220	180	250	370	250	300
Protein (gm.)	60	70	80	90	80	100	140	115	120
Fat (gm.)	50	70	80	100	80	130	165	130	145
Total food exchanges									
Milk	2	2	2	2	4	4	4	2	2
Vegetable A	†	†	†	†	†	†	†	†	†
Vegetable B	1	1	1	1	1	1	1	1	1
Fruit	3	3	3	4	3	4	6	4	4
Bread	4	6	8	10	6	10	17	12	15
Meat	5	6	7	8	5	7	10	10	10
Fat	1	4	5	8	3	11	15	12	15

*These diets contain more milk and are planned for children.
†As desired.

total calories required in the diet, the nutritionist may make an allocation of these calories among the various food exchange groups according to the general usage of these particular foods in the average diet.

Meal pattern. After having determined the total day's food exchanges from each of the food exchange groups, the next step is to distribute these total day's exchanges throughout the day to achieve the necessary distribution balance required.

Two things may be used to govern this distribution: (1) individual adaptation to work or home requirements for daily schedule and (2) the type of controls being used—insulin or other medication. In addition, a general listing of diets has been developed by the American Diabetes Association for the convenience of physicians who do not have nutritionists to care for patients and handle the diet management. These are called the ADA Meal Plans and vary in calories from 1,200 to 3,000, including several adapted for children. These may be used as general guidelines but require individual adaptation for practical usefulness. These ADA diets are given in Table 18-3.

Menu plans. Using this basic meal pattern, any number of menu plans may be developed. A variety of food choices can be made while still maintaining the necessary consistency of meal pattern for the required dietary balance. A number of meal plans can reflect a variety of life situation adaptation needs and practical problems. These may include not only situations at home and the routine work schedule, but also special situations, such as holiday meals, entertaining, eating out, travel, and special physical activity periods. Also variety can be worked in by counseling with the nutritionist and other members of the health team concerning marketing and food preparation.

PATIENT EDUCATION
Basis of successful control

The key to satisfactory management of diabetes lies in sound, realistic patient education. It must be initiated early on diagnosis of diabetes and followed up as needed for reevaluation, reinforcement, and support. It must include the patient and his family in planning the overall management program, especially the diet. Only then will the diet be realistic in terms of the life situation needs and personal goals of the individual patient. A general admonition to "stay away from starches and sweets" is wholly inadequate and may well lead to bizarre food choices. Wise teaching is based instead on a well-planned diet program with sound general nutrition education. Frequently the nutrition of the whole family improves when the home meals are planned around the well-balanced outline given the diabetic member. Also, because the patient has a flexible plan that allows for a variety of food choices in a variety of situations, he is far more likely to follow it and build the consistent food habits that will give better long-range diabetic control.

What the diabetic patient must know

Education of the diabetic patient should include a thorough knowledge of those factors that he must understand to care for his diabetes himself. These factors include the following:

1. The disease—general facts of diabetes, its nature, symptoms, and care
2. The diet—basic knowledge of food values, individual diet plan, and ways of using substitutes; practical guides in marketing and food preparation may be needed
3. Insulin or oral hypoglycemics—details of equipment or use of oral drugs; relation to food intake and exercise
4. Urine testing—methods of testing urine for sugar and acetone and recording of results
5. Exercise—its value in diabetic control and general health; its relation to balance with insulin and food
6. Skin care and hygiene—for control of infection and maintenance of good circulation
7. Insulin shock—recognition of symptoms and knowledge of action to counteract those symptoms
8. Diabetic acidosis—recognition of symptoms and the need for immediate medical care
9. Personal identification—the necessity for a card or tag identifying diabetic needs, especially if receiving insulin
10. Educational resources—reading materials and community organizations providing services

Diet instructions

Methods

INDIVIDUAL COUNSELING. Skilled personal diet counseling given to newly diagnosed diabetic patients is the most valuable means for initiating a stable course. Regulation of the diabetes depends on securing the necessary cooperation of the patient himself. He will be the one making the day-to-day decisions about his general health habits. Sound knowledge is the basis of wise action and consistent habits. Therefore the initial dietary interview and the planning of the diet *with* the patient to meet his individual needs are of primary importance.

FOLLOW-UP PROGRAM. The initial instruction is insufficient alone. The learning process requires follow-up of some kind. The follow-up program may include additional individual interviews at which adjustments in the diet may be made, new material introduced, and former knowledge corrected or reinforced. Emotional support is provided also for acceptance of the disease and the working out of personal adjustment to its care. These conferences may also involve other family members in discussions that strengthen the instructions and clarify home needs.

GROUP INSTRUCTION. Group instruction and discussion is a helpful adjunct to personal counseling. These may take the form of more structured class situations or more informal small group discussions. These group situations are regularly held in many clinics. Physicians, nurses, dietitians, and other members of the health team share in the teaching responsibilities or leading the group discussion. Such a group process often reinforces personal decisions, and the exchange of ideas and experiences provides resources for learning.

Teaching materials

VISUAL AIDS AND EQUIPMENT. A number of visual aid materials are available or can easily be constructed. Often such aids clarify the concepts that are important in diabetes and provide practical illustrations. Food models help to picture portion sizes. These may be wax or plastic models or flat cardboard picture models. Also different sizes of cups, glasses, and spoons may help the patient to determine standard portion sizes. Other charts, diagrams, and pamphlets help clarify factual material. Sometimes exhibits prepared around a basic facet of care provide additional background information. Filmstrips and slides are useful for group discussion. Also demonstration equipment for displaying the increasing variety of food products on the market or variety in food preparation may be used. Equipment may be provided also for practice in insulin administration and urine testing as needed.

PROGRAMED INSTRUCTION. Teaching machines are used in some clinics to assist the patient education program. Usually this teaching method is well accepted by the patient and is effective. Although it cannot replace the necessary personal instruction and is not intended to do so, it provides helpful reinforcement. Some clinics are also expanding their education program to include the use of closed-circuit television.

READING AND REFERENCE MATERIALS. A number of standard reference books have been provided for diabetic patients. Some of these are listed in the patient education references at the end of this chapter. Two are particularly useful: *A Modern Pilgrim's Progress With Further Revelations for Diabetics* by Duncan, and Danowski's clear and practical guide for self-care, covering all facets of diabetes.

Additional printed material may be available from various pharmaceutical firms or other groups. Such material needs to be evaluated carefully and used according to the need in a particular setting.

Community resources

American Diabetes Association. The American Diabetes Association is a national organization with local chapters in various communities. It is an important coordinating organization, developing resource materials, providing guidance for activities of local chapters, and conducting research. Local chapters are active in many communities with annual detection drives, conferences, and group meetings and classes, sometimes cooperatively sponsored by the community adult evening school.

Professional groups. Other professional community organizations, such as the American Dietetic Association and nursing associations, may also provide resource persons and material.

Medic Alert. An identification program for alerting medical personnel to the needs of persons with hidden health problems has been provided through the creative efforts of a California physician, Dr. Marion Collins. When his own daughter, a student nurse, suffered a near fatal reaction to horse serum given in a routine postinjury tetanus injection, he designed for her an identifying metal disc to protect her from such danger subsequently in the course of routine care. Afterward he began to prepare identifying disks for his patients who had drug allergies or other hidden medical problems. In 1956 his plan was officially endorsed by the American College of Surgeons and is now a nonprofit service foundation with more than 150,000 American members and affiliated groups in a number of foreign countries. This important community resource provides a small stainless steel medallion, worn on a bracelet or as a pendant, that carries the individual's assigned identification serial number, a brief warning of the medical problem, and a telephone number. The number may be called collect day or night to reach the central answering service in the foundation's Turlock, California, headquarters. Here all member's records are kept on file and are available to medical personnel.

The small membership fee is paid only once. It includes the stainless steel medallion and emblem and a supplemental wallet card. Additional information may be obtained by writing Medic Alert Foundation International, Turlock, California 95380.

PATIENT EDUCATION MATERIALS

ADA Forecast, published bimonthly by the American Diabetes Association, Inc., 18 E. 48th St., New York, N. Y. 10017.

ADA Meal Planning Booklet, American Diabetes Association, 18 E. 48th St., New York, N. Y. 10017; also, Diabetic Diet Card for Physicians.

ADA Meal Plans, No. 1-9, American Diabetes Association, 18 E. 48th St., New York, N. Y. 10017; Chicago, 1956, American Dietetic Association.

Behrman, M.: Cookbook for diabetics, New York, 1959, American Diabetes Association, Inc.

Danowski, T. S.: Diabetes as a way of life, ed. 2, New York, 1964, Coward-McCann, Inc.

Dolger, H., and Seeman, B.: How to live with diabetes, New York, 1958, W. W. Norton & Co., Inc., Publishers; New York, 1964, Pyramid Books.

Duncan, G. G., and Duncan, T. G.: A modern pilgrim's progress with further relevations for diabetics, ed. 2, Philadelphia, 1967, W. B. Saunders Co.

Gormican, A.: Controlling diabetes with diet, Springfield, Ill., 1971, Charles C Thomas, Publisher.

Mohammed, M. F. B., and others: You and your diabetes, (audiovisual programmed instruction), New York, 1971, New Century Press.

Prater, B., Denton, N., and Fisher, K.: Food and You: nutrition in diabetes, Intermountain Regional Medical Program, Salt Lake City, 1970, University of Utah.

Public Health Service, U. S. Department of Health, Education, and Welfare, Washington, D. C.: Are you related to a diabetic? (Pub. No. 726, rev. 1964); Diabetes, (Pub. No. 137, 1964); Diabetes mellitus, a guide for nurses (Pub. 861, 1963); Taking care of diabetes (Pub. No. 567, 1963).

Revel, D. T.: Gourmet recipes for diabetics, Springfield, Ill., 1971, Charles C Thomas, Publisher.

Rosenthal, H., and Rosenthal, J.: Diabetic care in pictures, Philadelphia, 1960, J. B. Lippincott Co.

Strachan, C. B.: The diabetic's cookbook, Houston, 1956, Medical Arts Publishing Foundation.

Stanford, E. D.: Feet first, Division of Nursing, Public Health Service, Washington, D. C., 1970, U. S. Government Printing Office.

Travis, L. B.: Juvenile diabetes mellitus: an instructional aid, Galveston, Tex., 1969, University of Texas Press.

CHAPTER 19 CARDIOVASCULAR DISEASES

Cardiovascular disease is a health problem of major proportions in most countries of Western society. Its incidence in the United States continues to increase, causing more deaths than all other diseases together. It accounts for cardiac symptoms in about 75% of all adult patients under care in general hospitals. The pattern is the same in other developed countries.

A number of conditions involve organs of the cardiovascular system—the heart, the blood vessels, and the blood itself. Three basic problems will be considered here: atherosclerosis, congestive heart failure, and hypertension. Diet modification plays a role in the basic therapy indicated for each one.

THE PROBLEM OF ATHEROSCLEROSIS
Multiple risk factors

Although much has been learned by tremendous research efforts in many areas of the world, the precise cause of cardiovascular disease is still obscure. Multiple risk factors have emerged as contributory components in the disease process. These multiple risk factors are summarized in Table 19-1.

Personal characteristics. The personal characteristics that seem to be involved in the incidence of cardiovascular disease include a strong family history of heart disease, higher occurrence in men than in women, and age ranges lower than those in previous generations for heart attacks, from approximately the ages of 30 to 55 years. The person is frequently overweight and is of a personality type more reactive to stress. He tends to be a "work addict," putting in long hours under considerable pressure and getting little sleep.

Behavior patterns. Various behavior patterns that seem involved in the incidence of cardiovascular disease include smoking, especially heavy cigarette smoking from an early age. Eating habits are also involved. These include using a greater amount of animal fats; sweets, especially sugar (sucrose); and salt. Larger amounts of food in general have often led to overweight. Also the behavior pattern includes little physical activity in a generally sedentary life situation.

Metabolic relationships. Certain disease situations of a metabolic nature seem to be involved with the incidence of heart disease. These include a relationship with diabetes, evidenced in some by an intolerance for carbohydrates, and elevated blood serum levels of various lipids, including triglycerides, lipoproteins, and cholesterol. Hypertension is also a frequent accompaniment and seems to be related in some way to increased use of salt in the diet, as well as to heredity. It seems to be associated with sex (occurring more in women) and with race (occurring more in blacks).

Definition of atherosclerosis

The term *atherosclerosis* is given to the basic underlying pathologic process in coronary heart disease. The word comes from

248

Table 19-1. Multiple risk factors in cardiovascular disease

PERSONAL CHARACTERISTICS	BEHAVIOR PATTERNS	METABOLIC RELATIONSHIPS
Family history Sex (higher incidence in men) Age (approximately 30 to 55 years) Overweight Stress (personality type: work addiction, with heavy pressures and limited sleep)	Smoking Eating habits (use of excess fats, sugar, salt, and quantity) Exercising (little or no physical activity)	Diabetes Hypertension Hyperlipidemia (elevated serum lipids—triglycerides, lipoproteins, cholesterol)

two Greek roots: *ather*, meaning porridge or chaff, and *sklerosis*, which means thickening or hardening. Thus the name is given to a condition characterized by hardening or thickening of the walls of major blood vessels by porridgelike deposits of material. These deposits are composed of fatty materials, which form plaques on the inside walls of the blood vessels. As this process continues, degeneration and thickening occur in the arterial walls, which in turn causes a narrowing of the vessel lumen and the development of blood clots. Eventually the blood vessel may be narrowed sufficiently to cut off the flow of blood at that point. This blockage of the blood vessel is called an occlusion. The tissue area serviced by the involved artery is therefore deprived of the blood supply that carries its vital oxygen and nutrient materials. This condition is called *ischemia* and causes cell death. The localized area of dying or dead tissue is called an *infarct*. When the artery involved is one supplying the cardiac muscle (myocardium), the result is an acute *myocardial infarction,* commonly called an *MI,* or a *heart attack.*

Relation of general lipid metabolism

The nature of the underlying disease process has focused attention on fat metabolism. Several fat-related materials or compounds are involved.

Cholesterol. The artery deposits and plaque formations are largely composed of cholesterol. Thus some relationship to the body's mechanisms for handling cholesterol seems to be involved.

Saturated fats. Large-scale studies have demonstrated a definite association between types of dietary fat and effect on elevated blood lipid levels. These elevated blood levels of fats are called *hyperlipidemia,* or *hypertriglyceridemia.* Hyperlipidemia seems to be linked to high fat intake with a large percent of that intake being animal, or saturated, fat. Dietary substitution of foods high in polyunsaturated fatty acids (pp. 252 and 253) for foods high in saturated fatty acids has produced a lowering effect on these blood lipids, especially blood cholesterol. However, the significance of these lowered blood lipid levels in terms of the disease process is unknown at this point. If the serum cholesterol value returns to normal, is further atherosclerosis prevented? Is the disease process reversed? These are the important questions to which answers have not been found, but the mass of clinical and experimental data does suggest some disorder related to lipid metabolism.

Lipoproteins. Lipoproteins are the major transport forms of lipids in the blood. Review carefully the discussion in Chapter 3 concerning fat metabolism. An increase in one or more of these plasma lipoproteins creates the condition called *hyperlipoproteinemia.* This increased concentration of certain lipoproteins in the blood plasma has been found in a number of studies to be associated with

Table 19-2. Characteristics of the classes of lipoproteins

	CHYLOMICRONS (NONMIGRATING)	PRE-BETA LIPOPROTEINS, VERY LOW DENSITY (VLDL)	BETA LIPOPROTEINS, LOW DENSITY (LDL)	ALPHA LIPOPROTEINS, HIGH DENSITY (HDL)
Size, density	Largest, lightest	Next largest, lightest	Smaller, heavier	Smallest, most dense, heaviest
Triglycerides	80% to 95% Diet, exogenous	60% to 80% Endogenous	13% to 15% Endogenous	10% to 13% Endogenous
Cholesterol	2% to 7%	15% to 20%	45% to 50%	20% to 25%
Phospholipids	3% to 6%	15% to 20%	20% to 25%	30% to 35%
Protein	1% to 2%	5% to 7%	25% to 30%	45% to 50%
Place of synthesis	Intestinal wall	Liver	Liver	Liver
Function	Transport of diet TG* to plasma and tissue	Transport of endogenous TG* to tissue	Unclear: catabolic residue of VLDL (?)	Unknown: bare, unloaded transport vehicle to take TG* from liver to tissues (?)

*TG—Triglycerides.

an increased risk of atherosclerotic heart disease.

CLASSES OF LIPOPROTEINS. The lipoproteins in the blood are produced in two places: (1) the intestinal wall after initial ingestion, digestion, and absorption of dietary fat and (2) in the liver from body fat sources. Four groups of these lipoproteins have been identified, varying from compounds carrying a large amount of fat from the meal just consumed, chylomicrons (p. 21), to alpha lipoproteins, carrying little fat. These four classes of lipoproteins are characterized in Table 19-2.

TYPES OF LIPID DISORDERS. On the basis of which type of lipoproteins is found to be elevated in the blood, five different types of lipid disorders involving these lipoproteins have been identified. Types II and IV are the most commonly encountered in clinical practice. The treatment of each is determined by the nature of the elevated lipids. These types of lipid disorders are summarized in Table 19-3.

Specific diet guides for each of these types of lipid disorders may be obtained from the National Institutes of Health. The source of these materials is listed in the patient education materials at the end of this chapter.

Patients will need brief and clear explanations of their particular diets and the rationale for them. Many misunderstandings may be arrived at from lay articles or public advertising of food products. These may have to be corrected and clarified. The food fat spectrum (p. 19) will be a useful tool in teaching.

Principles of diet therapy

Fat-controlled diets

AMOUNT OF FAT. The annual per capital consumption of fat in the United States is estimated to be about 100 pounds. About half the calories of the average American's diet is contributed by fat. The suggestion has been made that this be moderated to about 35% or lower if weight reduction is needed.

KIND OF FAT. About two thirds of the total fat in the American diet is of animal origin and therefore is mainly saturated fat. The remaining one third comes from vegetable sources and is mainly unsaturated fat. The fat-controlled diet reduces the animal fat and uses instead more plant fat, thus bringing the ratio of polyunsaturated fat calories to about half the total fat calories. A simplified fat-control diet list for general use is given on

Table 19-3. Types of lipid disorders*

TYPE	DIET	LIPID PATTERN	CLINICAL SIGNS	GENETIC DEFECT
I Rare Early childhood Familial	Low fat, 25 to 35 gm.; high carbohydrate; MCT	Increased chylomicrons	Abdominal pain Lipemia, retinalis, xanthoma Hepatosplenomegaly	Deficient enzyme: lipoprotein lipase
II Common All ages Genetic: autosomal, dominant	Low cholesterol Low saturated fat High unsaturated fat	Increased beta lipoproteins (50% cholesterol), LDL Increased cholesterol	Xanthoma (tendon) Corneal arcus Vascular disease Accelerated atherosclerosis	Defective plasma clearing on catabolism of LDL
III Relatively uncommon Adult When genetic, recessive, sporadic	Weight reduction Low cholesterol High unsaturated fat	Increased abnormal form beta LP Increased triglycerides Increased cholesterol	Xanthoma (palmar) Vascular disease	Unclear
IV Most common Adult Familial	Weight reduction Low carbohydrate, no alcohol Low cholesterol High unsaturated fat	Increased pre-beta LP, VLDL Increased triglycerides Sometimes carbohydrate induced	Usually no overt symptoms Abnormal glucose tolerance High uric acid Stress, obesity Accelerated atherosclerosis	Abnormal glucose tolerance Lipogenesis
V Uncommon Early adult Sporadic familial	Weight reduction Low fat and carbohydrate High protein	Increased chylomicrons Increased triglycerides Increased cholesterol	Abdominal pain Pancreatitis Hepatosplenomegaly	Unclear

*Data from Frederickson, D. S., Levy, R. I., and Lees, R. S.: Fat transport in lipoproteins—an integrated approach to mechanisms and disorders, N. Engl. J. Med. **276**:34, 1967.

pp. 252 and 253. If the diet is also to be low in cholesterol, food sources of cholesterol have to be controlled more strictly. These foods include egg yolk, organ meats, and shellfish. A list of some foods with their cholesterol content is included in Appendix B.

Diet therapy in acute phases. In the acute phases of cardiovascular disease additional dietary modification may be indicated. The basic therapeutic objective is cardiac rest. Hence the purpose of all care is to assure

this requirement for restoring the damaged heart to adequate functioning. The diet will be modified, therefore, in energy value and texture.

CALORIES. A brief period of undernutrition during the first few days after the attack is advisable. The metabolic demands for digestion, absorption, and utilization of food require a generous cardiac output. Small portions of food decrease the level of metabolic activity to one that the weakened heart

Fat-controlled diet—high polyunsaturated fatty acids diet

	FOODS ALLOWED	FOODS NOT ALLOWED
Soups	Made from bouillon cubes, vegetables, and broths from which fat has been removed; cream soups made with nonfat milk	Meat soups, commercial cream soups, and those made with whole milk or cream
Meat, fish, poultry	One or two servings daily (not to exceed a total of 4 oz.) lean muscle meat, broiled or roasted: beef, veal, lamb, pork, chicken, turkey, ham; organ meats (all visible fat should be trimmed from meat); all fish and shellfish	Bacon, pork sausage, luncheon and dried meat, and all fatty cuts; wieners, fish roe, duck, goose, skin of poultry, and TV dinners
Milk and milk products	At least 1 pt. nonfat milk or nonfat buttermilk daily; nonfat cottage cheese, sapsago cheese	Whole milk and cream; all cheeses (except nonfat cottage cheese), ice cream, imitation ice cream (except that containing safflower oil, ice milk, sour cream, commercial yogurt
Eggs	Egg whites	Egg yolks
Vegetables	All raw or cooked as tolerated (leafy green and yellow vegetables are good sources of vitamin A)	No restrictions
Fruits	All raw, cooked, dried, frozen, or canned; use citrus or tomatoes daily; fruit juices	Avocado and olives
Salads	All fruit, vegetable, and gelatin salads	
Cereals	All cooked and dry cereals; serve with nonfat milk or fruit; macaroni, noodles, spaghetti, and rice	
Breads	Whole wheat, rye, enriched white, and French bread; English muffins, graham and saltine crackers	Commercial pancakes, waffles, coffee cakes, muffins, doughnuts, and all other quick breads made with whole milk and fat; biscuit mixes and other commercial mixes, cheese crackers, pretzels
Desserts	Fruits; tapioca, cornstarch, rice, junket puddings, all made with nonfat milk and, without egg yolks; fruit whips made with egg whites; gelatin desserts; angel food cake; sherbet, ices, and special imitation ice cream containing safflower oil; cake and cookies made with nonfat milk, oil, and egg white; fruit pie (pastry made with oil)	Omit desserts and candies made with whole milk, cream, egg yolk, chocolate, cocoa butter, coconut, hydrogenated shortenings, butter, and other animal fats

---

Fat-controlled diet—high polyunsaturated fatty acids diet—cont'd

	FOODS ALLOWED	FOODS NOT ALLOWED
Concentrated fats	Corn oil, soybean oil, cottonseed oil, sesame oil, safflower oil, sunflower oil; walnuts and other nuts except cashew and those commercially fried or roasted Margarine made from above oils, such as Award, Mazola, Emdee, Fleishmann's, and Kraft Corn Oil Commercial French and Italian salad dressings if not made with olive oil Gravy may be made from bouillon cubes or fat-free meat stock thickened with flour and oil added if desired Freshly ground or old-fashioned peanut butter	Butter, chocolate, coconut oil, hydrogenated fats and shortenings, cashew nuts; mineral oil, olive oil, margarine, except as specified; commercial salad dressings, except as listed; hydrogenated peanut butter; gravy, except as noted
Sweets	Jelly, jam, honey, hard candy, and sugar	
Beverages	Tea, coffee, or coffee substitutes; tomato juice, fruit juice, cocoa prepared with nonfat milk	Beverages containing chocolate, ice cream, ice milk, eggs, whole milk, or cream

If the diet is also to be high in unsaturated fat it should include liberal amounts of the following:
1. Oils allowed that can be incorporated in salad dressings or added to soups, to nonfat milk, to cereal, to vegetables
2. Walnuts, almonds, Brazil nuts, filberts, pecans
3. Extra margarine in or on foods

---

can accommodate. Some physicians may simply request liquids or milk only for the first day or so and then prescribe more food as the patient improves. During the early recovery stages the calories may be limited to 800 to 1,200 to continue cardiac rest from metabolic loads. If the patient is overweight as is frequently the case this caloric level may be continued for a longer period to bring about desired weight losses.

TEXTURE. Early feedings may be soft or easily digested to avoid effort in eating and chewing. Smaller meals served more frequently may give needed nutrition without undue strain or pressure.

THE PROBLEM OF EDEMA CONTROL IN CONGESTIVE HEART FAILURE

In congestive heart failure the weakened heart muscle (myocardium) is unable to maintain an adequate cardiac output to sustain a normal blood circulation. The resulting fluid imbalances cause edema to develop, bringing problems in breathing and placing added stress on the laboring heart.

Causes of cardiac edema

Imbalance in capillary fluid shift mechanism. As the heart fails to pump out the returning blood fast enough, the venous return is retarded, and a disproportionate amount of blood accumulates in the vascular system concerned with the right side of the heart. As a result the venous pressure rises, overcoming the balance of filtration pressures necessary to maintain the normal capillary fluid shift mechanism. This mechanism is the main means of maintaining the normal flow of fluids throughout the body. Body fluids must travel from the blood vessels into the tissues to service the cells and then back into circulation in the vessels (p. 82). This important mechanism is discussed in Chapter 7.

In congestive heart failure as a result of

the failure of this mechanism to operate properly fluid that normally would flow between the tissue spaces and the blood vessels is held in the tissue spaces, rather than being returned to circulation. This accumulation of fluid in the tissues is called *edema*.

Hormonal mechanisms. Two basic hormonal mechanisms that normally control water balance in the body only contribute to the cardiac edema in congestive heart failure. These are the aldosterone and ADH mechanisms.

ALDOSTERONE MECHANISM. This mechanism, although intended as a lifesaving sodium- and hence water-conserving mechanism, in this instance only compounds the edema problem. As the heart fails to propel the blood circulation forward, the deficient cardiac output effectively reduces the blood flow through the kidney. The decreased renal blood pressure triggers the renin-angiotensin mechanism, which in turn causes the adrenals to produce aldosterone. Aldosterone is the hormone that causes the kidney to reabsorb more sodium and following it, water. As a result still more water is held in the tissues.

ADH MECHANISM. This water-conserving hormonal mechanism also adds to the edema. The cardiac stress and the reduced renal flow cause the release of ADH, the antidiuretic hormone from the pituitary gland. This hormone stimulates still more water reabsorption in the nephrons of the kidney.

Increased free cell potassium. As the reduced blood circulation depresses cell metabolism, cell protein is broken down and releases its bound potassium in the cell. As a result, the amount of free potassium is increased inside the cell, which increases osmotic pressure. Sodium ions in the fluid surrounding the cell then also increase to balance the increase within the cells and hence prevent cell dehydration. The larger amount of sodium then in time causes more water retention.

Review carefully the metabolism of sodium, potassium, and water in Chapter 7. These mechanisms are discussed there in greater detail with diagrams to help clarify the abnormal shifts and balances involved in cardiac edema. These abnormal shifts produce a serious dislocation in the body water compartments.

Principles of diet therapy— sodium-restricted diets

Because of the role of sodium in water balance, the diet used to treat cardiac edema restricts the sodium intake. Four levels of dietary sodium restrictions have been outlined by the American Heart Association and are in common use throughout the United States.

Sodium in the general diet. The taste for salt is an acquired one. Some persons salt food heavily and habituate their taste to high salt levels. Others acquire a taste for less salt and use smaller amounts. Common daily adult intakes of sodium range rather widely, according to habit, from about 3 or 4 gm. to as high as 10 to 12 gm. with heavy use.

Levels of sodium-restricted diets. The main source of dietary sodium is in sodium chloride, common table salt. Many other lesser used sodium compounds, such as baking powder and baking soda, contribute small amounts. Otherwise the remaining dietary source is the naturally occuring sodium in foods as one of their minerals. The four levels of sodium restricted diets increasingly delete food items or ways of food preparation.

MILD SODIUM RESTRICTION (2 TO 3 GM.). Salt may be used *lightly* in cooking, but no added salt is allowed. Obviously salty foods in which salt has been used as a preservative or a flavoring agent are omitted. These food items would include pickles, olives, bacon, ham, and potato chips. A list for mild sodium restriction is shown on p. 255.

MODERATE SODIUM RESTRICTION (1,000 MG.). There may be no salt used in cooking, no added salt, and no salty foods. Beginning with this level, some control of natural sodium foods is instituted. Vegetables that are higher in sodium are limited in use, salt-free canned vegetables are substituted for regular canned

---

Restrictions for a mild low-sodium diet (2 to 3 gm.)

DO NOT USE:

1. Salt at the table (use salt lightly in cooking)
2. Salt-preserved foods such as salted or smoked meat (bacon and bacon fat, bologna, dried or chipped beef, corned beef, frankfurters, ham, kosher meats, luncheon meats, salt pork, sausage, smoked tongue), salted or smoked fish (anchovies, caviar, salted and dried cod, herring, sardines), sauerkraut, olives
3. Highly salted foods, such as crackers, pretzels, potato chips, corn chips, salted nuts, salted popcorn
4. Spices and condiments, such as bouillon cubes,* catsup,* chili sauce,* celery salt, garlic salt, onion salt, monsodium glutamate, meat sauces, meat tenderizers,* pickles, prepared mustard, relishes, Worcestershire sauce, soy sauce
5. Cheese,* peanut butter*

---

*Dietetic low-sodium kind may be used.

---

ones, salt-free baked products are used, and meat and milk may be eaten in moderate portions.

STRICT SODIUM RESTRICTION (500 MG.). In addition to the deletions thus far, meat, milk, and eggs are allowed only in smaller portions. Milk is limited to 2 cups total in any form, meat to five or six ounces total daily, and eggs to no more than one. Vegetables with higher sodium content are deleted.

SEVERE SODIUM RESTRICTION (250 MG.). No regular milk may be used; low-sodium milk is substituted. Meat is limited to 2 to 4 ounces in all for the day and eggs to about three a week. It becomes more important, therefore, to devise ways of incorporating adequate low-sodium milk to ensure sufficient protein intake.

The 500 mg. low-sodium diet is given on pp. 256 to 258. It includes modifications for increasing it to a 1,000 mg. sodium diet or reducing it to a 250 mg. sodium diet.

THE PROBLEM OF HYPERTENSION

Hypertension is defined as persistent levels of blood pressure elevated above 150 systolic and 90 diastolic. About 20% of the population develops hypertension. About 95% of these have essential hypertension, that is, of no known cause. The remainder of persons with hypertension develop this blood pressure elevation from some specific cause asso-

ciated with other disease processes. Hypertension is a symptom complex that may be present in a number of disorders. It is a common clinical problem in cardiovascular disease.

Essential hypertension usually begins as an unstable, intermittent process in the age period of the late 30s to the early 50s. Sometimes it may appear abruptly and severely and take an accelerated course. Such factors as coffee, tobacco, and stimulating drugs, as well as emotional disturbances and obesity, seem to play a role. The disease is also strongly familial. It affects more women than men. However, among men, especially those of the black race, the disease is tolerated more poorly.

Clinical symptoms

No symptoms at all may occur, or severe symptoms may be present. Among these may be morning headaches, easy fatigue, irritability, and a feeling of nervousness. If the heart is involved, shortness of breath, edema, palpitations, and general discomfort may occur. There may be occasional transient attacks, such as dizziness and blackouts, indicating some central nervous system involvement.

Principles of diet therapy

Relation of diet to drug therapy. The major objective of treatment is the lowering of the

Low-sodium diet (500 mg.)

GENERAL DESCRIPTION:

1. All foods are to be prepared and served without the addition of salt, baking powder, or baking soda.
2. Take only those foods that are tolerated and in the amounts specified.
3. Read all food labels for the *addition of salt or sodium in any form.*
4. Avoid medications and laxatives unless approved by a physician.
5. The suggested menu pattern for 500 mg. sodium contains approximately 275 gm. carbohydrate, 85 gm. protein, 130 gm. fat, and 2,300 calories. All menu patterns meet the recommended allowances of vitamins and minerals.

	DAILY ALLOWANCE	FOODS TO AVOID
Milk	Limit to 2 cups daily—frozen, powdered, or canned or as 1 cup evaporated milk, used as beverage or in cooking; 2 tbsp. cream (1 oz.)	Malted milk, sour cream, buttermilk, condensed milk, milkshakes, chocolate milk, fruit flavored beverage powders, whipped toppings
Eggs	One daily	
Meat, poultry,	Six oz. cooked daily; fresh beef, lamb, liver, pork, veal, rabbit, chicken, duck, goose, quail, turkey, cod, halibut, filet of sole, tuna, salmon, or meats canned without salt, frozen meat containing no salt or sodium (beef or calf liver allowed not more than once in 2 weeks)	All meat, poultry, fish not listed; meat, fish, or poultry that is smoked, cured, canned, frozen containing salt or sodium, pickled, salted, or dried (bacon, ham, luncheon meats, sausages, salt pork, canned salmon and tuna, sardines), clams, crabs, lobsters, (oysters Eastern), scallops, shrimp, anchovies, salted dried cod, frozen fish filets, commercial meat pies, TV dinners
Cheese	Special dietetic low sodium cheese may be used as a meat substitute as part of the daily allowance	Any other
Fruit	Three servings daily, including one citrus—½ cup per serving, fresh, canned, or frozen	Dried figs, raisins containing sodium sulfite
Vegetables	Four servings daily (fresh, frozen, or dietetic canned vegetables only)—½ cup per serving; asparagus, green beans, wax beans, lima beans, navy beans, broccoli, cauliflower, corn, cucumber, endive, eggplant, lentils, onions, parsnips, peppers, radishes, rutabagas, cabbage, Brussels sprouts, lettuce, mushrooms, okra, soybeans, squash, tomatoes, unsalted tomato juice, turnip greens	Canned vegetables or juices containing salt (V-8 juice), sauerkraut, white turnips, beets, celery, carrots, artichokes; greens—beets, spinach, chard, dandelion, kale, mustard; frozen peas, frozen lima beans, frozen mixed vegetables
Potato or substitute	Two servings daily of potato, rice, macaroni, spaghetti, noodles, fresh sweet potatoes	Potato chips, corn chips

Low-sodium diet (500 mg.)—cont'd

	DAILY ALLOWANCE	FOODS TO AVOID
Cereal	One serving daily shredded wheat, puffed rice, puffed wheat, or cooked cereals that contain no added salt or sodium, such as regular Cream of Wheat, cornmeal, Malt-o-Meal, rice, Wheatena, Pettijohns, Ralston, oatmeal	Quick-cooking Cream of Wheat and all other ready-to-eat cereals not listed; self-rising flour
Breads	Low-sodium bread or unsalted matzos; low-sodium crackers	Potato chips, salted crackers, salted popcorn, pretzels, regular bread, rolls, biscuits, muffins, waffles, commercial mixes
Fats	Sweet butter, lard, salad oil, shortening, low-sodium salad dressing as desired; unsalted margarine (check label and brand)	Salted nuts, salted butter, bacon fat, margarine, salted peanut butter, gravies, and commercial salad dressings
Soup	Homemade soup cooked with allowed meat, vegetables, and milk	Broth, bouillon, consomme, and canned soups
Sweets	Jelly, jam, sugar, honey, gumdrops, marshmallows as desired; small amounts of brown sugar	Any commercial jam and jelly containing a sodium preservative, molasses, candy, candy bar
Desserts	Fruit, gelatin desserts made with plain gelatin and fruit juice, fruit pie made without salt; rice, tapioca, or cornstarch pudding made with low-sodium milk and/or fruit and fruit juices, desserts made with sodium-free baking powder	All others—ice cream, sherbet, desserts made with regular baking powder or baking soda, rennet tablets, pudding mixes; commercial gelatin desserts, pudding and cake mixes
Beverages	Tea, coffee, Postum, Sanka, cocoa, (except Dutch-process) made with low-sodium milk allowance, fruit juice	Instant cocoa mix, prepared beverage mixes
Condiments	Allspice, bay leaves, caraway seeds, cinnamon, curry powder, garlic, mace, marjoram, mustard powder, nutmeg, paprika, parsley, pimiento, rosemary, sage, sesame seeds, thyme, tumeric, ginger, pepper, vinegar; extracts of almond, lemon, vanilla, peppermint, walnut, maple	Celery salt, garlic salt, catsup, prepared mustard, salt, meat sauces, meat tenderizers, monosodium glutamate, soy sauce, pickles, relishes, olives, prepared horseradish, Worcestershire sauce, chili sauce, seasoning salts
Miscellaneous		Baking powder, baking soda, chewing tobacco

500 MG. SODIUM DIET SUGGESTED MENU PATTERN

Breakfast	*Lunch*	*Dinner*
1 fruit	3 oz. unsalted meat	3 oz. unsalted meat
1 egg	Unsalted potato	Unsalted potato
Low-sodium cereal	Low-sodium vegetable	Low-sodium vegetable
1 low-sodium bread	Low-sodium vegetable salad	Low-sodium salad
1 unsalted butter	1 low-sodium bread	1 low-sodium bread

Continued.

Low-sodium diet (500 mg.)—cont'd

500 MG. SODIUM DIET SUGGESTED MENU PATTERN—CONT'D

Breakfast	*Lunch*	*Dinner*
Jelly	1 pat unsalted butter	1 pat unsalted butter
½ cup milk	Jelly	Jelly
Coffee	1 fruit	1 cup milk
2 tbsp. cream (1 oz.)	½ cup milk	Coffee
	Coffee	Fruit

MODIFICATIONS FOR A 250 MG. SODIUM DIET

The 250 mg. sodium diet is essentially the same as the 500 mg. sodium diet except for the following:
1. Use low-sodium milk (2 or more glasses) instead of regular milk
2. Use only 5 oz. of meat instead of 6 oz.
3. Omit cream

MODIFICATIONS FOR A 1,000 MG. SODIUM DIET

One of the three following modifications may be used to raise the sodium content in the 500 mg. sodium diet to 1,000 mg.

Modification I
1. Two slices regular bread are allowed daily
2. 2 tsp. only regular butter (above this amount, unsalted butter must be used)
3. One serving (½ cup) is allowed daily of spinach, celery, carrots, beets, artichoke, white turnips

Modification II (high protein)
1. 10 oz. of meat are allowed instead of 6 oz.
2. One serving of prepared or milk dessert, such as ice cream, custard, gelatin, or 1 cup milk
3. Two eggs instead of 1
4. One serving of spinach, celery, carrots, beets, or artichoke is allowed

Modification III
1. Three slices regular bread may be used in place of the low-sodium bread (above this amount unsalted bread must be used)

---

blood pressure to normal levels with the hope of improving the symptoms and preventing the development of vascular damage. The main treatment involves drug therapy with a series of drugs being used currently to control blood pressure levels. Diuretic drugs are also used to remove some of the excess water in the tissues from the body. The action of these drugs causes some potassium loss. Thus potassium replacement in food and medication is usually a part of treatment.

The results of a number of studies have linked hypertension to a sensitivity to high salt use. Thus diet therapy in the main is aimed at reducing salt use. With the advent of the potent antihypertensive drugs, severe restriction of sodium in the diet is not necessary. However, the effectiveness of these drugs is enhanced and the hypertensive condition improved by moderate restriction of sodium to from 500 to 1,000 mg., depending on individual needs and responses. The 500 and 1,000 mg. sodium diets given on pp. 256 to 258 may be used.

Relation to obesity. Frequently the hypertensive patient is also overweight. In this case a weight reduction modification would also be used with the diet in an effort to bring the weight to an ideal level and maintain it. Guidelines for weight reduction diets have been included in the previous chapter and may be used for reference, along with the low–sodium food exchange groups (pp. 259 to 262).

Hypertension is considered controllable but not curable with present drugs and care.

Low–sodium food exchange groups

FOODS PERMITTED | FOODS TO AVOID

Group A vegetables

Raw, cooked, or canned, without salt or fat; may be eaten as desired; one serving contains little or no calories and 9 mg. sodium

FOODS PERMITTED	FOODS TO AVOID
Asparagus	Canned vegetables (unless packed without salt)
Beans, green	
Broccoli	
Brussels sprouts	The following vegetables are high in natural salt and must be omitted from the diet
Cauliflower	
Celery*	Beet greens
Cabbage, fresh	Swiss chard
Chicory	Kale
Cucumbers	Sauerkraut
Eggplant	
Endive	
Escarole	
Lettuce	
Mushrooms	
Okra	
Parsley	
Peppers	
Radishes	
Squash, summer	
Spinach*	
Tomatoes	
Salt-free tomato juice	
Watercress	

Group B vegetables

Only ½ cup of one of the following vegetables may be used per day; contain approximately 9 mg. sodium, 7 gm. carbohydrate, 2 gm. protein, and 35 calories per serving

FOODS PERMITTED	FOODS TO AVOID
Beets*	White turnips
Carrots*	Frozen peas
Onions	
Peas	
Pumpkin	
Artichoke	
Rutabaga	
Winter squash	

Fruits

Fresh, dried, cooked, or canned, without added sugar; this list shows the amount of fruit to use for one serving, containing 2 mg. sodium, 10 gm. carbohydrate, and 40 calories

FOODS PERMITTED		FOODS TO AVOID
Apple	1 small	Canned tomato juice or vegetable juices
Applesauce	½ cup	Fruit or fruit products that contain sodium
Apricots, fresh	2 medium	benzoate, maraschino cherries; dried fruit
Apricots, dried	4 halves	with sodium sulfate added: read label
Bananas	½ small	(use only sun dried fruits)
Blackberries	1 cup	
Raspberries	1 cup	
Blueberries	⅓ cup	
Strawberries	1 cup	

*Vegetables allowed once a day if sodium allowance is 1,000 mg.

Continued.

Low–sodium food exchange groups–cont'd

FOODS PERMITTED		FOODS TO AVOID
Fruits—cont'd		
Cantaloupe	¼ medium	
Cherries	10 large	
Dates	2	
Figs, fresh	2 large	
Watermelon	1 cup	
Grapefruit juice	½ cup	
Grapes	12	
Grape juice	¼ cup	
Honeydew melon	⅛ medium	
Oranges	1 small	
Orange juice	½ cup	
Peaches	1 medium	
Pears	1 small	
Pineapples	½ cup	
Pineapple juice	⅓ cup	
Plums	2 medium	
Prunes, dried	2 medium	
Tangerines	1 large	

Bread

One serving contains 15 gm. carbohydrate, 2 gm. protein, 70 calories, 5 mg. sodium (substitute the following for one slice salt-free bread)

Salt-free passover		Regular bread and rolls
matzo	½	Biscuits and popovers
Salt-free melba toast	3	Salted or soda crackers
Low sodium toast		Pastries and cakes
(Nabisco)	2	Prepared muffins, waffles, cakes
Cooked cereals		Pancake and pastry mixes
(without salt)	½ cup	Self-rising flour
Pearl barley		Cornmeal
rice, noodles	½ cup	Quick cooking (5-minute) hot cereals
Macaroni, spaghetti	½ cup	Dry cereals, except those listed
Lima beans, fresh	½ cup	Pretzels, potato chips
Navy beans, dried	½ cup	Salted popcorn
Soybeans, cowpeas	½ cup	Frozen lima beans
Potato (white)	1 small	
Potato (sweet)	¼ cup	
Parsnips	⅔ cup	
Corn (fresh, frozen,		
or canned, unsalted		
or 1 small ear)	⅔ cup	
Puffed wheat,		
puffed rice	¾ cup	
Shredded wheat	1 biscuit	
Popcorn, unsalted	1 cup	

Low–sodium food exchange groups–cont'd

FOODS PERMITTED		FOODS TO AVOID

Meats

One oz. contains 7 gm. protein, 5 gm. fat, 25 mg. sodium, 75 calories; substitute the following for one oz. salt-free meat (baked, broiled, stewed, or panbroiled)

FOODS PERMITTED		FOODS TO AVOID
Fresh or frozen beef, lamb, liver, pork, rabbit, veal, or tongue	1 oz.	All smoked, processed, or canned meats, fish, or fowl, such as anchovies, caviar, herring, salted dried cod, bacon, oysters
Fresh fish (except shellfish)	1 oz.	Cold cuts
		Corned beef or chipped beef
Fresh or frozen chicken, duck, turkey, or quail	1 oz.	Frankfurters or sausages
		Brain, kidney
		Ham, smoked tongue, sausage
Canned salt-free tuna or salmon	¼ cup	All cheese, except salt-free
		Frozen fish filets, clams, crab, lobster, shrimp, sardines, oysters, kosher meats
Salt-free peanut butter	1 tbsp.	Peanut butter, except salt-free
Salt-free American cheese	1 oz.	
Salt-free cottage cheese (dry curd)	¼ cup	
Egg (no more than one a day)		

Fats

One serving contains 5 gm. fat, little or no sodium, and 45 calories; substitute the following for 1 tsp. salt-free butter

FOODS PERMITTED		FOODS TO AVOID
Butter, salt-free	1 tsp.	Salted butter, oleomargarine
Cream, light (sweet or sour)	2 tbsp.	Commercial mayonnaise or French dressing
Cream, heavy	1 tbsp.	Bacon fat and other salty meat drippings, olives
Avocado	⅛	Salted nuts
French dressing, salt-free	1 tbsp.	Salt pork
Mayonnaise, salt-free	1 tsp.	
Oil or cooking fat	1 tsp.	
Nuts, unsalted	6 small	

Seasonings

FOODS PERMITTED	FOODS TO AVOID
Allspice	Rennet tablets
Baking yeast	Salt in any form
Caraway	Baking soda and baking powder
Cinnamon	Prepared mustard, catsup, meat sauces, chili sauce, horseradish
Curry powder	
Garlic	Bouillon or canned soups
Ginger	Olives, pickles, relishes
Herbs	Celery salt, celery seed, onion salt, garlic salt
Horseradish (fresh grated)	

Continued.

Low–sodium food exchange groups–cont'd

FOODS PERMITTED	FOODS TO AVOID
Seasonings—cont'd	
Lemon juice or extract	
Mace	Accent, Zest, Tok
Mustard, dry	Salted meat tenderizers
Nutmeg	Prepared horseradish
Paprika	Worchestershire sauce
Parsley	Meat extracts
Peppermint extract	Meat sauces
Sage	
Saccharine	
Thyme	
Tumeric	
Vanilla extract	
Walnut extract	
Pepper, black	
Pepper, red	
Pepper, white	
Vinegar	

Thus treatment at present must continue indefinitely. Therefore the education of the patient should involve not only instruction about drug therapy—the kinds of drugs, their general action, and mode of use—and his diet but also the reasons for continuing the treatment program even after his blood pressure has come down and is being held at acceptable levels. Sometimes this is difficult for patients to realize when they feel well and see no overt symptoms as a reason to continue the treatment.

PATIENT EDUCATION

Since cardiovascular disease assumes a more or less chronic nature, an important responsibility of all the members of the health team is education of the patient and his family concerning *continuing* needs for health care. Such teaching should not wait for "discharge instructions" from the hospital but should begin early in the convalescence and give the patient a clear knowledge of positive needs. Such an approach will provide practical resources for self-care within the limits of individual capacity and help avoid the negative apprehension of becoming a "cardiac cripple."

Many excellent resources for patient education are provided by the American Heart Association through their national and regional offices. Practical discussions with patients and their families have to center on food buying and preparation to make the diet palatable and acceptable to the patient. This is especially true with the sodium modified diets, since salt tastes are pronounced and food without salt needs alternative seasonings. Many helpful suggestions are included in the American Heart Association booklet and in the cookbooks listed at the end of the chapter. A survey of local markets will give guidance concerning commercial products. Label reading on all commercial products should become a habit. The new nutrient labeling regulations currently being adopted by the FDA and mandatory throughout the food industry by 1974 should help give more specific information to the patient and his family concerning the fat and salt content in various food products. For those patients who must continue a calorie-restricted as well as low-sodium diet, a listing of the low–sodium food exchange groups is given on pp. 259 to 262. These low–sodium food exchange group listings of specific foods may be used with the 800- to 1,500-calorie diet plans in the previous chapter on weight control (p. 233) to make food choices and general diet guidelines for a combination low-calorie, low-sodium diet.

PATIENT EDUCATION MATERIALS

American Heart Association, New York City (or local heart association)
  Booklets
    Planning fat-controlled meals for unrestricted calories, 1962.
    Planning fat-controlled meals for 1,200 and 1,800 calories, rev. 1966.
    Your sodium-restricted diet: 500 mg., 1,000 mg., and mild restriction, 1958.
  Foldout charts
    Sodium-restricted diet, 500 mg., 1965.
    Sodium-restricted diet, 1000 mg., 1966.
    Sodium-restricted diet, mild, 1967.
    Recipes for fat-controlled low cholesterol meals, 1968.

The way to a man's heart: a fat-controlled low cholesterol meal plan to reduce the risk of heart attack, 1968.

Haferkorn, V.: Assessing individual learning needs as a basis for patient teaching, Nurs. Clin. North Am. 6:199, 1971.

Heap, B., and others: Simplifying the sodium-restricted diets, J. Am. Diet. Assoc. 49:327, 1966.

Keys, A., and Keys, M.: Eat well and stay well, Garden City, N. Y., 1963, Doubleday & Co., Inc.

National Institutes of Health, National Heart and Lung Institute: The dietary management of hyperlipoproteinemia, Bethesda, Md., 1971, NIH.

Payne, A. S., and Callahan, D.: The low-sodium, fat-controlled cookbook, Boston, 1965, Little, Brown & Co.

Public Health Service: The food you eat and heart disease, Pub. 537, 1963, U. S. Department of Health, Education, and Welfare.

Stead, E. S., and Warren, G. K.: Low-fat cookery, New York, 1959, McGraw-Hill Book Co., Inc.

Waldo, M.: Cooking for your heart and health, New York, 1961, G. P. Putnam's Sons, Inc.

CHAPTER 20 RENAL DISEASES

BASIC RENAL FUNCTIONS AND STRUCTURES
Renal functions

An understanding of the basic functions of the kidney is necessary to understand interferences with these functions in disease states. The basic functional unit of the kidney is the nephron. The diagram of the nephron in Fig. 20-1 should be studied carefully.

The nephron is an exquisite example of a highly complex, minute tissue unit. It is adapted in fine detail to its vital function—maintaining an internal fluid environment compatible with life. These vital units of the kidney are the master chemists of our bodies. We have the kind of body fluids and tissues that we have not merely because of what the mouth takes in but because of what the kidneys keep. Only because they work in the way they do has it become possible for us to have specific tissues of specific natures to do specific tasks.

Each kidney contains some one million nephrons. As the body fluid flows through these finely structured units, the nephrons perform four significant functions to support life:

1. *Filtration* of most constituents from the entering blood except red cells and proteins
2. *Reabsorption* of needed substances as the filtrate continues along the winding tubules
3. *Secretion* of additional ions to maintain acid-base balance
4. *Excretion* of unneeded materials in a concentrated urine

Nephron structures

Specific nephron structures perform unique metabolic tasks to maintain body balance. Each of these may be identified in Fig. 20-1.

Glomerulus. At the head of the nephron the blood enters in a single capillary and then branches into a group of collateral capillaries. This tuft of collateral capillaries is held closely applied in a cup-shaped membrane. This cup-shaped capsule is named *Bowman's capsule* for the young English physician Sir William Bowman, who in 1843 first clearly established the basis of plasma filtration and consequent urine secretion on this intimate relationship of blood-filled glomeruli and enveloping membrane. The filtrate formed here is cell free and virtually protein free. Otherwise it carries the same constituents as does the entering blood.

Tubules. Continuous with the base of Bowman's capsule the nephron tubule winds in a series of convolutions toward its terminal in the kidney pelvis. Specific reabsorption functions are performed by the four sections of the tubule: the proximal tubule, the loop of the Henle, the distal tubule, and the collecting tubule.

PROXIMAL TUBULE. In the first section nearest the glomerulus major nutrient reabsorption occurs. Essentially 100% of the glucose and amino acids and 80% to 85% of the water, sodium, potassium, chloride, and most other substances are reabsorbed. Only 15% to 30% of the filtrate remains to enter the next section, the loop of Henle.

LOOP OF HENLE. This is the midsection of

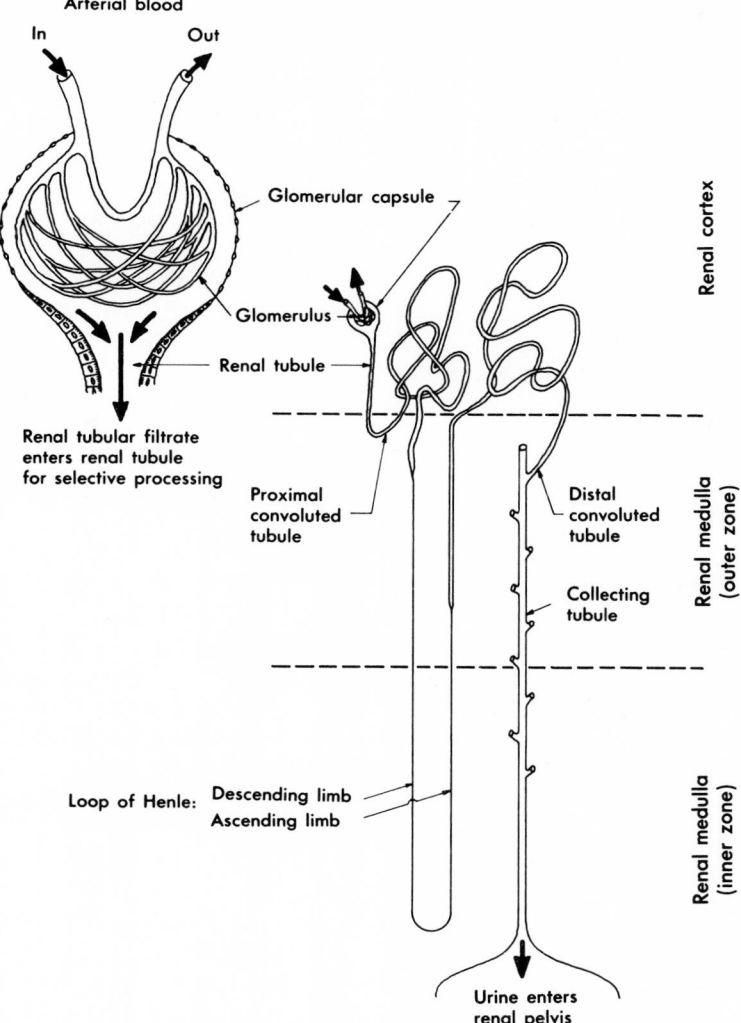

Arterial blood

In   Out

Glomerular capsule

Glomerulus

Renal tubule

Renal tubular filtrate
enters renal tubule
for selective processing

Proximal
convoluted
tubule

Distal
convoluted
tubule

Collecting
tubule

Loop of Henle: Descending limb
Ascending limb

Urine enters
renal pelvis

Renal cortex

Renal medulla
(outer zone)

Renal medulla
(inner zone)

Fig. 20-1. The nephron—functional unit of the kidney.

the renal tubule. Here the tubule narrows, and its thin loop dips into the central renal medulla. Through a balanced system of water and sodium exchange in the limbs of the loop, important fluid density is created surrounding the loop. This area of increased density is important to concentrate the urine by osmotic pressure as it later passes through this same area of the kidney in the collecting tubule.

DISTAL TUBULE. The latter portion of the tubule functions primarily in acid-base balance through secretion of ionized hydrogen. It also conserves sodium by reabsorbing it under the influence of aldosterone (p. 254).

COLLECTING TUBULE. In the final section of the tubule water is absorbed under the influence of the hormone ADH and the osmotic pressure of the more dense surrounding fluid. The resulting volume of urine now concentrated and excreted is only 0.5% to 1% of the original filtered water.

PROBLEMS OF KIDNEY DISEASE

Various inflammatory and degenerative diseases may involve the kidney diffusely, covering entire nephrons and nephron segments. In such conditions the normal functions of the nephron are disrupted, and nutritional disturbances in the metabolism of protein, electrolytes, and water follow. The main function disrupted in these diseases is that of filtration and reabsorption. Several of these diseases are given here as representative of such conditions. These include acute glomerulonephritis, the nephrotic syndrome, and chronic renal failure.

Acute glomerulonephritis

Usually some streptococcal infection has preceded and is related to the onset of glomerulonephritis. It has a more or less sudden onset, and after a brief course in the majority of cases, especially among children, recovery is complete. In others the disease may progress or become latent only to develop later into chronic glomerulonephritis. The disease process involves primarily the glomeruli. As a result of loss of glomerular function, specifically filtration function, degeneration of the tubules adjoining follows.

Clinical symptoms. Classic symptoms include blood and protein in the urine and varying degrees of edema, hypertension, and renal insufficiency. Oliguria (diminished urine output) or anuria (no urine output) may occur because of acute or chronic renal failure.

Diet therapy

PROTEIN. Controversy exists concerning the use of a low-protein diet. Studies seem to indicate, however, that no advantage is found in restricting protein. In short-term acute cases in children, pediatricians and nutritionists in general favor overall optimum nutrition with adequate protein unless renal failure develops. This complication usually lasts no more than 2 or 3 days and is managed by conservative treatment.

SODIUM. Salt also is not restricted unless complications of edema, hypertension, or renal output become dangerous. In such cases a 500 to 1,000 mg. sodium diet may be used (pp. 256 to 258). In most patients, especially children with acute poststreptococcal glomerulonephritis, diet modifications are not crucial. Treatment centers mainly on bed rest and drugs. The diet should simply be an optimum one, including basic nutrition for healing.

WATER. Water intake should be adjusted to output as a rule, including losses in vomiting or diarrhea. During periods of diminished urine output the intake of water may be only 500 to 700 ml. a day.

Nephrotic syndrome

The primary degenerative defect in nephrosis is in the capillary basement membrane of the glomerulus. As this degeneration continues, the effect on the tissue is to create large enough "pores" to permit the escape of large amounts of protein into the filtrate. The subsequent tubular changes are probably secondary then to the high-protein concentration in the filtrate with some protein uptake from the tubule lumen. Thus both filtration and reabsorption functions may be disrupted in nephrosis.

Clinical symptoms. The primary symptom in nephrosis is massive albumin in the urine. Other findings include additional protein losses in the urine, including globulins and specialized binding proteins for thyroid and iron. The loss of these proteins sometimes produces signs of hypothyroidism and anemia. Blood levels of plasma proteins drop as a result of this loss, and serum cholesterol levels rise.

As the serum protein losses continue, tissue proteins are broken down in an effort to supply the body's need, and general malnutrition ensues. Fatty tissue changes in the liver, sodium retention, and edema occur. Severe fluid accumulation in the abdomen and legs may mask the gross tissue wasting that is occurring.

Diet therapy. Treatment is directed toward control of the major symptoms. These include edema, malnutrition, and massive protein losses.

PROTEIN. Replacement of the prolonged nitrogen deficit from the protein loss is a fundamental and immediate need. The plasma albumin level may have been reduced to 20% or less of its normal value. This is the major factor in causing the water retention and resultant tissue swelling. (See p. 81.) Daily protein allowances of 100 to 150 gm. or more will be needed in the diet.

CALORIES. To ensure protein use for tissue synthesis sufficient calories must always be given. High calorie intakes daily of 50 to 60 calories per kilogram of body weight are essential. Every effort must be made to ensure that the patient actually consumes the diet. His appetite is usually poor, so that much encouragement and support are needed. The food must be appetizing and in the form most easily tolerated.

SODIUM. To combat the massive edema sodium levels in the diet must be sufficiently low. Usually the 500 mg. sodium diet (pp. 256 to 258) is satisfactory to help initiate diuresis.

The dietary management is similar to that given for hepatitis (pp. 218 and 219), with even more need for sodium restriction. Use of low-sodium milk is indicated to help maintain the desired high-protein intake and yet restrict sodium to the more severe levels.

Chronic renal failure—uremia

Progressive degenerative changes in renal tissue bring marked depression of all renal functions. Eventually few functioning nephrons may remain, and these slowly deteriorate. Uremia is the term given the symptom complex of advanced renal insufficiency. Although the name derives from the common finding of elevated blood urea levels, the symptoms result not so much from uremia concentrations per se as from disturbances in acid-base balance and in fluid and electrolyte metabolism and from accumulation of other obscure toxic substances not clearly identified.

Clinical symptoms. Individual patients vary in degree of symptoms. Each one must be managed according to individual laboratory test indications of renal function. Usually anemia, weakness, loss of weight, and hypertension are present. Sometimes aching and pain in bones and joints occur. Later signs of progressive illness include skin, oral, and gastrointestinal bleeding caused by increased capillary fragility; muscle twitching; uremic convulsions; Cheyne-Stokes respiration (an irregular, cyclic type of breathing); ulceration of the mouth; and fetid breath. Resistance to infection is low.

Diet therapy

TREATMENT OBJECTIVES. Treatment aims at correction of individual nutrient imbalances according to the progression of the illness and the patient's response to the treatment being used. In general, however, overall treatment has several basic objectives:

1. To reduce and minimize protein breakdown
2. To avoid dehydration or overhydration
3. To correct acidosis carefully
4. To correct electrolyte depletions and avoid excesses
5. To control fluid and electrolyte losses from vomiting and diarrhea
6. To maintain nutrition and weight
7. To maintain appetite and morale
8. To control complications such as hypertension, bone pain, and central nervous system abnormalities

GENERAL PROTEIN AND ELECTROLYTE CONTROL. The knotty problem is to provide sufficient protein to prevent tissue protein breakdown, yet avoid an excess that would elevate urea levels. A number of years ago Borst, an English physician, proposed a nonprotein, nonpotassium plan composed of butter, sugar, and cornstarch, served as soup, pudding, or butterballs. However, the diet is drastic and intolerable and is rarely administered except in extreme cases.

With more recent advances in the use of hemodialysis, some kidney treatment centers have outlined a more liberal moderate-protein intake for their patients undergoing di-

Table 20-1. Basic pattern for a controlled protein, sodium, and potassium diet*

FOOD	PROTEIN (GM.)	SODIUM (MG.)	POTASSIUM (MG.)	CALORIES	WATER (ML.)
Breakfast					
Scrambled egg (1 medium)	6.0	61.0	64.5	80	36.9
Puffed wheat (1 oz. or substitute from cereal list)	4.0	1.1	95.2	102	1.0
Whole milk (⅓ cup)	3.0	40.5	117.1	53	71.1
Unsalted bread (1 slice)	2.0	5.2	7.2	60	8.2
Unsalted butter (2 tsp.)		7.6	3.2	70	2.2
Jam or preserves (1 tbsp. or substitute from sweets list)		2.4	17.6	54	5.8
Noon meal					
Roast beef (3 oz. or substitute from meat list)	22.0	51.0	314.5	245	46.5
Green beans, low-sodium canned (½ cup or substitute from vegetable list)	1.5	2.0	95.0	25	58.3
Rice, cooked (½ cup or substitute from rice list)	1.7	0.5	23.5	92	60.9
Unsalted bread (1 slice)	2.0	5.2	7.2	60	8.2
Unsalted butter (2 tsp.)		7.6	3.2	70	2.2
Jelly (1 tbsp. or substitute from sweets list)		3.4	15.0	55	5.8
Apricots, canned (4 halves or substitute from fruit list)	0.4	0.6	142.7	52	46.9
Evening meal					
Broiled chicken (3 oz. substitute from meat list)	20.0	56.0	233.0	185	60.4
Mixed vegetables, frozen (½ cup or substitute from vegetable list)	2.4	40.5	146.0	48	63.2
Unsalted bread (1 slice)	2.0	5.2	7.2	60	8.2
Unsalted butter (2 tsp.)		7.6	3.2	70	2.2
Apple, fresh (1 2 in. diameter or substitute from fruit list)	0.2	1.0	110.0	70	126.6
Sugar (6 tsp.)		0.2	0.4	92	Trace
Fat, cooking (4 tbsp.)				442	
Total	67.2	298.6	1,405.7	1,985	614.6

*From Jordan, W. L., Cimino, J. E., Grist, A. C., McMahon, G. E., and Doyle, M. M.: Basic pattern for a controlled protein, sodium, and potassium diet, J. Am. Diet. Assoc. **50:**138, 1967.

Table 20-2. Food exchange lists for use with controlled protein, sodium, and potassium diet*

FOOD	PROTEIN (GM.)	SODIUM (MG.)	POTASSIUM (MG.)	WATER (ML.)
Meat list—two items daily				
Beef				
Ground, commercial (2 oz.)	14.0	26.7	255.1	30.4
Loin roast (3 oz.)	20.0	51.0	314.5	37.3
Pot roast (3 oz.)	22.0	51.0	314.5	46.5
Rib roast (3 oz.)	17.0	51.0	314.5	34.0
Cheese, low-sodium dietetic (2 oz.)	17.0	7.0	17.5	22.5
Chicken				
Broiled (3 oz.)†	20.0	56.0	233.0	60.4
Dark meat, boned, no skin (2½ oz.)	22.0	62.3	233.8	45.1
White meat, no skin (2 oz.)	18.01	38.4	244.9	38.2
Lamb				
Leg roast (3 oz.)	20.0	59.5	246.5	42.8
Loin chops, without bone (3 oz.)	16.5	58.5	243.6	35.0
Shoulder roast (3 oz.)	18.0	59.5	246.5	39.3
Perch, breaded (3 oz.)†	17.0	57.8	195.5	50.0
Pork				
Chops, without bone (2½ oz.)	16.0	45.5	272.9	29.4
Roast (2 oz.)	13.0	36.6	221.3	25.3
Turkey roast (2 oz.)	17.4	42.0	147.0	31.0
Veal roast or cutlet (2 oz.)	15.0	45.3	283.3	32.9
Vegetable list—two items daily				
Asparagus				
Canned, low-sodium (1½ oz.)	1.3	1.5	79.5	39.3
Fresh (1½ oz.)	0.9	0.4	80.0	39.3
Frozen (1½ oz.)	1.4	0.4	96.3	38.9
Beans				
Green, canned, low-sodium (½ cup)	1.5	2.0	95.0	58.3
Lima, canned, low-sodium (¼ cup)	2.3	1.6	88.8	30.2
Beets				
Canned, low-sodium (½ cup)	0.7	37.9	138.0	74.1
Fresh, cooked (¼ cup)	0.5	17.8	85.8	37.5
Broccoli, fresh, cooked (¼ cup)	1.2	3.8	100.0	34.2
Brussels sprouts				
Fresh, cooked (¼ cup)	1.4	3.3	88.5	28.7
Frozen (¼ cup)	1.1	4.5	96.5	29.0
Cabbage				
Cooked (½ cup)†	0.9	11.0	128.0	90.2
Raw (½ cup)	0.7	10.0	117.0	46.0
Carrots				
Canned, low-sodium (½ cup)	0.6	28.3	87.0	67.4
Fresh, cooked (¼ cup)	0.4	11.9	81.0	33.1
Raw (half, 1 oz.)	0.3	11.7	85.5	24.7
Cauliflower				
Fresh, cooked (½ cup)	1.4	5.4	124.0	55.7
Frozen (½ cup)	1.1	6.0	124.0	56.4
Celery (1 stalk, 8 × 1½ in.)	0.4	50.4	136.0	37.6

*From Jordan, W. L., Cimino, J. E., Grist, A. C., McMahon, G. E., and Doyle, M. M.: Basic pattern for a controlled protein, sodium and potassium diet, J. Am. Diet. Assoc. 50:138, 1967.
†If these items (highest in fluid in each list) are selected, fluid intake for the day will be approximately 1,000 ml.

Continued.

Table 20-2. Food exchange lists for use with controlled protein, sodium, and potassium diet—cont'd

FOOD	PROTEIN (GM.)	SODIUM (MG.)	POTASSIUM (MG.)	WATER (ML.)
Vegetable list—select two items daily—cont'd				
Corn, fresh, cooked (¼ cup)	2.1	Trace	105.5	48.9
Cucumber, raw (1½ oz.)	0.3	3.1	82.4	40.9
Endive or escarole (1 oz.)	0.5	3.9	83.7	26.5
Kale, fresh, cooked (½ cup)	2.5	23.6	121.5	50.1
Lettuce (⅛ head, 1 oz.)	0.2	2.5	48.1	26.3
Mixed vegetables, frozen (½ cup)	2.4	40.5	146.0	63.2
Okra				
Fresh (8 pods, 3 oz.)	1.7	1.7	147.9	77.4
Frozen (8 pods, 3 oz.)	1.9	1.7	139.4	75.1
Onions, mature, cooked (½ cup)†	1.3	7.4	115.5	96.4
Peas				
Early June, canned, low-sodium (¼ cup)	3.0	1.9	60.0	50.1
Fresh (¼ cup)	2.2	0.4	78.4	32.6
Frozen (¼ cup)	2.0	46.0	54.0	32.8
Spinach, fresh, cooked (¼ cup)	1.3	22.5	146.0	41.4
Squash				
Summer, fresh, cooked (¼ cup)	0.5	0.5	74.0	50.1
Winter, fresh, cooked (¼ cup)	0.6	0.5	132.3	46.2
Tomatoes				
Canned, low-sodium (¼ cup)	0.6	1.8	131.5	56.9
Raw (¼ of 2 × 2½ in.)	0.4	1.2	91.5	35.1
Turnips, fresh, cooked (½ cup)	0.6	26.0	145.7	73.0
Fruit list—two items daily				
Apples				
Juice, canned (⅓ cup)	0.1	0.7	77.1	73.0
Raw (1 small, 2-in. diameter)†	0.2	1.0	110.0	126.6
Apricots, canned, heavy syrup (4 halves)	0.4	0.6	142.7	46.9
Blackberries				
Canned, heavy syrup (½ cup)	1.0	1.3	136.0	92.6
Raw (½ cup)	0.9	0.7	122.4	60.8
Blueberries				
Canned, heavy syrup (½ cup)	0.5	1.3	68.8	72.3
Raw (½ cup)	0.5	0.7	56.7	58.2
Cherries				
Raw, sweet or sour (½ cup)	0.7	1.1	108.8	45.8
Royal Ann, canned, heavy syrup (¼ cup)	0.6	0.6	78.1	48.4
Grapefruit sections, syrup pack (¼ cup)	0.4	0.6	84.0	50.5
Grapes				
Juice, canned (⅓ cup)	0.4	0.8	134.5	70.5
Juice (½ cup)	1.0	2.3	120.9	62.4
Peach, raw (1 small, 2 in. diameter)	0.3	0.6	115.0	101.6
Pears				
Canned (2 halves)	0.2	1.2	98.3	93.4
Raw (1 small, 3 × 2½ in.)†	0.6	1.8	118.0	151.4
Pineapple				
Canned, heavy syrup (2 slices)	0.4	1.2	117.0	97.5
Juice, canned (⅓ cup)	0.3	0.7	110.8	71.4
Raw (½ cup)	0.3	0.7	102.0	59.7

Table 20-2. Food exchange lists for use with controlled protein, sodium, and potassium diet—cont'd

FOOD	PROTEIN (GM.)	SODIUM (MG.)	POTASSIUM (MG.)	WATER (ML.)
Fruit list—two items daily—cont'd				
Plums				
Greengage, raw (½ cup)	0.5	1.3	105.0	99.1
Other than Damson (1 raw, 2-in. diameter)	0.3	0.6	102.0	51.9
Raisins, dried, seedless (2 tbsp.)	0.4	4.0	144.0	1.8
Raspberries				
Black, raw (½ cup)	0.9	0.6	123.0	50.1
Red, raw (½ cup)	0.7	0.6	104.0	50.1
Strawberries				
Frozen (2½ oz.)	0.3	0.7	74.0	49.9
Raw (½ cup)	0.5	0.7	122.2	66.9
Tangerine (1 small, 2½ in. diameter, 5 oz.)	0.9	2.3	144.0	99.2
Cereal list—one item daily				
Corn grits, cooked (1 cup)†	3.0		26.6	210.8
Cornflakes (½ oz.)	1.0	140.5	16.8	0.5
Farina, enriched, uncooked, unsalted (1 oz.)	3.4	0.6	24.9	23.4
Oatmeal, cooked, unsalted (¾ cup)	3.4	0.5	84.5	152.2
Puffed wheat, low-sodium (1 oz.)	4.0	1.1	95.2	0.9
Shredded Wheat, low-sodium (1 oz.)	3.0	0.8	97.4	1.8
Rice list—one item daily				
Macaroni, cooked, unsalted (½ cup)	2.5	0.7	42.7	50.4
Noodles, cooked, unsalted (½ cup)	3.5	1.6	35.2	56.3
Rice, cooked, unsalted (½ cup)	1.7	0.5	23.5	60.9
Spaghetti, cooked, unsalted (½ cup)†	2.5	0.7	42.7	82.8
Sweets list—two items daily				
Cookie, plain, assorted (one)	1.0	91.0	16.8	1.6
Honey (1 tbsp.)†	Trace	1.0	10.7	3.6
Jams or preserves (1 tbsp.)†	Trace	2.4	17.6	5.8
Jelly (1 tbsp.)†	0	3.4	15.0	5.8
Sugar, powdered (¼ cup)	0	0.3	0.9	Trace

alysis for chronic uremia. Such a diet plan is given in Table 20-1. Basic food exchange lists for use with this diet plan are given in Table 20-2.

Individual patient adjustments may be made from such a plan. For example, salt may be added if increased sodium chloride is needed. Protein food allowances may be decreased and low-protein bread used if less protein is desired. Carbohydrate foods may be increased if added calories and a protein-sparing effect is required. The intake of the major electrolytes, sodium and potassium, as well as water, is carefully controlled according to individual kidney function and laboratory tests of each item. Thus careful records of total water intake and output are necessary.

A summary of the average dietary needs in chronic renal failure includes the following:

1. Protein—30 to 70 gm.
2. Carbohydrate—300 to 400 gm.
3. Fat—70 to 90 gm.
4. Calories—2,000 to 2,500
5. Sodium—400 to 2,000 mg. (4 gm. salt)
6. Potassium—1,300 to 1,900 mg.

THE LOW-PROTEIN–ESSENTIAL AMINO ACID

Food plan for the modified Giordano-Giovannetti diet

1 egg

6 oz. milk or one additional egg

Low-protein bread (one loaf), approximately ½ lb., 650 calories, and 1.5 gm. protein

Fruit—two to four servings

Vegetables—two to four servings

Fruit and vegetable choices to total 3 to 12 gm. of protein and 1,300 to 1,900 mg. of potassium

Free-food list—use as desired for extra calories; this list includes food containing little or no protein, such as butter, oil, jelly, honey; condiments such as herbs and spices; beverages such as tea, coffee, Sanka, carbonated beverages, hard candy, sugar, cornstarch, tapioca, etc.

Nutrient supplements as prescribed; these may contain an amino acid supplement—formula of minimum adult requirements of essential amino acids or only 0.5 gm. methionine if additional food source is given in milk and eggs, a multivitamin supplement, and an iron supplement

---

DIET (MODIFIED GIORDANO-GIOVANNETTI REGIMEN). The separate work of the two Italian physicians Carmelo Giordano at the University of Naples and Sergio Giovannetti at the University of Pisa has given an encouraging dietary base to sustain patients with uremia and alleviate many of their difficult symptoms. The basis of the diet is the principle of feeding only essential amino acids to fulfill the extremely low-protein restriction of about 20 gm. This causes the body to use its own excess urea nitrogen to synthesize the nonessential amino acids needed for tissue protein production.

The foods used in various clinical settings in different countries to fulfill the diet principle relate to cultural food choices. The general features of the food plan developed for use in the United States for the modified Giordano-Giovannetti diet is given above. The animal sources of protein in the food plan, one egg and 6 ounces of milk, supply minimal requirements of all the essential amino acids except methionine; thus an amino acid supplement, especially of methionine, is generally also used with the diet. Practical diet plans, food exchange lists, recipes, and food preparation suggestions have helped to make the diet useful in the home situation.*

---

*For a detailed outline of the modified Giovannetti diet, including a basic food plan and food exchange lists, consult Williams, S. R.: Nutrition and diet therapy, ed. 2, St. Louis, 1973, The C. V. Mosby Co., pp. 563-567.

Careful instruction must be given the patient and his family, with much follow-up, help, and support to carry out the plan in a practical manner.

The diet has been effective with a number of patients in reducing the clinical symptoms. Blood urea concentrations decrease, nitrogen balance becomes positive, and clinical symptoms such as loss of appetite, vomiting, fatigue, and muscle twitching disappear or improve. The diet has effectively reduced the production of protein breakdown materials and prevented wastage of the body protein. A number of patients have been able to return to their usual work situations while awaiting further dialysis treatments or kidney transplants.

RENAL CALCULI
Causes

Although the basic cause of kidney stones is unknown, many factors contribute directly or indirectly to their formation. These factors relate to the nature of the urine itself or to the conditions of the urinary tract environment.

Concentration of urinary constituents

CALCIUM. By far the majority of kidney stones—about 96%—are composed of calcium compounds. These compounds may combine calcium with phosphorus or with oxalate. Excessive urinary calcium may result from prolonged use of high-calcium foods such as milk and dairy products, from alkali therapy for peptic ulcer, or from continued use of a hard water supply. In addition, excess vitamin D may cause increased calcium absorption from the intestine, as well as increased calcium withdrawal from the bone. Prolonged immobilization such as occurs in body casting, long-term illness, or disability may lead to withdrawal of bone calcium and increase concentrations in the urine (p. 66). Excessive activity of the parathyroid gland may also cause excess excretion of both calcium and phosphorus.

URIC ACID. Excess uric acid excretion may be caused by increased breakdown of purines as in gout. Purines are nucleoproteins found in a number of animal protein sources, espe-cially organ meats. Excess uric acid may also result from rapid breakdown of tissue protein, such as in wasting diseases. It may also occur with prolonged use of fad diets for weight control that recommend high intakes of protein and restrictive amounts of carbohydrates.

CYSTINE. Cystine is an amino acid that accumulates in the urine because of a hereditary metabolic defect in the renal tubular reabsorption of the acid. This accumulation in the urine is a condition called cystinuria.

Urinary tract conditions. Several physical changes in the urine may predispose susceptible persons to stone formation. These include a concentration of urine resulting from a reduced water intake or from excess water loss

---

Low-calcium diet (approximately 400 mg. calcium)

	FOODS ALLOWED	FOODS NOT ALLOWED
Beverages*	Carbonated, coffee, tea	Chocolate flavored drinks, milk, milk drinks
Bread	White and light rye bread or crackers	Dark breads
Cereals	Refined	Oatmeal, whole grain cereals
Desserts	Cake, cookies, gelatin, pastries, pudding, sherbets, all made without chocolate, milk, or nuts; if egg yolk is used, it must be from 1 egg allowance	
Fat	Butter, cream, 2 tbsp. daily; French dressing, margarine, salad oil, shortening	Butter and cream, except in amounts allowed, mayonnaise
Fruit	Canned, cooked, or fresh fruit or juice except rhubarb	Dried fruit, rhubarb
Meat, eggs	8 oz. daily of any meat, fowl, or fish except clams, oysters, or shrimp; not more than 1 egg daily, including those used in cooking	Clams, oysters, shrimp, cheese
Potato or substitute	Potato, hominy, macaroni, noodles, refined rice, spaghetti	Whole grain rice
Soup	Broth, vegetable soup made from allowed vegetables	Bean or pea soup, cream or milk soups
Sweets	Honey, jam, jelly, sugar	
Vegetables	Any canned, cooked, or fresh vegetables or juice except those listed	Dried beans, broccoli, green cabbage, celery, chard, collards, endive, greens, lettuce, lentils, okra, parsley, parsnips, dried peas, rutabagas
Miscellaneous	Herbs, pickles, popcorn, relishes, salt, spices, vinegar	Chocolate, cocoa, milk gravy, nuts, olives, white sauce

*Depending on calcium content of local water supply; in instances of high-calcium content, distilled water may be indicated.

Low-calcium test diet (200 mg. calcium)

	GM.	MG. CALCIUM
BREAKFAST		
Orange juice, fresh	100	19.00
Bread (toasted), white	25	19.57
Butter	15	3.00
Rice Krispies	15	3.70
Cream, 20% butterfat	35	33.95
Sugar	7	0.00
Jam	20	2.00
Distilled water, coffee, or tea*		0.00
		81.22
LUNCH		
Beefsteak, cooked	100	10.00
Potato	100	11.00
Tomatoes	100	11.00
Bread	25	19.57
Butter	15	3.00
Honey	20	1.00
Applesauce	20	1.00
Distilled water, coffee, or tea		0.00
		56.57
DINNER		
Lamb chop, cooked	90	10.00
Potato	100	11.00
Frozen green peas	80	10.32
Bread	25	19.57
Butter	15	3.00
Jam	20	2.00
Peach sauce	100	5.00
Distilled water, coffee, or tea		0.00
		60.89
Total		198.68 mg. calcium

*Use distilled water only for cooking and for beverages.

Food sources of oxalates

FRUITS	VEGETABLES
Currants	Beans, green and wax
Concord grapes	Beets
Figs	Beet greens
Gooseberries	Chard
Plums	Endive
Raspberries	Okra
Rhubarb	Spinach
	Sweet potatoes
	Tomatoes

NUTS	BEVERAGES
Almonds	Chocolate
Cashews	Cocoa
	Tea

Low-purine diet (approximately 125 mg. purine)

GENERAL DIRECTIONS
1. During acute stages use only list 1
2. After acute stage subsides and for chronic conditions use the following schedule:
   a. Two days a week but not consecutively use list 1 entirely
   b. The remaining days add foods from lists 2 and 3 as indicated
   c. Avoid list 4 entirely
3. Keep diet moderately low in fat

TYPICAL MEAL PATTERN

BREAKFAST	LUNCH	DINNER
Fruit	Egg or cheese dish	Egg or cheese dish
Refined cereal and/or egg	Vegetables as allowed	Cream of vegetable soup
White toast	(cooked or in salad)	if desired
Butter, 1 tsp.	Potato or substitute	Starch (potato or substitute)
Sugar	White bread	Colored vegetable as allowed
Coffee	Butter, 1 tsp.	White bread and butter,
Milk if desired	Fruit or simple dessert	1 tsp. if desired
	Milk	Salad as allowed
		Fruit or simple dessert
		Milk

FOOD LIST 1—THE FOLLOWING CONTAIN AN INSIGNIFICANT AMOUNT OF PURINES
AND MAY BE USED AS DESIRED

Beverages
  Carbonated
  Chocolate
  Cocoa
  Coffee
  Fruit juices
  Postum
  Tea
Butter*
Breads—white and crackers, corn bread
Cereals and cereal products
  Corn
  Rice
  Tapioca
  Refined wheat
  Macaroni
  Noodles
Cheese of all kinds*
Eggs
Fats of all kinds* (moderate amount)
Fruits of all kinds
Gelatin, Jell-O
Milk—buttermilk, evaporated, malted, sweet
Nuts of all kinds*
  Peanut butter*
Pies* (except mincemeat)
Sugar and sweets
Vegetables
  Artichokes
  Beets
  Beet greens

Vegetables—cont'd
  Broccoli
  Brussels sprouts
  Cabbage
  Carrots
  Celery
  Corn
  Cucumber
  Eggplant
  Endive
  Kohlrabi
Lettuce
  Okra
Parsnips
Potato—white and sweet
Pumpkin
  Rutabagas
  Sauerkraut
  String beans
  Summer squash
  Swiss chard
  Tomato
  Turnips

*High in fat.

Low-purine diet (approximately 125 mg. purine)—cont'd

FOOD LIST 2—ONE ITEM FOUR TIMES A WEEK: FOODS THAT CONTAIN A MODERATE AMOUNT (UP TO 75 MG.) OF PURINE IN 100 GM. SERVING

Asparagus	Herring	Oysters
Bluefish	Kidney beans	Peas
Bouillon	Lima beans	Salmon
Cauliflower	Lobster	Shad
Chicken	Mushrooms	Spinach
Crab	Mutton	Tripe
Finnan haddie	Navy beans	Tuna fish
Ham	Oatmeal	Whitefish

FOOD LIST 3—ONE ITEM ONCE A WEEK: FOODS THAT CONTAIN A LARGE AMOUNT (75 TO 150 MG.) OF PURINE IN 100 GM. SERVING

Bacon	Lentils	Quail
Beef	Liver sausage	Rabbit
Calf tongue	Meat soups	Sheep
Carp	Partridge	Shellfish
Chicken soup	Perch	Squab
Codfish	Pheasant	Trout
Duck	Pigeon	Turkey
Goose	Pike	Veal
Halibut	Pork	Venison

FOOD LIST 4—AVOID ENTIRELY: FOODS THAT CONTAIN LARGE AMOUNTS (150 TO 1,000 MG.) OF PURINE IN 100 GM. SERVING

Sweetbreads	825 mg.
Anchovies	363 mg.
Sardines (in oil)	295 mg.
Liver (calf, beef)	233 mg.
Kidneys (beef)	200 mg.
Brains	195 mg.
Meat extracts	160 to 400 mg.
Gravies	Variable

such as that occurring in prolonged sweating, fever, vomiting, or diarrhea. Sometimes persons exposed to hot temperatures or climates for prolonged periods may suffer from such a concentration of urine. Also the degree of urine acidity may change to a more acid or a more alkaline state. These changes may be influenced by diet or altered by the ingestion of acid or alkaline medication.

Changes in the epithelial tissue of the urinary tract may also provide a nucleus for the formation of stones. These include bacterial masses from recurrent urinary tract infections and degeneration of tissue caused by vitamin A deficiency.

Clinical symptoms

Severe pain and numerous urinary symptoms may result. General weakness and sometimes fever occur. Laboratory examination of the urine and chemical analysis of any stone that is passed help to determine treatment.

Principles of diet therapy

Fluid intake. A large fluid intake produces a more dilute urine and helps to prevent concentration of the stone constituents.

Elements of stone composition

CALCIUM STONES. A low-calcium diet of about 400 mg. daily is usually given. This is about half that of an average adult intake of 800

Acid and alkaline ash food groups

ACID ASH	ALKALINE ASH	NEUTRAL
Meat	Milk	Sugars
Whole grains	Vegetables	Fats
Eggs	Fruit (except	Beverages (coffee and tea)
Cheese	cranberries,	
Cranberries	prunes, and plums)	
Prunes		
Plums		

Acid ash diet

The purpose of this diet is to furnish a well-balanced diet in which the total acid ash is greater than the total alkaline ash each day. It lists the following:

   I. Unrestricted foods
   II. Restricted foods
   III. Foods not allowed
   IV. Sample of a day's diet

I. UNRESTRICTED FOODS; YOU MAY EAT ALL YOU WANT OF THE FOLLOWING FOODS:
1. Breads: any, preferably whole grain; crackers, rolls
2. Cereals: any, preferably whole grain
3. Desserts: angle food or sunshine cake; cookies made without baking powder or soda; cornstarch pudding, cranberry desserts, custards, gelatin, ice cream, sherbet, plum or prune desserts; rice or tapioca pudding
4. Fats: any, such as butter, margarine, salad dressings, Crisco, Spry, lard, salad oils, olive oil, etc.
5. Fruits: cranberries, plums, prunes
6. Meat, egg, cheese; any meat, fish, or fowl, two servings daily; at least one egg daily
7. Potato substitutes: corn, hominy, lentils, macaroni, noodles, rice, spaghetti, vermicelli
8. Soup: broth as desired; other soups from foods allowed
9. Sweets: cranberry or plum jelly; sugar, plain sugar candy
10. Miscellaneous: cream sauce, gravy, peanut butter, peanuts, popcorn, salt, spices, vinegar, walnuts

II. RESTRICTED FOODS: DO NOT EAT ANY MORE THAN THE AMOUNT ALLOWED EACH DAY
1. Milk: 1 pt. daily (may be used other than as beverage)
2. Cream: ⅓ cup or less daily
3. Fruits: one serving daily (in addition to those listed previously); certain fruits listed below are not allowed at any time
4. Vegetables, including potato: two servings daily; certain vegetables listed below are not allowed at any time

III. FOODS NOT ALLOWED
1. Carbonated beverages, as ginger ale, Coca Cola, root beer
2. Cake or cookies made with baking powder or soda
3. Fruits: dried apricots, bananas, dates, figs, raisins, rhubarb
4. Vegetables: dried beans, beet greens, dandelion greens, carrots, chard, lima beans
5. Sweets: chocolate or candies other than those in group I; syrups
6. Miscellaneous: other nuts, olives, pickles

IV. SAMPLE MENU

BREAKFAST	LUNCH	DINNER
Grapefruit	Creamed chicken	Broth
Wheatena	Steamed rice	Roast beef, gravy
Scrambled eggs	Green beans	Buttered noodles
Toast, butter, plum jam	Bread, butter	Sliced tomato
Coffee, cream, sugar	Stewed prunes	Mayonnaise
	Milk	Bread, butter
		Vanilla ice cream

Summary of diet therapy principles in renal stone disease		
STONE CHEMISTRY	NUTRIENT MODIFICATION	DIETARY ASH (URINARY pH)
Calcium	Low calcium (400 mg.)	Acid ash Acid ash
phosphate	Low phosphorus (1,000 to 1,200 mg.)	
oxalate	Low oxalate	
Uric acid	Low purine	Alkaline ash
Cystine	Low methionine	Alkaline ash

mg. This lower level of calcium intake may be achieved mainly by a removal of milk and dairy products. An outline for such a low-calcium diet is given on p. 273. Sometimes a test diet of only 200 mg. of calcium may be used to rule out hyperparathyroidism as a causative factor (p. 274).

In addition to calcium restriction, the material composing the calcium compound would also be restricted. For example, if the stone is of calcium oxalate composition, food sources of oxalates are also eliminated. A list of such foods is given on p. 274. If the stone is of calcium phosphate composition, foods high in phosphorus are also curtailed. Since the major food sources of phosphorus are the same as those for calcium, the low-calcium diet usually suffices with one added restriction. Meat is the other major source of phosphorus. Thus it would have to be curtailed in quantity.

URIC ACID STONES. About 4% of total kidney stones are uric acid stones. Since uric acid is a metabolic product of purines, dietary control of purines is indicated. Purines are found in active tissues such as glandular meat, other lean meat, meat extractives, and, in lesser amounts, in plant sources such as whole grains and legumes. A low-purine diet is outlined on pp. 275 and 276.

CYSTINE STONES. About 1% of the total stones produced are cystine. Their occurrence is relatively rare. Cystine is a nonessential amino acid produced from the essential amino acid methionine; thus a diet low in methionine is used. Since methionine is an essential amino acid, it is found mainly in the complete protein foods—milk, meat, and eggs. Thus the low-methionine diet restricts meat to 2 oz. daily and eliminates milk (soy milk is substituted) and eggs.

Urinary acidity. An attempt to control the solubility factor is made by changing the urinary pH to an increased acidity or alkalinity, depending on the chemical composition of the stone formed. For example, since calcium stones have an alkaline chemistry, an acid ash diet may also be used to create a urinary environment less conducive to precipitation of the basic stone elements. On the other hand, since uric acid stones and cystine stones are both of acid composition, an alkaline ash diet would be used for the same purpose. A listing of foods leaving an acid ash and foods leaving an alkaline ash are given on p. 277. An acid ash diet applying these food groups is shown on the same page. Cranberry juice seems to have a urinary acidifying effect or bacteriostatic value and is frequently used as a dietary adjunct.

A summary of the diet therapy principles in renal stone disease is given above for review.

CHAPTER 21 NUTRITIONAL CARE OF A SURGERY PATIENT

Surgery places great physiologic and psychologic stress on the body. Nutritional demands are greatly increased. Deficiencies can easily develop and sooner or later lead to serious clinical problems. Thus careful attention to preoperative preparation of the patient and to his postoperative therapeutic needs reduces complications and provides resources for better wound healing and a more rapid recovery.

PREOPERATIVE NUTRITIONAL CARE
Nutrient stores

When time permits, in cases of elective surgery rather than emergency situations, nutritional preparation of the patient for surgery should correct any nutrient deficiencies that exist. The diet should also provide optimum reserves for the period of surgery itself and for the time immediately afterward, when no oral feedings can be taken. These nutrient stores particularly demand protein, calories, vitamins, and minerals.

Protein. The most common nutritional deficiency in surgical patients is that of protein. Tissue and plasma reserves are imperative to fortify the patient for blood losses during surgery and for tissue breakdown in the immediate postoperative period.

Calories. If protein is to be used for its building purposes, sufficient nonprotein calories must always be provided for energy demands. If underweight is present to any degree, sufficient extra calories have to be provided to build the weight up to maintenance level. Glycogen stores in the liver are necessary to spare protein for tissue synthesis. If the patient is overweight, some weight reduction is indicated to reduce surgical risk.

Vitamins and minerals. Tissue stores of vitamins are needed for the added metabolism of carbohydrates and proteins. Any deficiency state such as anemia should be corrected. Electrolytes and fluids should be in balance and correction made of any dehydration acidosis or alkalosis.

Immediate preoperative period

In the usual preparation for surgery, nothing is given by mouth for at least 8 hours prior to surgery. This assures that the stomach has no retained food at the time of the operation. Food in the stomach may be vomited and aspirated during anesthesia or recovery from it. Also any food present may increase the possibility of postoperative gastric retention or expansion or interfere with the surgical procedure itself.

If the surgery is of an emergency nature, no time is available for building up nutritional reserves. This is all the more reason for maintaining an optimum nutrient reserve supply constantly through an optimum daily diet.

POSTOPERATIVE NUTRITIONAL CARE
Nutritional demands for healing

Therapeutic nutrition becomes all the more significant as a means of aiding recovery from surgery. In surgical disease and related procedures losses are greatly increased, whereas at the same time replacement from food is diminished or even absent for a period of time. Several nutrients demand particular attention.

Protein. Adequate protein intake in the postoperative recovery period is of primary therapeutic concern to replace losses and supply increased demands. A negative nitrogen balance of as much as 20 gm. a day may occur. This represents an actual loss of tissue protein of over a pound a day. In addition to protein losses from tissue breakdown, added loss of plasma proteins occurs through hemorrhage, wound bleeding, and exudates. Increased metabolic losses of protein result also from extensive tissue destruction and inflammation or from infection and trauma. If any degree of prior malnutrition or chronic infection existed, the patient's protein deficit may actually become severe and cause serious complications. There are a number of reasons for this increased protein demand.

TISSUE SYNTHESIS IN WOUND HEALING. Tissue protein can only be synthesized by essential amino acids brought to the tissue by the circulating blood. The eight essential amino acids (p. 30) must come either from diet protein or by intravenous injection. Tissue protein deficiencies are best met by oral feedings. As early as possible an intake of 100 to 200 gm. daily should be attempted to restore lost protein tissues and synthesize new tissue at the wound site.

AVOIDANCE OF SHOCK. A reduction in blood volume, a loss of plasma protein, and a decrease in circulating red blood cell volume contribute to the potential danger of shock. When protein deficiencies exist, this danger is enhanced.

CONTROL OF EDEMA. When the serum protein level is low, edema develops as a result of the loss of the colloidal osmotic pressure required to maintain the normal shift of fluid between the capillaries and the surrounding interstitial tissues (p. 83). This general edema may affect heart and lung action. Local edema at the surgical site also delays closure of the wound and hinders normal healing processes.

BONE HEALING. In orthopedic surgery in which extensive bone healing is involved, protein is essential for proper callus formation and calcification. A sound protein matrix is mandatory for the anchoring of mineral matter to form bone tissue.

RESISTANCE TO INFECTION. Amino acids are necessary constituents of the proteins involved in body defense mechanisms. These defense agents include antigens, antibodies, blood cells, hormones, and enzymes. Tissue integrity itself is a defense barrier against infection.

LIPID TRANSPORT. Proteins are necessary for the transport of lipids in the body and therefore for the protection of the liver (p. 18). The liver is a main site of fat metabolism. Protein present in the liver to combine with fat helps convert the fat and remove it from the liver, thus avoiding the danger of fatty infiltration. Protein provides essential lipotropic agents to form lipoproteins, the transport form of fat in the body.

It is evident, therefore, that multiple clinical problems may easily develop when protein deficiences exist. There may be poor wound healing and rupture of suture lines (dehiscence), delayed healing of fractures, anemia, depressed lung and heart function, reduced resistance to infection, extensive weight loss, liver damage, and increased mortality risks.

Water. Water balance is a vital concern after surgery. Adequate fluid therapy is necessary to prevent dehydration. During the postoperative period large water losses may occur from vomiting, hemorrhage, exudates, diuresis, or fever. When drainage is involved, as is common in many surgeries, there is still more fluid loss. Intravenous therapy will supply initial needs, but oral intake should begin as soon as possible and be maintained in sufficient quantity. In complicated cases or seriously ill patients cases with extensive drainage, for example, as much as 7 liters of fluid daily may be required.

Calories. As is always the case when increased protein is demanded for tissue rebuilding, sufficient nonprotein calories must be supplied for energy to protect the protein. Carbohydrate and fat must therefore be in sufficient supply in the total diet. As protein is increased, the total calories must be increased to a minimum of 2,800 calories per day before protein can be used for tissue repair and not be converted in part to provide energy. In acute stress, as in extensive radical surgery or burns, for example, when protein needs are as high as 250 gm. daily, as much as 4,000 to 6,000 calories are required. In addition to its protein-sparing action, carbohydrate also helps avoid liver damage from depletion of glycogen reserves. Fat calories must be adequate but not excessive. Excessive body fat is to be avoided, since fatty tissue heals poorly and is more susceptible to infection, hematoma, and serum collection.

Vitamins. Vitamin C is imperative for wound healing. Its presence is necessary for formation of cementing material in the ground substance of connective tissue, in capillary walls, and in the building up of new tissue. Extensive tissue regeneration, such as in burns or mastectomy, may require as much as 1 gm. or more of vitamin C daily. This is about fifteen to twenty times the normal requirement. As calories and protein are increased, the B vitamins—thiamine, riboflavin, and niacin—must also be increased to provide essential coenzyme factors to metabolize the carbohydrate and protein. Other B-complex vitamins—folic acid, B_{12}, pyridoxine, and pantothenic acid—also have important metabolic roles to play in stress situations and in the formation of hemoglobin. Vitamin K is essential to the blood-clotting mechanism.

Minerals. Replacement of mineral deficiencies and continued adequacy is essential. In the destruction of tissue, potassium and phosphorus are lost. Electrolyte imbalances of sodium and chloride result from water losses. Iron-deficiency anemia may be developed from blood loss or from faulty iron absorption.

Diet management

Oral vs. intravenous feeding. In some patients the gastrointestinal tract cannot be used, and intravenous feeding is the only way to sustain the patient. In such cases solutions of hydrolyzed protein (amino acids and polypeptides) may be used. Some fat emulsions are available for intravenous therapy but are more difficult to use. However, the majority of patients can and should progress to oral feedings as soon as possible to provide adequate nutrition and to stimulate action of the gastrointestinal tract. As soon as bowel sounds return, food by mouth can be used. A comparison of the nutritive value of an intravenous solution with oral feedings will make it evident that intravenous feeding cannot supply nutrient needs. It can only compete with starvation. For example, 1 liter of a 5% dextrose solution contains 50 gm. of sugar with an energy value of 200 calories; therefore 3 liters a day which is the most that can be administered, at best can supply only 600 calories. The basal energy requirement is about 700 calories, to say nothing of the increased metabolic demand of the stress of surgical illness. Therefore a rapid return to regular eating should be encouraged and maintained.

Hyperalimentation. In cases of major tissue trauma or damage or when a patient is unable to obtain sufficient nutrients orally, hyperalimentation is used as a feeding process. This is sometimes called an "elemental diet." It provides intravenous nutritional support with more concentrated solutions of the needed nutrient elements. For example, the solution used may contain a high percentage of glucose (20% to 50%), hydrolysates of amino acids, electrolytes, minerals, and vitamins. Intravenous hyperalimentation is usually done through a cutdown in the inferior or superior vena cava because there is danger of thrombosis if the solution is injected into a peripheral vein.

Postoperative diets. As rapidly as possible the patient should progress from clear to full liquids and then to a soft or regular diet. Giving the initial liquids as soon as possible stimulates normal gastrointestinal function and an early return to a full diet. These routine house diets are given in Table 15-1 (p. 192). Individual tolerance will be the guide, but encouragement and help should be supplied to enable the patient to eat as soon as possible.

NUTRITIONAL CARE OF THE PATIENT WITH GASTROINTESTINAL SURGERY
Mouth, throat, or neck surgery

Surgery involving the mouth, throat, or neck will require a modification in the manner of feeding. The patient usually cannot chew or swallow normally.

Oral liquid feedings. Concentrated feedings in liquid form should be planned to secure sufficient nutrition in less volume of food. Protein hydrolysates and added carbohydrate can enrich such a mixture. Milk-based beverages, soups, fruit juices with lactose or other sugar, and eggnogs can supply frequent reinforced nourishment. A concentrated milk shake formula, for example, as given on p. 199, can be supplemented with skimmed-milk powder or a protein concentrate such as Casec. Such a concentrated milk shake can supply 20 gm. of protein and 400 calories.

Tube feedings. Tube feedings are indicated in cases in which the patient cannot chew or swallow normally at all. This is the case after radical neck or facial surgery or when the patient is comatose or severely debilitated. Usually a nasogastric tube is used. However, in cases of esophageal obstruction the tube is inserted into an opening made in the abdominal wall. This procedure is called a gastrostomy. The formula will be prescribed according to need and tolerance of the indi-

vidual patient, and small amounts will be given initially with a gradual increase. Usually 2 liters of formula are sufficient for a 24-hour period. Each feeding should not exceed 8 to 12 ounces in each 3- to 4-hour interval. Two general types of formula are used: prepared formula and a calculated and blended food mixture.

PREPARED FORMULA. A variety of commercial preparations are available for simple dilution with water or milk. These include nutrient materials in powdered form, such as Sustagen, a protein hydrolysate, or Lonalac, a low-sodium product. These are simple to use when mixed with water in the desired proportions. However, in the higher calorie formula requirements the amount of the nutrient material needed to fulfill the calorie requirement renders too concentrated an amount of carbohydrate. Diarrhea may result. In such cases the planned formula of balanced ingredients may provide a more desirable ratio of nutrients.

CALCULATED AND BLENDED FOOD MIXTURE. In cases in which a more desirable ratio is needed, an individual formula may be calculated and mixed in a blender. For example, a planned formula such as that given in Table 21-1 would give a 3,000-calorie tube feeding with a balanced ratio of nutrient ingredients. In comparison, a 3,000-calorie formula using Sustagen alone would require about 5 cups of this powder to 2,500 ml. of water. This would render a nutrient ratio of 180 gm. of protein, 500 gm. of carbohydrate, and 30 gm. of fat. Often this much carbohydrate causes gastrointestinal discomfort and diarrhea.

Other mixtures of food may be liquefied in a blender and sometimes are preferred by patients because they not only tolerate them better, but also they feel that they are getting regular foods. Any that will liquefy can be used, or strained baby food may be used to simplify the mixing. The usual ingredients include a milk base with additions of egg, strained meat, vegetable, fruit, fruit juice, nonfat dry milk, cream, brewer's yeast, and

Table 21-1. Sample tube feeding formula (2,500 ml., 3,000 calories)

INGREDIENTS	AMOUNT	PROTEIN	FAT	CARBOHYDRATE
Homogenized milk	1 qt.	32	40	48
Eggs	3	21	16	
Apple juice	400 ml.			55
Vegetable oil	30 ml.		30	
Strained baby food (4 oz. jars)				
Beef liver	4 cans	56	12	14
Beets	2 cans	3		20
Peaches	2 cans	1	1	59
Sustagen	1½ cups	52	7	150
	(225 gm.)			
(Water as needed to total 2,500 ml.)		___	___	___
Totals		165	106	346
Total calories	2,998			

Table 21-2. Types of tube feedings

INGREDIENTS	CALORIES	PROTEIN (GM.)	FAT (GM.)	CARBOHYDRATE (GM.)
Regular tube feeding				
6 eggs	452	36.6	33.0	
1 qt. homogenized milk	666	34.2	38.1	47.8
1 cup nonfat milk solids	434	42.7	1.2	61.7
½ cup Karo syrup	468			122.0
1 tablet brewers' yeast				
75 mg. ascorbic acid				
¼ tsp. salt				
1,500 ml.	2,020	113.5	72.3	231.5
Sustagen				
3 cup Sustagen	1,755	105.0	15.0	300.0
4 cup water				
1,200 ml.				
600 gm. Sustagen	2,300	140.0	20.0	400.0
(4 cup)				
1,200 ml. water				
1,400 ml.				
Add for banana Sustagen:				
2 tsp. banana flakes	88	1.2		23.0
or				
1 mashed banana				
Low-calcium tube feeding				
6 cans strained meat	540	80.4	25.2	
1 qt. fruit juice	432	0	2.0	108.0
Karo syrup ¼ cup	234			61.0
Ascorbic acid				
Brewers' yeast				
1,800 ml.				
Totals	1,206	80.4	27.2	169.0

Continued.

Table 21-2. Types of tube feedings—cont'd

INGREDIENTS		CALORIES	PROTEIN (GM.)	FAT (GM.)	CARBOHYDRATE (GM.)
Low-sodium tube feeding					
1 qt. low-sodium milk		666	34.2	38.1	47.8
Casec, 90 gm. (3 oz.) 18 tbsp.		306	75.0		
Karo syrup, ¼ cup 1,000 ml.		234			61.0
	Totals	1,206	109.2	38.1	108.8

ascorbic acid. These formulas may be compared with other sample mixtures given in Table 21-2. A number of products are available that provide prepared tube feeding materials. These products may also be used for oral feedings when this route is possible. These substances are used according to the nutrient adjustment required or the avoidance of residue needed.

Stomach surgery

Immediate postoperative period. A number of nutritional problems may develop after gastric surgery, depending on the type of surgical procedure and the patient's individual response. Care must be taken in planning the diet after any degree of gastric resection, but especially after a total gastrectomy. Otherwise, serious nutritional deficits will develop. When a vagotomy is performed also, increased gastric fullness and distention may result. The stomach becomes atonic and empties poorly, so that food fermentation follows, producing flatus and diarrhea. After gastric surgery about 50% of patients fail to regain weight to optimum levels.

Generally, however, after gastric surgery oral feedings are *gradually* resumed according to the individual patient's tolerances. A typical pattern of dietary progression is given on p. 285. A diet pattern of this type will cover about a 2-week period following surgery. The basic principles of diet therapy for this postgastrectomy period are (1) to keep meals small and frequent and (2) to eat only simple, easily digested, mild, low-bulk foods.

Later "dumping syndrome." The "dumping syndrome" is a complication sometimes encountered after initial recovery from a gastrectomy when the patient begins to eat food in greater volume and variety. He may experience increasing discomfort after meals. About 10 to 15 minutes after he has eaten, he has a cramping, full feeling, his pulse is rapid, and he feels a wave of weakness, cold sweating, and dizziness. Frequently he becomes nauseated and vomits. Such a distressing reaction to food intake increases his anxiety, and he eats less and less. He continues to lose weight and becomes increasingly malnourished. This postgastrectomy complex of symptoms may be termed more precisely the *jejunal hyperosmolic syndrome*. It is more likely to occur in patients who have had total gastrectomies.

The symptoms of shock described here result when a meal containing a high proportion of readily soluble carbohydrates rapidly enters the jejunum, the second section of the small intestine, which has been attached to the small remaining portion of the stomach during the surgery. This rapidly entering food mass is a concentrated hyperosmolar solution in relation to the surrounding circulating blood. To achieve an osmotic balance, therefore, water is drawn from the blood into the intestine, causing a rapid shrinking of the vascular fluid compartment. As a result the blood pressure drops, and signs of cardiac insufficiency appear—rapid pulse, sweating, weakness, and tremors.

A second sequence of events may follow

Postgastrectomy diet pattern

First 24 to 48 hours	Nothing by mouth, intravenous therapy
Days 2 to 4	Ice chips, sips of water (temperature adjusted to patient response; some tolerate warm water better)
Day 5	1 to 2 oz. water every even hour, and 1 to 2 oz. milk each odd hour
Day 6	Same feedings—increased to 3 oz. each
Day 7	Same feedings—increase to 4 oz. each
Day 8	Same feedings—soft-cooked egg added at 8 A.M. and 6 P.M. feedings
Days 9 to 16	Water as desired; progress to a six-feeding ulcer-type diet
Day 16	Full bland diet; small meals with interval snacks

Diet for postoperative gastric dumping syndrome

GENERAL DESCRIPTION

1. Five or six small meals daily
2. Relatively high-fat content to retard passage of food and help maintain weight
3. High-protein content (meat, egg, cheese) to rebuild tissue and maintain weight
4. Relatively low-carbohydrate content to prevent rapid passage of quickly utilized foods
5. No milk; no sugar, sweets, or desserts; no alcohol or sweet carbonated beverages
6. Liquids between meals only; avoid fluids for at least one hour before and after meals
7. Relatively low roughage foods; raw foods as tolerated

MEAL PATTERN

Breakfast	2 scrambled eggs with 1 or 2 tbsp. butter or margarine
	½ to 1 slice bread with butter or margarine or small serving cereal
	2 crisp bacon slices
	1 serving solid fruit*
Midmorning sandwich	1 slice bread
	Butter or margarine
	2 oz. lean meat
Lunch	4 oz. lean meat with 1 or 2 tbsp. butter or margarine
	Green or colored vegetable† with butter or margarine
	½ to 1 slice bread with butter or margarine
	½ banana or other solid fruit*
Midafternoon	Same snack as midmorning
Dinner	4 oz. lean meat with 1 or 2 tbsp. butter or margarine
	Green or colored vegetable† with butter or margarine
	½ to 1 slice bread with butter or margarine (or small serving starchy vegetable substitute)
	1 serving solid fruit*
Bedtime	2 oz. meat, 2 eggs, or 2 oz. cheese or cottage cheese
	1 slice bread or 5 crackers
	Butter or margarine

*Fruit choice: applesauce, baked apple, canned fruit (drained), banana, orange or grapefruit sections.
†Vegetable choice: asparagus, spinach, green beans, squash, beets, carrots, peas.

about 2 hours later. The concentrated solution of carbohydrate is rapidly digested and absorbed. This causes a consequent rise in the blood glucose. The glucose load in the blood then stimulates an overproduction of insulin, which in turn leads to an eventual drop in the blood sugar below normal fasting levels. Symptoms of mild hypoglycemia result.

Dramatic relief of these distressing symptoms and gradual regain of lost weight follows careful control of the diet. Characteristics of this diet are listed on p. 285.

Gallbladder surgery

For patients suffering with acute gallbladder disease or gallstones the treatment is usually surgical removal of the gallbladder. Review of discussions of gallbladder disease in Chapter 16, pp. 220 to 223, and the role of vitamin K in Chapter 6 may be helpful.

After the surgical removal of the gallbladder (cholecystectomy) control of dietary fat remains essential to wound healing and comfort. The presence of fat in the duodenum continues to stimulate the cholecystokinin mechanism, which causes contraction and pain in the surgical area. There is also a period of adjustment to the more watery supply of liver bile for the preparation of fats for digestion. Depending on individual toleration and response, a relatively low-fat diet may have to be followed for as long as a month with moderate habits of fat use thereafter. The low-fat diet outlined on pp. 222 and 223 for gallbladder disease may serve as a guide.

Intestinal surgery—ileostomy and colostomy

In cases of intestinal lesion or obstruction or when chronic ulcerative colitis involves the entire colon, the treatment of choice is usually resection of the intestine and establishment of a permanent *ileostomy* with removal of the diseased colon. The end of the remaining small intestine, the ileum, is attached to an opening in the abdominal wall, and a stoma (small permanent opening) is formed to provide for discharge of intestinal

contents. In a *colostomy* the left side of the colon is resected, and a stoma is made with the descending colon attached to the opening in the abdominal wall.

Therefore an ileostomy and a colostomy produce different problems in management. The intestinal contents at the point of the ileum are unformed, irritating, more liquid in texture, and even erosive to the skin. The ileostomy drains freely, almost continuously, and should never be irrigated. Thus establishment of controlled functioning is difficult, although many patients do develop a reasonable degree of regularity in relation to food intake. Some kind of appliance is necessary to hold the discharge.

A colostomy is more manageable. The normal contents of the intestine at this point in the colon are solid or semisolid because it is further down the intestinal tract and more absorption of water and electrolytes has taken place in the first part of the colon. The consistency of the discharge, therefore, is more formed and less irritating and hence creates fewer control problems. Often the sigmoid (lower portion of the colon) colostomy can be adequately controlled by simple dietary measures and periodic irrigation so that in many cases no protective appliance is required.

Dietary measures may include the use of a low-residue diet immediately after surgery. However, as soon as possible the diet should be advanced to a regular pattern of food to provide optimum nutrition and physical rehabilitation. This use of regular food provides an additional means of psychologic support. Individual tolerances for specific foods may be accommodated in the diet, and the patient can avoid these few foods that may cause him individual discomfort.

Rectal surgery

For a brief period after rectal surgery (hemorrhoidectomy) a clear fluid or nonresidue diet may be indicated to delay initial bowel movement until healing has begun. Sometimes a residue-free elemental diet formula is used, such as Vivonex. The basic foods used subsequently are almost completely digested and absorbed in the small intestine, leaving minimal residue for elimination by the colon.

NUTRITIONAL CARE OF THE PATIENT WITH BURNS

The burned patient, especially one with extensive burns, presents a tremendous nutritional challenge. His nutritional care is often the determining factor in his survival and healing. His feeding program is adjusted to individual needs and follows three distinct periods after the injury.

Immediate shock period (days 1 to 3)

A massive flooding edema occurs at the burn site during the first hours after the second day. Loss of enveloping skin surface and exposure of tissue fluids lead to immediate loss of water and electrolytes, mainly sodium, and large protein depletion. In an effort to balance this loss the water shifts from the other tissue spaces in the body but only adds to the continuous loss at the burn site. As a result the water circulating in the blood is withdrawn, thus decreasing the blood volume and pressure. A concentration of blood and diminished urine output occur as a result. Cell dehydration follows as cell water is drawn out to balance the tissue fluid losses. Cell potassium is also withdrawn, and circulating serum potassium levels rise.

Immediate intravenous fluid therapy seeks to replace three constituents (1) *colloid (protein)* through blood or plasma transfusion or by plasma expanders such as Dextran, (2) the *electrolytes* sodium and chlorine by use of a saline lactated Ringer's solution, and (3) *water* (dextrose solution) to cover additional involuntary losses. The rate of flow should be carefully monitored. Half the calculated fluid and electrolytes has to be given during the first 8 hours, one fourth during the second 8 hours, and one fourth during the third 8 hours. During the second 24-hour period the patient will require about half the amount of fluid given during the first 24 hours.

Recovery period (days 3 to 5)

As the initial replacement fluid and electrolytes are gradually reabsorbed into the general circulation, balance is established, and the pattern of massive tissue loss is reversed. At this point a sudden diuresis occurs, indicating successful therapy. Intravenous therapy should then be discontinued and oral solutions of water and electrolytes used. One such oral solution is Holdrane's solution. It is made up of 3 to 4 gm. (½ teaspoon) salt, 1½ to 2 gm. (1½ teaspoon) sodium bicarbonate (baking soda), and 1,000 ml. (1 quart) water, flavored with lemon juice and chilled. A careful check of fluid intake and output is essential, and constant checks for signs of dehydration and overhydration should be made.

Secondary feeding period (days 6 to 15)

Despite the patient's depression and lack of appetite at this point, his life may well depend on rigorous nutritional therapy during this secondary feeding period. He may need to be fed by a tube, but oral feeding should be encouraged and supported as much as possible. He needs a high-protein intake, 150 to as high as 400 gm., to counteract tissue destruction by the burn and tissue breakdown afterward with continued nitrogen losses and to fulfill the increased metabolic demands of infection or fever. From 3,500 to 5,000 calories with a high percentage of carbohydrate is necessary to meet these demands. Extra vitamin C therapy, 1 to 2 gm., is needed for tissue regeneration. Increased thiamine, riboflavin, and niacin are necessary to supply oxidative enzyme systems to metabolize extra carbohydrate and protein loads. Optimum tissue health is necessary for the subsequent grafting to be successful. Since these nutritional needs are so vital, a careful record of protein and calorie intake and the amount of food consumed is a necessary tool for planning care. After initial liquid feedings using concentrated protein hydrolysates a soft to regular diet will probably be taken by the second week or so. Much continued support and effort is needed to encourage the patient to eat, supplying items he likes.

Follow-up reconstruction period (weeks 2 to 5 and afterward)

Grafting and plastic surgery may follow at this point. Continued optimum nutrition is essential to maintain tissue integrity for successful results of reconstructive efforts. In the rehabilitation period that follows, the patient needs continued physical, nutritional, and personal care to minimize or avoid any possible disfigurement or disability.

APPENDIXES

A FOOD VALUES*

	APPROXIMATE MEASURE	CALORIES	PROTEIN (GM.)	FAT (GM.)	CARBO-HYDRATE (GM.)
Beverages					
Coca-Cola	1 bottle (6 oz.)	78	0	0	20.4
Ginger ale	1 glass (6 oz.)	60	0	0	15.3
Chocolate milk shake	1 regular (8 oz. milk)	421	11.2	17.8	58.0
Chocolate malted milk	1 regular (8 oz. milk)	502	13.1	19.5	72.1
Cider, sweet	1 glass (6 oz.)	94	0.2	0	25.8
Cocoa, all milk	1 cup (6 oz. milk)	174	6.9	8.5	20.3
Eggnog	1 glass (6 oz. milk)	233	12.5	12.6	17.7
Lemonade	1 large glass, 1 oz. lemon juice	104	0.2	0	27.2
Milk, buttermilk	½ pt.	86	8.5	0.2	12.4
Milk, chocolate	½ pt.	185	8.0	5.5	26.5
Milk, skim	½ pt.	87	8.6	0.2	12.5
Milk, whole	½ pt.	166	8.5	9.5	12.0
Soda, ice cream, vanilla	1 regular	261	2.3	7.1	48.7
Soda, ice cream chocolate	1 regular	255	2.7	8.3	46.0
Breads					
Bread, corn	1 piece (2 in. square)	93	3.2	3.2	13.1
Bread, rye	1 slice	57	2.1	0.3	12.1
Bread, white enriched	1 slice	63	2.0	0.7	11.9
Bread, whole wheat	1 slice	55	2.1	0.6	11.3
Biscuit, baking powder	1 average (2 in. diam.)	109	2.4	4.1	14.9
Bun, cinnamon, plain	1 average	158	3.1	4.8	25.6
Doughnut, cake type, plain	1 average	135	2.2	6.5	17.5
Doughnut, sugared or iced	1 average	151	2.2	6.5	21.7
Muffin, white	1 average, 12 from 2 cups flour	120	3.2	4.3	17.1
Muffin, whole wheat	1 average, 12 from 2 cups flour	120	3.4	4.3	17.1
Pancake, various flours	1 average (4 in. diam.)	62	2.3	1.2	10.7
Roll, white, soft	1 Parker House	81	2.1	1.6	13.6

*From Church, C. F., and Church, H. N.: Food values of portions commonly used, ed. 11, Philadelphia,
Abbreviations: diam., diameter; gm., gram; I.U., international unit; lb., pound; mcg., microgram; mg.,
data inadequate to give a specific figure; 0—none.
Equivalents: 1,000 mcg. = 1 mg., 1,000 mg. = 1 gm.; 28.34 gm. = 1 oz.

CALCIUM (MG.)	IRON (MG.)	VITAMIN A (I.U.)	THIAMINE (MCG.)	RIBOFLAVIN (MCG.)	NIACIN (MG.)	ASCORBIC ACID (MG.)
0	0	0	0	0	0	0
0	0	0	0	0	0	0
363	0.9	687	120	547	0.5	4
420	1.3	891	186	655	0.5	4
11	0.9	75	37	56	Trace	2
224	0.9	295	80	334	0.3	2
242	1.5	843	123	451	0.2	2
4	Trace	0	20	Trace	Trace	15
288	0.2	10	90	430	0.3	3
272	0.2	230	80	400	0.2	2
303	0.2	10	90	440	0.3	3
288	0.2	390	90	420	0.3	3
69	0.1	295	24	106	0.1	1
75	0.7	297	30	127	0.2	1
29	0.7	229	90	102	0.7	(0)
17	0.4	0	40	20	0.4	(0)
18	0.4	0	60	40	0.5	0
22	0.5	0	70	30	0.7	0
19	0.5	20	86	70	0.6	0
27	0.9	205	85	87	0.8	0
12	0.6	41	72	63	0.5	Trace
12	0.6	41	72	63	0.5	Trace
30	0.7	193	78	95	0.6	0
33	0.7	193	88	85	0.5	0
96	0.3	44	30	53	0.2	0
19	0.5	73	72	64	0.5	0

1970, J. B. Lippincott Co.
milligram; oz., ounce; tbsp., tablespoonful, level; tsp., teaspoonful, level; (   ), tentative data; −,

Continued.

FOOD VALUES—cont'd

	APPROXIMATE MEASURE	CALORIES	PROTEIN (GM.)	FAT (GM.)	CARBO-HYDRATE (GM.)
Breads–cont'd					
Roll, white, sweet	1 average commercial	178	4.7	4.3	29.6
Waffle, plain, average	1 waffle (5½ in. diam.)	232	5.1	14.0	21.4
Cereals and cereal products					
Cheerios	1 oz. (1⅛ cups)	104	4.1	2.0	19.7
Cornflakes	1 oz. (1⅓ cups)	105	2.1	0.1	24.4
Cream of Wheat, cooked	¾ cup	102	3.5	0.3	21.7
Grapenuts	1 oz. (¼ cup)	110	2.8	0.2	24.0
Macaroni, cooked	½ cup (1 in. pieces)	105	3.6	0.4	21.2
Macaroni and cheese, baked	1 cup	506	18.9	25.0	45.3
Noodles, egg, enriched, cooked	¾ cup	81	2.7	0.75	15.3
Oatmeal, cooked	¾ cup	111	4.0	2.1	19.5
Popcorn	1 cup	54	1.8	0.7	10.7
Post Toasties	1¼ cups (1 oz.)	100	2.1	0.1	24.0
Rice, white, cooked	¾ cup	103	2.1	0.15	22.5
Rice Krispies	1 cup	107	1.6	0.1	25.1
Rice, puffed	1 cup	107	1.8	0.1	24.7
Spaghetti, cooked	¾ cup	162	5.5	0.6	33.0
Spaghetti, Italian-style	1 average serving with meat sauce	396	12.7	20.7	39.4
Sugar Crisp	1 oz. (individual package)	110	1.9	0.3	25.0
Wheat, shredded	1 large biscuit (4 × 2¼ in.)	106	3.2	0.5	22.1
Cracker, graham	1 (2½ in. sq.)	28	0.5	0.7	5.0
Cracker, Ritz	1	16	0.2	0.8	2.0
Cracker, saltine	1	14	0.3	0.3	2.3
Matzo	1 piece (6 in. diam.)	78	2.1	0.2	17.3
Pretzels	7 average thin sticks	37	0.9	0.3	7.5
Ry-Krisp	1 double-squared wafer	20	0.7	0.1	4.1
Zwieback	1 piece (61 to 1 lb.)	31	0.9	0.7	5.3
Dairy products					
Butter	1 tsp.	36	0	4.1	0
Butter	1 tbsp.	100	0.1	11.3	0.1
Cheese, cheddar, American	1 oz. (1 slice ¼ in. thick)	113	7.1	9.1	0.6
Cheese, cottage	½ cup	107	22.0	0.55	2.2

*Vitamin A and D values for butter and cream are average year-round figures; vitamin A and D content

CALCIUM (MG.)	IRON (MG.)	VITAMIN A (I.U.)	THIAMINE (MCG.)	RIBOFLAVIN (MCG.)	NIACIN (MG.)	ASCORBIC ACID (MG.)
35	0.3	0	30	70	0.6	0
59	0.9	178	122	159	0.8	Trace
47	2.1	(0)	325	56	0.6	0
2	0.5	(0)	120	20	0.6	0
10	1.1	0	17	17	0.2	0
—	1.0	(0)	130	—	1.5	0
7	0.75	(0)	120	75	1.0	0
407	2.0	970	220	450	2.0	Trace
4	0.6	45	165	75	1.35	0
15	1.2	(0)	165	38	0.3	0
(2)	(0.4)	(0)	(50)	(20)	(0.3)	0
—	0.4	(0)	110	—	0.5	0
7	0.2	(0)	20	8	0.5	0
7	0.5	(0)	110	10	2.0	0
4	0.5	(0)	125	11	1.5	0
10	1.2	(0)	186	113	0.5	0
27	2.1	901	120	117	3.0	(24)
3	0.5	(0)	14	—	0.7	0
13	1.0	(0)	60	30	1.3	0
1	0.1	(0)	20	10	0.1	0
1	0.1	(0)	—	—	—	0
1	0.1	(0)	Trace	Trace	Trace	0
—	—	0	—	—	—	0
1	0.1	0	1	4	0.1	0
3	0.2	0	20	10	0.1	0
8	0.1	0	—	—	—	0
1	0	165*	Trace	Trace	Trace	0
3	—	460*	Trace	Trace	Trace	0
206	0.3	400	10	120	Trace	(0)
108	0.35	25	20	345	0.1	(0)

varies with the seasons.

Continued.

FOOD VALUES—cont'd

	APPROXIMATE MEASURE	CALORIES	PROTEIN (GM.)	FAT (GM.)	CARBO-HYDRATE (GM.)
Dairy products–cont'd					
Cheese, cream	2 tbsp.	106	2.6	10.5	0.6
Cream, light	1 tbsp.	30	0.4	3.0	0.6
Cream, heavy, sweet or sour	1 tbsp.	50	0.3	5.2	0.5
Cream, heavy, whipped	1 heaping tbsp., sweetened	52	0.3	5.2	1.3
Milk, whole	½ pt.	166	8.5	9.5	12.0
Milk, chocolate	½ pt.	185	8.0	5.5	26.5
Milk, skim	½ pt.	87	8.6	0.2	12.5
Milk, buttermilk	½ pt.	86	8.5	0.2	12.4
Desserts					
Vanilla blancmange	½ cup	152	4.2	4.7	23.8
Brownies	1 (2 × 2 × ¾ in.)	141	1.8	8.4	16.6
Cake, angel	1 piece ($^1/_{10}$ of average cake)	145	3.4	0.1	33.0
Cake, chocolate, 2 layer, white icing	1 piece ($^1/_{12}$ of cake)	356	3.1	7.7	45.0
Cake, white, 2 layer, chocolate icing	3 in. section	314	4.0	10.4	52.6
Cake, sponge	1 piece ($^1/_{10}$ of average cake)	145	3.2	2.3	28.1
Cookies, oatmeal	1 large (3½ in. diam.)	114	1.6	4.4	17.5
Cookies, sugar	1 cookie (3½ in. diam.)	64	1.0	2.6	9.1
Custard, baked	1 (4 from 1 pt. milk)	205	8.8	9.1	22.8
Fig bars, commercial	1 small, average	56	0.7	0.8	12.1
Gingerbread, made with hot water and 1 egg	1 small piece (2 in. cube)	206	2.2	9.9	26.9
Ice cream, vanilla	¼ of 1 pt.	147	2.8	8.9	14.6
Jell-O, plain	1 serving (5 to 1 package)	65	1.6	0	15.1
Jell-O with whipped cream	1 serving, 1 tbsp. cream	117	1.8	5.4	16.4
Pie, apple	$^1/_6$ of medium pie	377	3.8	14.3	60.2
Pie, blueberry	$^1/_6$ of medium pie	372	3.9	15.4	56.9
Pie, cherry	$^1/_6$ of medium pie	360	4.3	12.4	59.6
Pie, chocolate	$^1/_6$ of medium pie	294	6.9	13.7	37.7
Pie, custard	$^1/_6$ of medium pie	266	7.6	12.1	32.7

*Vitamin A and D values for butter and cream are average year-round figures; vitamin A and D content

CALCIUM (MG.)	IRON (MG.)	VITAMIN A (I.U.)	THIAMINE (MCG.)	RIBOFLAVIN (MCG.)	NIACIN (MG.)	ASCORBIC ACID (MG.)
19	0.1	(410)	Trace	60	Trace	(0)
15	0	120*	4	20	Trace	Trace
12	0	220*	Trace	20	Trace	Trace
12	0	220*	Trace	20	Trace	Trace
288	0.2	(390)	90	420	0.3	3
272	0.2	230	80	400	0.2	2
303	0.2	(10)	90	440	0.3	3
(288)	0.2	10	90	430	0.3	1
144	0.1	195	45	210	0.1	1
11	0.5	226	38	41	0.2	(0)
3	0.1	(0)	3	66	0.1	0
24	0.5	265	17	70	0.1	(0)
88	0.4	390	20	70	0.2	(0)
12	0.6	220	24	59	0.1	(0)
12	0.5	27	59	36	0.2	(0)
5	0.2	25	32	27	0.2	(0)
163	1.1	607	82	315	0.1	(0)
11	0.2	0	3	10	0.1	(0)
45	1.4	69	66	54	0.5	0
87	0.1	369	29	135	0.1	1
(0)	(0)	(0)	(0)	(0)	(0)	(0)
12	(0)	212	4	16	Trace	Trace
11	0.5	156	46	26	0.4	1
14	0.7	166	25	29	0.4	5
16	0.6	601	41	26	0.4	2
118	0.8	325	30	128	0.2	(0)
111	0.8	305	63	215	0.2	(0)

varies with the seasons.

Continued.

FOOD VALUES—cont'd

	APPROXIMATE MEASURE	CALORIES	PROTEIN (GM.)	FAT (GM.)	CARBO-HYDRATE (GM.)
Desserts–cont'd					
Pie, lemon meringue	⅙ of medium pie	281	3.8	9.8	45.3
Pie, mince	⅙ of medium pie	398	3.9	10.9	71.8
Pie, raisin	⅙ of medium pie	437	4.6	12.4	81.2
Pie, pumpkin	⅙ of medium pie	330	6.7	10.7	53.5
Sherbet, average serving	½ cup commercial	118	1.4	0	28.8
Shortcake, biscuit, strawberries	1 cup berries, 1 medium biscuit	399	4.8	8.9	61.2
Pudding, cornstarch, chocolate	½ cup	219	4.5	6.6	37.1
Pudding, cornstarch, vanilla	½ cup	152	4.2	4.7	23.8
Pudding, tapioca, cream	½ cup	133	4.9	5.0	17.3
Eggs					
Egg, boiled	1 medium	77	6.1	5.5	0.3
Egg, fried	1 medium, 1 tsp. margarine	110	6.1	9.2	0.3
Egg, omelet, plain	1 medium	120	6.6	9.8	1.0
Egg, omelet, Spanish	2 eggs, 4 tbsp. sauce	329	14.6	26.9	7.6
Egg, scrambled	1 medium, 1 tbsp. milk, 1 tsp. fat	120	6.6	9.8	1.0
Fats and oils					
Butter	1 tsp.	36	Trace	4.1	Trace
Butter	1 tbsp.	100	0.1	11.3	0.1
Dressing, commercial mayonnaise	1 tbsp.	58	0.2	5.5	2.1
Dressing, commercial French	1 tbsp.	59	0.1	5.3	3.0
Dressing, homemade mayonnaise	1 tbsp.	92	0.2	10.1	0.4
Dressing homemade French	1 tbsp.	86	0.0	9.2	0.7
Dressing, Thousand Island	1 rounded tbsp.	98	0.3	10.0	2.4
Margarine	1 tsp.	36	Trace	4.1	Trace
Margarine	1 tbsp.	100	0.1	11.3	0.1
Fish					
Flounder or sole, baked	¼ lb.	204	16.9	20.0	0
Haddock, fried	1 filet (3 × 3 × ½ in.)	214	23.5	9.0	8.1
Halibut steak, cooked	1 serving (4 to 1 lb.)	205	21.0	12.2	0
Herring, pickled	2 small	223	20.4	15.1	0
Oysters, fried	6	412	15.1	29.6	18.2

CALCIUM (MG.)	IRON (MG.)	VITAMIN A (I.U.)	THIAMINE (MCG.)	RIBOFLAVIN (MCG.)	NIACIN (MG.)	ASCORBIC ACID (MG.)
13	0.5	260	29	52	0.1	1
35	3.4	12	106	55	0.5	1
47	2.0	27	98	53	0.5	(0)
103	2.2	2,278	58	163	0.5	(0)
48	0	0	20	70	0	(0)
73	2.0	429	167	207	1.3	(89)
147	0.2	196	45	217	0.2	(0)
144	0.1	195	45	210	0.1	(0)
105	0.5	313	46	186	0.1	1
26	1.3	550	40	130	Trace	0
27	1.3	702	40	130	Trace	0
44	1.3	726	46	153	Trace	0
103	3.4	2,008	110	260	1.0	13
44	1.3	726	56	165	Trace	0
1	0	165	Trace	Trace	Trace	0
3	0	460	Trace	Trace	Trace	0
1	0.1	20	Trace	Trace	(0)	(0)
Trace	Trace	0	0	0	0	0
2	0.1	34	3	3	Trace	0
Trace	Trace	(0)	(0)	(0)	(0)	0
3	0.2	109	9	5	0.1	1
1	0	165	(0)	(0)	(0)	(0)
3	0	460	(0)	(0)	(0)	(0)
69	0.9	—	49	54	1.6	0
44	1.4	139	69	134	2.6	—
15	0.8	497	55	61	8.8	—
22	1.1	—	—	—	—	0
134	6.4	1,539	134	274	1.2	0

Continued.

FOOD VALUES—cont'd

	APPROXIMATE MEASURE	CALORIES	PROTEIN (GM.)	FAT (GM.)	CARBO-HYDRATE (GM.)
Fish–cont'd					
Oysters, raw	½ cup (6 to 9 medium)	100	11.8	2.5	6.7
Oysters, escalloped	1 serving of 6	356	15.9	18.0	31.6
Salmon, pink	⅔ cup	143	20.5	6.2	0
Salmon, red	⅔ cup	173	20.2	9.6	0
Scallops, fried	5 to 6 medium	426	23.8	28.4	19.3
Scallops, raw	2 or 3 (12 to 1 lb.)	78	14.8	0.1	3.4
Shrimp, canned	4 to 6 shrimp	64	13.4	0.7	0
Tuna, canned	⅝ cup solids	198	29.0	8.2	0
Fruits					
Apple, baked, unpared	1 large, 2 tbsp. sugar	213	0.6	0.8	64.9
Apple, raw	1 small (2¼ in. diam.)	50	0.3	0.4	13.0
Apple, raw	1 large (3 in. diam.)	117	0.6	0.8	30.1
Applesauce, canned	½ cup, sweetened	92	0.3	0.2	25.0
Applesauce, canned	½ cup	50	0.3	0.3	13.1
Apricots, raw	2 or 3 medium	51	1.0	0.1	12.9
Apricots, canned in syrup	4 halves, 2 tbsp. juice	80	0.6	0.1	21.4
Apricots, canned in water	4 halves	32	0.5	0.1	8.1
Avocado	½ small pear	245	1.7	26.4	5.1
Banana, raw	1 small	88	1.2	0.2	23.0
Banana, raw	1 medium	132	1.8	0.3	34.5
Banana, raw	1 large	176	2.4	0.4	46.0
Blueberries, canned in syrup	½ cup	123	0.5	0.5	32.4
Blueberries, canned in water	½ cup	45	0.5	0.5	10.9
Blueberries, frozen, no sugar	⅝ cup	61	0.6	0.6	15.1
Cantaloupe, diced	½ cup	24	0.7	0.2	5.5
Cherries, sweet, canned in syrup	½ cup red	105	0.6	0.1	28.5
Cherries, canned in water	½ cup red	51	0.8	0.4	12.6
Cherries, maraschino	1 cherry	19	Trace	Trace	5.2
Cranberry jelly	1 rounded tbsp.	47	Trace	Trace	13.0
Cranberry sauce	1 rounded tbsp.	40	Trace	0.1	10.3
Dates, dried and fresh	3 or 4 pitted	85	0.6	0.2	22.6
Figs, canned in syrup	3 with 2 tbsp. juice	113	0.8	0.3	30.0
Figs, dried	2 small	81	1.2	0.4	20.5
Fruit cocktail, canned	6 tbsp. fruit and juice	70	0.4	0.2	18.6

CALCIUM (MG.)	IRON (MG.)	VITAMIN A (I.U.)	THIAMINE (MCG.)	RIBOFLAVIN (MCG.)	NIACIN (MG.)	ASCORBIC ACID (MG.)
113	6.7	385	175	240	1.4	—
158	7.0	894	143	277	1.5	0
187	0.8	70	30	180	8.0	(0)
259	1.2	230	40	160	7.3	(0)
41	3.1	0	91	173	2.3	(0)
26	1.8	0	(40)	100	1.4	—
58	1.6	30	5	15	1.1	(0)
(8)	1.4	80	50	120	12.8	(0)
12	0.6	(180)	40	45	0.3	(2)
5	0.3	80	33	27	0.1	4
12	0.6	180	80	60	0.4	9
5	0.5	40	25	15	0.1	1 to 2
5	0.5	35	25	10	0.1	1 to 2
16	0.5	2,790	30	50	0.8	7
10	0.3	1,350	20	20	0.3	4
10	0.3	1,350	20	20	0.3	4
10	0.6	290	60	130	1.1	16
8	0.6	430	40	50	0.7	10
12	0.9	645	60	75	1.0	15
16	1.2	860	80	100	1.4	20
14	0.6	50	15	15	0.3	17
14	0.6	50	15	15	0.3	16
16	0.8	240	20	20	0.3	14
20	0.5	4,104	60	48	0.6	40
11	0.3	430	30	20	0.1	3
11	0.3	120	30	20	0.1	3
1	Trace	35	(3)	(2)	Trace	Trace
Trace	Trace					
(2)	(0.1)	(6)	(4)	(4)	Trace	Trace
22	0.6	18	27	30	0.7	(0)
35	0.4	50	30	30	0.4	Trace
56	0.9	24	48	36	0.5	(0)
9	0.4	160	10	10	0.4	2

Continued.

FOOD VALUES—cont'd

	APPROXIMATE MEASURE	CALORIES	PROTEIN (GM.)	FAT (GM.)	CARBO-HYDRATE (GM.)
Fruits–cont'd					
Grapefruit, raw	½ small	40	0.5	0.2	10.1
Grapefruit, raw	½ large (5 in. diam.)	100	1.3	0.5	25.3
Grapes, green seedless	60	66	0.8	0.4	16.7
Grapes, Tokay	22	66	0.8	0.4	16.7
Honeydew melon	¼ of 5 in. diam. melon	32	0.5	0	8.5
Lemons, raw	1 medium	32	0.9	0.6	8.7
Limes, raw	1 large	37	0.8	0.1	12.3
Olives, green	1 large	7	0.1	0.7	0.2
Olives, ripe	1 large or 2 small	7	0.1	0.7	0.2
Orange, whole	1 small (2½ in. diam.)	45	0.9	0.2	11.2
Orange, whole	1 large (3⅜ in. diam.)	106	2.1	0.5	26.3
Orange sections	½ cup	44	0.9	0.2	10.8
Peaches, raw	1 medium-large	46	0.5	0.1	12.0
Peaches, raw	1 cup, sliced	77	0.8	0.2	20.2
Peaches, canned in syrup	2 halves, 1 tbsp. juice	68	0.4	0.1	18.2
Peaches, canned in water	2 halves, 2 tbsp. juice	27	0.5	0.1	6.8
Peaches, frozen	½ cup, scant	78	0.4	0.1	20.2
Pears, raw	1 medium pear	63	0.7	0.4	15.8
Pears, canned in syrup	2 halves, 1 tbsp. juice	68	0.2	0.1	18.4
Pears, canned in water	2 halves, 1 tbsp. juice	31	0.3	0.1	8.2
Pineapple, canned in syrup	½ cup, crushed	102	0.5	0.2	27.5
Pineapple, canned in syrup	1 large or 2 small slices, 1 tbsp. juice	78	0.4	0.1	21.1
Pineapple, canned in juice	1 large or 2 small slices, 2 tbsp. juice	55	0.5	0.1	14.5
Plums, raw	2 medium	50	0.7	0.2	12.9
Plums, canned in syrup	2 medium, 2 tbsp. juice	76	0.4	0.1	20.4
Prunes, raw, dried	3 medium or 4 small	67	0.6	0.2	17.8
Prunes, cooked, no sugar	4 medium, 2 tbsp. juice	86	0.7	0.2	22.7
Prunes, cooked, with sugar	4 medium, 2 tbsp. juice	119	0.7	0.2	31.2
Raisins	1 tbsp.	27	0.2	0.1	7.2
Raisins	1 cup	429	3.7	0.8	113.9

CALCIUM (MG.)	IRON (MG.)	VITAMIN A (I.U.)	THIAMINE (MCG.)	RIBOFLAVIN (MCG.)	NIACIN (MG.)	ASCORBIC ACID (MG.)
22	0.2	Trace	40	20	0.2	40
55	0.5	Trace	100	50	0.5	100
17	0.6	80	60	40	0.2	4
17	0.6	80	60	40	0.2	4
(17)	(0.4)	40	50	30	0.2	23
40	0.6	0	40	Trace	0.1	50
(40)	0.6	0	(40)	Trace	(0.1)	27
5	0.1	16	Trace	—	—	—
5	0.1	3	Trace	Trace	—	—
33	0.4	(190)	80	30	0.2	49
78	0.9	(447)	188	71	0.5	115
32	0.4	(180)	75	25	0.3	48
8	0.6	880	20	50	0.9	8
13	1.0	1,478	34	84	1.5	13
5	0.4	450	10	20	0.7	4
5	0.4	450	10	20	0.7	4
6	0.4	520	10	30	0.5	4
13	0.3	20	20	40	0.1	4
8	0.2	Trace	10	20	0.1	2
8	0.2	Trace	10	20	0.1	2
38	0.8	105	100	20	0.2	12
29	0.6	80	70	20	0.2	9
29	0.6	80	70	20	0.2	9
17	0.5	350	60	40	0.5	5
8	1.1	230	30	30	0.4	1
14	1.0	473	25	40	0.2	Trace
17	1.3	545	22	45	0.4	Trace
17	1.3	545	22	45	0.4	Trace
8	0.3	5	15	8	0.1	—
125	5.3	80	240	130	0.8	Trace

Continued.

FOOD VALUES—cont'd

	APPROXIMATE MEASURE	CALORIES	PROTEIN (GM.)	FAT (GM.)	CARBO-HYDRATE (GM.)
Fruits–cont'd					
Raspberries, black, raw	⅔ cup	74	1.5	1.6	15.7
Raspberries, red, raw	¾ cup	57	1.2	0.4	13.8
Rhubarb, cooked, sweetened	½ cup fruit and syrup	137	0.3	0.1	35.1
Strawberries, raw	10 large	37	0.8	0.5	8.3
Strawberries, frozen, sweetened	½ cup, scant	106	0.6	0.4	26.6
Watermelon	½ cup cubes	28	0.5	0.2	6.9
Watermelon	1 slice (6 in. diam., 1½ in. thick)	168	3.0	1.2	41.4
Fruit juices					
Apple juice, canned	2 tbsp.	16	0.03	0	4.3
Apple juice, canned	3 fl. oz.	48	0.1	0	13.8
Apricot juice	3 fl. oz.	44	0.5	0.4	10.2
Grape juice, commercial	3 fl. oz.	67	0.4	0	18.2
Grapefruit juice, fresh	3¼ fl. oz.	36	0.5	0.1	9.2
Grapefruit juice, canned	3¼ fl. oz., sweetened	52	0.5	0.1	13.7
Grapefruit juice, canned	3¼ fl. oz.	38	0.5	0.1	9.8
Lemon juice, fresh	1 tbsp.	4	0.1	Trace	1.2
Orange juice, fresh	3¼ fl. oz.	44	0.8	0.2	11.0
Orange juice, canned	3¼ fl. oz., sweetened	54	0.6	0.2	13.9
Orange juice, canned	3⅛ fl. oz.	44	0.8	0.2	11.1
Pineapple juice, canned	3¼ fl. oz.	49	0.3	0.1	13.0
Prune juice, canned	3 fl. oz.	63	0.3	0	17.4
Tomato juice, canned	3 fl. oz.	21	0.9	0.2	4.3
Meats					
Bacon	1 strip, drained (6 in.)	48	1.8	4.4	0.2
Bacon, Canadian, cooked	1 slice (2¼ in. diam., ³/₁₆ in. thick)	57	6.6	3.1	0.1
Beef brisket, raw	3 pieces (2 × 1 × 1 in.)	338	15.8	30.0	0
Beef chuck, pot roast	1 slice (2 in. × 1½ in. × ½ in.)	93	7.8	6.6	0
Beef, hamburger, medium-cooked	1 small patty (2 oz.)	118	12.9	7.1	0
Beef, hamburger, medium-cooked	1 medium patty (5 to 1 lb.)	246	14.6	20.4	0

*Calcium may not be available because of high oxalic acid content.

CALCIUM (MG.)	IRON (MG.)	VITAMIN A (I.U.)	THIAMINE (MCG.)	RIBOFLAVIN (MCG.)	NIACIN (MG.)	ASCORBIC ACID (MG.)
40	0.9	0	20	(70)	(0.3)	(24)
40	0.9	130	20	(70)	(0.3)	24
26*	0.2	16	2	—	Trace	2
28	0.8	60	30	70	0.3	60
22	0.6	40	20	50	0.2	41
7	0.2	590	50	50	0.2	6
42	1.2	3,540	300	300	1.2	36
2	0.2	12	6	9	Trace	Trace
6	0.5	40	20	30	Trace	1
10	0.3	—	40	50	0.2	Trace
8	0.3	Trace	40	20	0.2	40
8	0.3	Trace	30	20	0.2	35
8	0.3	Trace	30	20	0.2	35
2	Trace	0	6	Trace	Trace	8
19	0.2	(190)	80	30	0.2	49
10	0.3	(100)	70	20	0.2	42
10	0.3	(100)	70	20	0.2	42
15	0.5	80	50	20	0.2	9
(24)	(1.5)	—	27	72	0.3	Trace
(6)	(0.3)	978	48	27	0.6	15
3	0.2	(0)	40	22	0.3	0
4	1.0	(0)	164	67	1.4	0
0	2.4	(0)	100	130	4.4	0
3	0.9	(0)	15	60	1.2	0
7	1.9	(0)	38	102	2.6	0
8	2.2	0	43	115	3.0	0

Continued.

FOOD VALUES—cont'd

	APPROXIMATE MEASURE	CALORIES	PROTEIN (GM.)	FAT (GM.)	CARBO-HYDRATE (GM.)
Meats–cont'd					
Beef, hamburger, medium-cooked	1 large patty (4 to 1 lb.)	300	18.2	24.6	0
Beef, hamburger on bun	1 average, plain	332	17.1	21.9	15.4
Beef, porterhouse, broiled	1 large steak with gravy (5 oz.)	513	34.5	40.5	0
Beef, rib, roasted	1 slice (3 × 2¼ × ¼ in.)	96	7.2	7.2	0
Beef, round, cubed, cooked	1 piece, 3 oz. (4 × 3 × ⅜ in.)	214	24.7	12.0	0
Beef, rump, pot roast	1 slice (5 × 3½ × ¼ in.)	320	17.8	27.2	0
Beefsteak, club, broiled	1 large (4 oz.)	410	27.6	32.4	0
Beef stew with potatoes, carrots, onions, gravy	3 oz. chuck, 2 small potatoes, 1 small carrot, 1 onion	529	28.1	19.6	56.1
Beef tongue, medium-cooked	3 slices, 2 oz. (3 × 2 × ⅛ in.)	160	11.6	12.2	0.2
Chili con carne (no beans)	½ cup, scant, 60% meat	200	10.3	14.8	5.8
Frankfurter, cooked	1 average (5½ in. long × ¾ in. diam.)	124	7.0	10.0	1.0
Ham, smoked, cooked	1 slice, 1 oz. (4 × 2½ × ⅛ in.)	119	6.9	9.9	(0.1)
Lamb chop, rib, cooked	1	128	7.9	(10.5)	0
Lamb, ground, cooked	1 patty, 2 oz. (2 in. diam., ½ in. thick)	130	8.2	10.5	0
Lamb, leg, roasted	1 slice, 1 oz. (3 × 2¾ × ⅛ in.)	82	7.2	5.7	0
Liver, beef, fried	1 slice, 1½ oz. (3 × 2¼ × ⅜ in.)	86	8.8	2.9	5.6
Liver, calf, cooked	1 slice, 1⅓ oz. (3 × 2¼ × ⅜ in.)	74	8.1	3.6	1.7
Liver, chicken, cooked	1 medium-large	74	8.8	3.6	1.0
Meat loaf, beef and pork	1 slice, 2⅓ oz. (4 × 3 × ⅜ in.)	264	10.4	19.2	11.5
Meat gravy	1 tbsp.	41	0.3	3.5	2.0
Pork chop, loin, fried	1 medium (2⅓ oz.)	233	16.1	18.2	0
Pork, loin, roasted	1 slice, 1 oz. (3 × 2½ × ¼ in.)	100	6.9	7.8	0
Pork, spareribs, roasted	Meat from 6 average ribs (3 oz.)	246	15.4	(20.0)	0
Veal chop, loin, fried	1 medium (3 oz.)	186	21.8	9.4	0

CALCIUM (MG.)	IRON (MG.)	VITAMIN A (I.U.)	THIAMINE (MCG.)	RIBOFLAVIN (MCG.)	NIACIN (MG.)	ASCORBIC ACID (MG.)
11	2.7	0	54	144	3.7	0
23	2.4	0	63	145	3.3	0
17	4.5	(0)	90	270	7.1	0
3	0.9	(0)	18	54	1.9	0
10	3.1	(0)	74	202	5.1	0
7	2.1	(0)	34	128	2.6	0
13	3.6	(0)	72	216	5.6	0
86	5.0	5,590	255	280	5.5	(20)
4	(1.5)	(0)	(30)	(130)	(1.5)	0
38	1.4	150	20	120	2.2	0
3	0.6	(0)	80	90	1.2	0
3	0.9	(0)	162	63	1.3	0
4	1.1	(0)	45	80	1.9	0
4	1.0	(0)	85	150	2.7	0
3	0.9	(0)	42	75	1.5	0
4	2.9	18,658	90	1,283	5.1	(10)
3	4.5	9,565	63	1,193	5.9	(8)
6	3.0	12,880	56	886	4.7	(4)
26	1.7	50	118	111	2.0	(0)
Trace	(0.1)	0	(10)	(7)	Trace	—
8	2.1	(0)	580	168	3.5	(0)
3	0.9	(0)	249	72	1.5	0
8	2.2	(0)	400	150	2.8	0
10	3.0	(0)	110	265	6.7	0

Continued.

FOOD VALUES—cont'd

	APPROXIMATE MEASURE	CALORIES	PROTEIN (GM.)	FAT (GM.)	CARBO-HYDRATE (GM.)
Meats–cont'd					
Veal cutlet, breaded, baked	1 average serving, 3 oz.	217	23.8	9.4	8.0
Veal, leg, roasted	1 slice, 1 oz. (3 × 2 × ⅛ in.)	70	8.4	3.8	0
Veal, stew, carrots, onions	½ cup	121	8.8	7.8	3.6
Sausages					
Bologna	1 slice, 1 oz. (4½ in diam., ⅛ in. thick)	66	4.4	4.8	1.1
Liver sausage	1 slice, 1 oz. (3 in. diam., ¼ in. thick)	79	5.0	6.2	0.5
Luncheon meat	1 slice (1 oz.)	81	4.6	6.8	0.5
Salami	1 slice, 1 oz. (3¾ diam., ¼ in. thick)	130	7.2	11.0	0
Nuts					
Almonds, chocolate	5 medium	84	2.0	6.9	5.1
Cashew nuts, roasted	6 to 8	88	2.8	7.2	4.1
Coconut, shredded, dried	2 tbsp.	83	0.5	5.9	8.0
Peanut butter	1 tbsp., scant	86	4.0	7.2	3.2
Peanuts, roasted	15 to 17	84	4.0	6.6	3.5
Pecans, shelled	12 halves or 2 tbsp., chopped	104	1.4	11.0	2.0
Poultry					
Chicken, broiler, fried	¼ chicken, no bone	232	22.4	13.61	3.1
Chicken, canned	⅓ cup boned meat	169	25.0	6.8	0
Chicken, creamed	½ cup, scant	208	17.6	12.1	6.6
Chicken, fryer, fried	½ breast (4 oz. raw)	232	26.8	11.9	3.1
Chicken, fryer, leg, fried	1 small	64	10.5	5.3	1.5
Chicken, hen, stewed	1 medium thigh or ½ breast	207	26.5	10.4	0
Chicken pie with peas, potatoes	2 in. square serving, 4 oz.)	230	9.6	12.1	20.2
Chicken, roasted	3 slices (3½ × 2½ × ¼)	198	28.3	(8.6)	0
Duck, roasted	3 slices (3½ × 3 × ¼ in.)	310	22.8	23.6	0
Goose	3 slices (3½ × 3 × ¼ in.)	322	28.1	22.4	0
Turkey	3 slices (3½ × 2½ × ¼ in.)	200	30.9	(7.6)	0

CALCIUM (MG.)	IRON (MG.)	VITAMIN A (I.U.)	THIAMINE (MCG.)	RIBOFLAVIN (MCG.)	NIACIN (MG.)	ASCORBIC ACID (MG.)
22	3.0	(0)	102	256	6.5	0
4	1.1	(0)	40	95	2.4	0
16	1.5	1,627	34	83	1.5	(0)
(3)	1.6	(0)	54	57	0.8	0
3	1.6	1,725	51	36	1.4	(0)
6	0.4	(0)	110	54	1.1	(0)
4	1.1	(0)	75	63	0.9	0
28	0.5	0	(27)	(75)	(0.5)	Trace
7	0.8	—	95	29	0.3	0
6	0.5	0	Trace	Trace	Trace	(0)
11	0.3	0	18	20	2.4	(0)
11	0.3	0	45	20	2.4	(0)
11	0.4	8	108	17	0.1	Trace
18	1.8	230	74	168	9.7	(0)
12	1.5	(0)	32	136	5.4	0
83	1.1	328	(40)	180	3.8	Trace
19	1.3	460	67	101	10.2	0
9	1.0	161	43	113	2.4	0
16	1.6	(0)	52	150	6.0	(0)
19	1.2	143	87	68	2.3	(6)
20	2.1	(0)	80	180	9.0	(0)
19	5.8	(0)				
10	4.6	(0)				
30	5.1	0 to 20	81	173	9.8	0

Continued.

FOOD VALUES—cont'd

	APPROXIMATE MEASURE	CALORIES	PROTEIN (GM.)	FAT (GM.)	CARBO-HYDRATE (GM.)
Salads					
Coleslaw	⅔ cup	68	2.3	3.5	7.9
Carrot and raisin	3 heaping tbsp. on lettuce leaf	153	1.9	5.8	27.9
Chicken with celery	½ cup, lettuce leaf	185	16.1	10.9	5.7
Gelatin with fruit	1 square, ¼ head lettuce	139	2.1	5.7	21.6
Gelatin with chopped vegetables	1 square, ¼ head lettuce	115	2.2	5.7	15.1
Lettuce with French dressing	1 wedge	133	1.4	10.8	6.9
Potato with onion, parsley	½ cup potato with French dressing	184	1.9	10.8	21.2
Prunes, stuffed with peanut butter	4 prunes	414	13.4	28.5	32.9
Sandwiches					
Bacon, lettuce, and tomato	1 sandwich	282	6.3	15.6	28.8
Cream cheese and jelly	1 sandwich	368	6.6	16.0	50.4
Chicken, hot, with gravy	1 sandwich, 3 tbsp. gravy	356	21.9	15.3	29.8
Chicken salad	1 sandwich	245	14.3	8.6	26.6
Chicken, sliced, lettuce	1 sandwich	303	15.8	14.4	26.6
Club (bacon, chicken, and tomato)	1 average, 3 slices toast, lettuce	590	35.6	20.8	41.7
Egg salad on white bread	1 average	279	10.5	12.5	30.6
Peanut butter	1 average	328	11.8	19.5	30.0
Roast beef, hot, with gravy	1 average, 3 tbsp. gravy	429	19.3	24.5	29.8
Tuna fish salad	1 average, white bread	278	11.0	14.2	25.8
Soups					
Asparagus, cream (Campbell's)	⅞ cup (3 to 1 can)	131	5.9	6.4	12.8
Bean, homemade	¾ cup	195	6.1	11.0	18.6
Beef noodle (Campbell's)	⅞ cup	52	3.3	2.4	4.5
Celery, cream (Campbell's)	⅞ cup	146	4.9	8.6	12.2
Chicken, cream (Campbell's)	⅞ cup	145	6.5	9.9	7.7
Chicken gumbo (Campbell's)	⅞ cup	51	1.9	0.9	8.8

CALCIUM (MG.)	IRON (MG.)	VITAMIN A (I.U.)	THIAMINE (MCG.)	RIBOFLAVIN (MCG.)	NIACIN (MG.)	ASCORBIC ACID (MG.)
53	0.5	200	50	85	0.2	(12)
48	1.5	4,708	83	81	0.5	(6)
32	1.3	290	53	130	3.4	(5)
23	0.5	391	42	50	0.3	16
24	0.5	1,977	37	58	0.3	(8)
22	0.5	540	40	80	0.2	8
21	0.8	243	70	38	0.8	(16)
63	2.3	800	110	140	7.9	5
53	1.5	870	160	142	1.6	13
60	1.1	575	120	140	1.0	2
49	2.4	(0)	178	209	6.5	0
50	1.5	10	142	140	3.2	1
52	1.8	320	162	172	4.6	2
103	4.3	1,705	384	410	10.2	27
68	2.4	580	160	210	1.0	2
61	1.0	165	96	80	5.4	(0)
43	2.9	(0)	166	209	4.9	(3)
48	1.2	231	142	113	4.1	1
(126)	(0.1)	(171)	(40)	(182)	(0.1)	(1)
52	1.9	1,364	120	70	0.5	(0)
(126)	(0.1)	(171)	(40)	(182)	(0.1)	(1)
(126)	(0.1)	(171)	(43)	(182)	(0.1)	(1)

Continued.

FOOD VALUES—cont'd

	APPROXIMATE MEASURE	CALORIES	PROTEIN (GM.)	FAT (GM.)	CARBO-HYDRATE (GM.)
Soups–cont'd					
Chicken noodle (Campbell's)	⅞ cup	56	3.1	19.0	6.6
Chicken rice (Campbell's)	⅞ cup	36	2.7	1.3	3.5
Clam chowder (Campbell's)	⅞ cup	64	2.2	2.4	8.3
Green pea (Campbell's)	⅞ cup	110	5.4	1.9	17.9
Oyster stew, homemade	1 serving, 8 oz. milk, 4 oysters	321	15.0	22.2	15.7
Scotch broth (Campbell's)	⅞ cup	96	5.8	2.8	11.8
Split pea, homemade	1 serving, ¾ cup	201	7.1	11.1	19.4
Tomato (Campbell's)	⅞ cup	141	5.6	6.1	15.9
Vegetable (Campbell's)	⅞ cup	68	2.9	1.5	10.9
Vegetable beef (Campbell's)	⅞ cup	77	5.9	2.1	7.9
Syrups and sugars					
Honey, strained	1 tbsp.	62	0.1	0	16.7
Molasses	1 tbsp.	50	—	0	13.0
Sorghum syrup	1 tbsp.	52	—	0	13.4
Sugar, brown	1 tbsp.	52	(0)	0	13.4
Sugar, powdered	1 tbsp.	42	(0)	0	10.9
Sugar, white, granulated	1 tbsp.	48	(0)	0	12.4
Sweets					
Caramels, plain	1 medium	42	0.3	1.2	7.8
Chocolate creams	1 average (35 to 1 lb.)	51	0.5	1.8	9.4
Chocolate fudge, made with milk	1 piece, 1¼ in. square (15 to 1 lb.)	118	0.5	3.1	23.7
Chocolate mints	1 medium (20 to 1 lb.)	87	0.9	3.1	15.8
Gumdrops	1 large or 8 small	33	0	0	8.6
Hershey's milk chocolate	1 bar, plain, small (1 oz.)	154	2.4	9.5	15.8
Hershey's Mr. Goodbar	1 bar	158	4.2	10.4	12.9
Jelly beans	10	66	0	0	16.7
Mars candy bar	1 bar, 1⅜ oz.	177	2.4	8.3	24.2
Mars, Forever Yours	1 bar	122	1.1	1.6	26.7
Mars, Milky Way	1 bar	121	1.2	2.0	24.8
Mars, Snickers	1 bar	122	1.9	3.0	22.8

CALCIUM (MG.)	IRON (MG.)	VITAMIN A (I.U.)	THIAMINE (MCG.)	RIBOFLAVIN (MCG.)	NIACIN (MG.)	ASCORBIC ACID (MG.)
352	3.8	1,058	188	550	1.1	(3)
44	1.6	1,446	139	81	1.0	(2)
(126)	(0.1)	(171)	(43)	(182)	(0.1)	(1)
1	0.2	(0)	Trace	10	Trace	1
33	0.9	—	14	12	Trace	—
30	2.4	—	—	—	—	—
11	0.4	(0)	(0)	(0)	(0)	(0)
—	—	(0)	(0)	(0)	(0)	(0)
—	—	(0)	(0)	(0)	(0)	(0)
13	0.2	17	2	14	Trace	Trace
—	—	—	—	—	—	—
14	0.2	64	3	19	Trace	Trace
—	—	—	—	—	—	—
(0)	(0)	0	0	0	0	0
57	0.7	43	27	145	0.1	Trace
34	0.5	36	47	72	2.0	Trace
52	0.4	0	17	121	0.27	Trace
22	0.2	0	15	53	0.14	Trace
29	0.2	0	15	107	0.13	Trace
27	0.1	0	10	102	0.08	Trace

Continued.

FOOD VALUES—cont'd

	APPROXIMATE MEASURE	CALORIES	PROTEIN (GM.)	FAT (GM.)	CARBO-HYDRATE (GM.)
Sweets–cont'd					
Mars, Three Musketeers	1 bar	147	0.8	0.9	35.1
Marshmallow, plain	1 average (60 to 1 lb.)	25	0.2	0	6.2
Mints, cream	10 (½ in. cubes	53	0	0	13.7
Peanut brittle	1 piece (2½ × 2½ × ⅜ in.)	110	2.1	3.9	18.2
Preserves and jellies					
Assorted jams, commercial	1 tbsp.	55	0.1	0.1	14.2
Assorted jellies	1 tbsp.	50	0	0	13.0
Vegetables					
Asparagus, canned	6 medium stalks	21	2.4	0.2	3.9
Beans, dry, with pork and tomato sauce	½ cup	147	7.5	2.7	24.0
Beans, green limas, cooked	½ cup	76	4.0	0.3	14.7
Beans, green limas, frozen	½ cup	109	6.4	0.7	19.9
Beans, green, canned	1 cup	27	1.8	0.2	5.9
Beans, green, frozen	½ cup	35	2.4	0.2	7.7
Beans, yellow canned	1 cup	27	1.8	0.2	5.9
Beets, canned	½ cup	34	0.8	0.1	8.1
Broccoli, cooked	⅔ cup	29	3.3	0.2	5.5
Brussels sprouts, cooked	½ cup (5 or 6)	33	3.1	0.4	6.2
Cabbage, raw	½ cup	12	0.7	0.1	2.7
Cabbage, cooked	½ cup	20	1.2	0.2	4.5
Carrots, cooked	½ cup	35	0.6	0.5	7.5
Cauliflower, cooked	½ cup	15	1.5	0.1	3.0
Celery, raw	1 large outer stalk (8 in. long)	7	0.5	0.1	1.5
Celery, raw	1 cup, diced	18	1.3	0.2	3.7
Celery, cooked	½ cup	12	0.9	0.2	2.4
Corn, canned	½ cup	70	2.3	0.6	16.7
Cucumber, raw	½ medium (6 to 8 slices)	6	0.4	0	1.4
Garlic bulbs, peeled	5	9	0.4	Trace	2.0
Kale, cooked	½ cup	20	2.0	0.3	3.6
Lettuce wedge	Small	15	1.0	0.3	2.7
Mushrooms, fresh	10 small or 4 large	16	2.4	0.3	4.0
Mushrooms, canned	½ cup	14	1.7	0.3	4.5
Parsley, raw	10 small sprigs	5	0.4	0.1	0.9

*Calcium may not be available because of the presence of oxalic acid.

CALCIUM (MG.)	IRON (MG.)	VITAMIN A (I.U.)	THIAMINE (MCG.)	RIBOFLAVIN (MCG.)	NIACIN (MG.)	ASCORBIC ACID (MG.)
15	0.2	0	6	43	0.04	Trace
(0)	(0)	(0)	(0)	(0)	0	0
10	0.5	7	22	12	1.2	0
2	0.1	2	4	4	0.04	1
(2)	(0.1)	(2)	(4)	(4)	(0.04)	1
23	2.1	760	90	120	1.1	18
53	2.3	110	165	45	0.6	3
23	1.4	230	110	70	0.9	12
53	1.9	220	110	70	0.8	17
45	2.1	620	40	70	0.5	7
65	1.1	450	70	100	0.6	11
45	2.1	150	40	70	0.5	7
18	0.6	15	15	35	0.2	5
130	1.3	3,400	70	150	0.8	74
24	0.9	280	28	84	0.4	33
23	0.3	40	30	25	0.2	25
39	0.4	75	40	40	0.3	27
27	0.8	14,760	30	25	0.4	3
13	0.7	54	35	50	0.3	17
20	0.2	0	20	20	0.2	3
50	0.5	0	50	40	0.4	7
33	0.3	0	25	20	0.2	3
4	0.5	190	30	50	0.8	5
5	0.2	0	20	20	0.1	4
1	0.2	—	—	—	—	3
113	1.1	4,190	35	115	0.9	26
22	0.5	540	40	80	0.2	8
9	1.0	0	100	440	4.9	5
(9)	(1.0)	0	20	300	2.4	(0)
19*	0.4	823	11	28	0.1	19

Continued.

FOOD VALUES—cont'd

	APPROXIMATE MEASURE	CALORIES	PROTEIN (GM.)	FAT (GM.)	CARBO-HYDRATE (GM.)
Vegetables–cont'd					
Parsnips, cooked	½ cup	47	0.8	0.4	10.7
Peas, green, cooked	½ cup	73	3.6	0.5	13.8
Peppers, green, raw	1 tbsp. chopped	3	0.1	Trace	0.6
Pepper, shell, baked	1 shell, no filling	17	0.8	0.1	3.9
Pickles, sour	1 large, (4 in. diam. × 1¾ in.)	15	0.7	0.3	3.0
Pickles, sweet	1 pickle (2 × ⅝ in.)	11	0.1	Trace	2.6
Pimento, canned	1 medium	9	0.3	0.2	2.0
Potatoes, white baked	1 medium (2½ in. diam.)	98	2.4	0.1	22.5
Potatoes, white, boiled	1 medium (2¼ in. diam.)	83	2.0	0.1	19.1
Potatoes, white, French fried	10 pieces (2 × ½ × ½ in.)	197	2.7	9.6	26.0
Potatoes, white, mashed with milk and margarine	½ cup	123	2.1	6.0	15.9
Potato chips	10 pieces (2 in. diam.)	108	1.3	7.4	9.8
Radish, red, raw	1 small	2	0.1	Trace	0.4
Sauerkraut, canned	⅔ cup	22	1.4	0.3	4.4
Spinach	½ cup	23	2.8	0.6	3.3
Squash, summer, cooked	½ cup, scant	16	0.6	0.1	3.9
Squash, winter, baked	½ cup	47	1.9	0.4	11.0
Sweet potatoes, baked	1 medium, peeled (5 × 2 in.)	183	2.6	1.1	41.3
Sweet potatoes, candied	1 halves (3¾ × 2¼ in.)	358	3.0	7.2	72.4
Tomatoes, raw	1 small	20	1.0	0.3	4.0
Tomatoes, canned	½ cup	23	1.2	0.2	4.7
Tomato catsup	1 tbsp.	17	0.3	0.1	4.2
Miscellaneous					
Cocoa, dry	1 tbsp.	21	(0.6)	1.7	3.4
Cornstarch	1 tbsp.	29	0	0	7.0
Gelatin, dry, plain	1 tbsp.	34	8.6	0	0
Postum	1 tsp.	4	0.06	Trace	0.8
Tapioca	1 tbsp.	36	0.06	Trace	8.6
Alcoholic beverages†				ALCOHOLIC GM.	
Beer, average	8 oz.	112	1.4	8.9	10.6

*Calcium may not be available because of the presence of oxalic acid.

†Calories in alcoholic beverages are derived from the alcohol content.

CALCIUM (MG.)	IRON (MG.)	VITAMIN A (I.U.)	THIAMINE (MCG.)	RIBOFLAVIN (MCG.)	NIACIN (MG.)	ASCORBIC ACID (MG.)
44	0.6	0	45	80	0.1	10
26	1.7	535	95	50	0.8	8
1	Trace	63	4	7	Trace	12
7	0.3	481	26	46	0.3	64
34	1.6	420	Trace	90	Trace	8
2	0.1	11	(0)	2	Trace	1
2	0.5	805	7	21	0.1	33
13	0.8	20	110	50	1.4	17
11	0.7	20	90	30	1.0	14
15	1.0	25	90	55	1.7	14
37	0.6	260	80	50	0.8	7
(6)	(0.4)	(10)	(40)	(20)	(0.6)	2
4	0.1	3	3	2	Trace	8
36	(0.5)	40	30	60	0.1	16
111*	1.8	10,600	70	180	0.6	27
15	0.4	260	40	70	0.6	11
24	0.8	6,190	50	150	0.6	7
44	1.1	11,410	120	80	0.9	28
72	1.8	12,500	80	80	1.0	18
11	0.6	1,100	60	40	0.5	23
(13)	0.7	1,260	72	36	0.8	19
2	0.1	(320)	15	12	0.4	2
9*	0.8	2	8	27	0.2	(0)
(0)	(0)	(0)	(0)	(0)	(0)	(0)
(0)	(0)	(0)	(0)	(0)	(0)	(0)
1	Trace	—	—	—	—	—
1	0.1	(0)	(0)	(0)	(0)	(0)
10	0.0	(0)	Trace	72	0.5	0

Continued.

FOOD VALUES—cont'd

	APPROXIMATE MEASURE	CALORIES	PROTEIN (GM.)	ALCO-HOLIC (GM.)	CARBO-HYDRATE (GM.)
Alcoholic beverages–cont'd					
Eggnog, Christmas type	1 punch cup	335	3.9	15.0	18.0
Gin, dry	1 jigger (1½ oz.)	105	—	15.1	
Highball	1 glass	166	—	24.0	
Manhattan	1 cocktail	164	Trace	19.2	7.9
Martini	1 cocktail	140	0.1	18.5	0.3
Old-fashioned	1 glass	179	—	24.0	3.5
Rum	1 jigger (1½ oz.)	105	—	15.1	0
Tom Collins	1 cocktail	180	—	21.5	9.0
Whiskey, bourbon	1 jigger (1½ oz.)	119	—	17.2	0
Whiskey, Scotch	1 jigger (1½ oz.)	105	—	15.1	0
Wine, California, red	1 wineglass (3⅓ oz.)	72	0.2	10.0	0.5
Wine, port	1 wineglass (3⅓ oz.)	158	0.2	15.0	14.0

CALCIUM (MG.)	IRON (MG.)	VITAMIN A (I.U.)	THIAMINE (MCG.)	RIBOFLAVIN (MCG.)	NIACIN (MG.)	ASCORBIC ACID (MG.)
44	0.7	84	35	113	Trace	Trace
—	—	—	—	—	—	—
—	—	—	—	—	—	—
1	Trace	35	3	2	Trace	(0)
5	0.1	4	Trace	Trace	Trace	(0)
—	—	—	—	—	—	—
—	—	—	—	—	—	—
—	—	—	—	—	—	—
—	—	—	—	—	—	—
—	—	—	—	—	—	—

B CHOLESTEROL CONTENT OF FOODS

Foods of plant origin, such as fruits, vegetables, cereal grains, legumes, and nuts, do not have cholesterol. The following list indicates the *approximate* amount in some foods of animal origin.

FOOD	AMOUNT IN COMMON SERVING	CHOLESTEROL (MG.)
Milk, nonfat		—
Nuts		—
Vegetable oils		—
Cottage cheese, creamed	½ cup	15
Bacon fat	1 tbsp.	25
Butter	2 tsp.	
Cheese, cheddar	1 oz.	
Cream (half and half)	3 tbsp.	30
Cream cheese	2 tbsp.	
Ice cream	½ cup	
Milk, whole	1 cup	
Beef		
Fish	3 oz., cooked, including lean and fat	70
Lamb		
Pork		
Poultry		
Caviar or fish roe	1 oz.	80
Shrimp	2 oz.	80
Crab meat	2 oz. About ⅓ cup	80
Lobster	2 oz.	120
Oysters	2 oz.	120 or more
Liver	2 oz., cooked	250
Kidney	2 oz., cooked	250
Egg yolk	1	300
Brains	2 oz. cooked	1,350 or more

C CALORIE VALUES OF SOME COMMON SNACK FOODS

FOOD	WEIGHT (GM.)	APPROXIMATE MEASURE	CALORIES
Beverages			
Carbonated, cola type	180	1 bottle, 6 oz.	70
Malted milk	405	1 regular (1½ cups)	420
Chocolate milk (made with skim milk)	250	1 cup	190
Cocoa	200	1 cup	235
Soda, vanilla ice cream	242	1 regular	260
Cake			
Angel food	40	2-inch section	110
Cupcake, chocolate, iced	50	1 cake, 2¾ in. diam.	185
Fruitcake	30	1 piece, 2 × 2 × ½ in.	115
Candy and popcorn			
Butterscotch	15	3 pieces	60
Candy bar, plain	57	1 bar	295
Caramels	30	3 medium	120
Chocolate-coated creams	30	2 average	130
Fudge	28	1 piece	115
Peanut brittle	30	1 oz.	125
Popcorn with oil added	14	1 cup	65
Cheese			
Camembert	28	1 oz.	85
Cheddar	28	1 oz.	105
Cream	28	1 oz.	105
Swiss (domestic)	28	1 oz.	105
Cookies			
Brownies	30	1 piece, 2 × 2 × ¾ in.	140
Cookies, plain and assorted	25	1 cooky, 3 in. diam.	120
Crackers			
Cheese	18	5 crackers	85
Graham	14	2 medium	55
Saltines	16	4 crackers	70
Rye	13	2 crackers	45
Dessert type cream puff and doughnuts			
Cream puff, custard filling	105	1 average	245
Doughnut, cake type, plain	32	1 average	125
Doughnut, jelly	65	1 average	225
Doughnut, raised	30	1 average	120

Continued.

CALORIE VALUES OF SOME COMMON
SNACK FOODS—cont'd

FOOD	WEIGHT (GM.)	APPROXIMATE MEASURE	CALORIES
Miscellaneous			
Hamburger and bun	96	1 average	330
Ice cream, vanilla	62	3½ oz. container	130
Sherbet	96	½ cup	120
Jams, jellies, marmalades, preserves	20	1 tbsp.	55
Syrup, blended	80	¼ cup	240
Waffles	75	1 waffle, 4½ × 5½ × ½ in.	210
Nuts			
Mixed, shelled	15	8 to 12	95
Peanut butter	16	1 tbsp.	95
Peanuts, shelled, roasted	144	1 cup	840
Pie			
Apple	135	4 in. section	345
Cherry	135	4 in. section	355
Custard	130	4 in. section	280
Lemon meringue	120	4 in. section	305
Mince	135	4 in. section	365
Pumpkin	130	4 in. section	275
Potato chips	20	10 chips, 2 in. diam.	115
Sandwiches			
Bacon, lettuce, tomato	150	1 sandwich	280
Egg salad	140	1 sandwich	280
Ham	80	1 sandwich	280
Liverwurst	90	1 sandwich	250
Peanut butter	85	1 sandwich	330
Soups, commercial canned			
Bean with pork	250	1 cup	170
Beef noodle	250	1 cup	70
Chicken noodle	250	1 cup	65
Cream (mushroom)	240	1 cup	135
Tomato	245	1 cup	90
Vegetable with beef broth	250	1 cup	80

D COMPOSITION OF BEVERAGES—ALCOHOLIC AND CARBONATED NONALCOHOLIC PER 100 GRAMS*

	FOOD ENERGY	PROTEIN	CARBO-HYDRATE	CALCIUM	PHOS-PHORUS	IRON	THIAMINE	RIBO-FLAVIN	NIACIN
Beverages									
Alcoholic									
Beer, alcohol 4.5% by volume (3.6% by weight)	42	.3	3.8	5	30	Trace	Trace	.03	.6
Gin, rum, vodka, whisky									
80-proof (33.4% alcohol by weight)	231	—	Trace	—	—	—	—	—	—
86-proof (36.0% alcohol by weight)	249	—	Trace	—	—	—	—	—	—
90-proof (37.9% alcohol by weight)	263	—	Trace	—	—	—	—	—	—
94-proof (39.7% alcohol by weight)	275	—	Trace	—	—	—	—	—	—
100-proof (42.5% alcohol by weight)	295	—	Trace	—	—	—	—	—	—
Wines									
Dessert, alcohol 18.8% by volume (15.3% by weight)	137	.1	7.7	8	—	—	.01	.02	.2
Table, alcohol 12.2% by volume (9.9% by weight)	85	.1	4.2	9	10	.4	Trace	.01	.1
Carbonated, nonalcoholic									
Carbonated waters									
Sweetened (quinine sodas)	31	—	8	—	—	—	—	—	—
Unsweetened (club sodas)	—	—	—	—	—	—	—	—	—
Cola type	39	—	10	—	—	—	—	—	—
Cream sodas	43	—	11	—	—	—	—	—	—
Fruit-flavored sodas (citrus, cherry, grape, strawberry, Tom Collins mixer, other) (10% to 13% sugar)	46	—	12	—	—	—	—	—	—
Ginger ale, pale dry and golden	31	—	8	—	—	—	—	—	—
Root beer	41	—	10.5	—	—	—	—	—	—
Special dietary drinks with artificial sweetener (less than 1 calorie per ounce)	—	—	—	—	—	—	—	—	—

*From Watt, B. K., and Merrill, A. L.: Composition of foods—raw, processed, prepared, U. S. Department of Agriculture, Agriculture Handbook, No. 8, Dec., 1963.

E FOOD AND NUTRITION BOARD, NATIONAL ACADEMY OF SCIENCES–NATIONAL RESEARCH COUNCIL RECOMMENDED DAILY DIETARY ALLOWANCES,[1]
revised 1973
Designed for the maintenance of good nutrition of practically all healthy people in the United States

	AGE (YR.)	WEIGHT (KG.)	WEIGHT (LB.)	HEIGHT (CM.)	HEIGHT (IN.)	ENERGY (KCAL)[2]	PROTEIN (GM.)	FAT-SOLUBLE VITAMINS			
								VITAMIN A ACTIVITY (RE)[3]	VITAMIN A ACTIVITY (I.U.)	VITA-MIN D (I.U.)	VITA-MIN E ACTIVITY[5] (I.U.)
Infants	0.0 to 0.5	6	14	60	24	Kg. × 117	Kg. × 2.2	420[4]	1,400	400	4
	0.5 to 1.0	9	20	71	28	Kg. × 108	Kg. × 2.0	400	2,000	400	5
Children	1 to 3	13	28	86	34	1,300	23	400	2,000	400	7
	4 to 6	20	44	110	44	1,800	30	500	2,500	400	9
	7 to 10	30	66	135	54	2,400	36	700	3,300	400	10
Men	11 to 14	44	97	158	63	2,800	44	1,000	5,000	400	12
	15 to 18	61	134	172	69	3,000	54	1,000	5,000	400	15
	19 to 22	67	147	172	69	3,000	52	1,000	5,000	400	15
	23 to 50	70	154	172	69	2,700	56	1,000	5,000		15
	51+	70	154	172	69	2,400	56	1,000	5,000		15
Women	11 to 14	44	97	155	62	2,400	44	800	4,000	400	10
	15 to 18	54	119	162	65	2,100	48	800	4,000	400	11
	19 to 22	58	128	162	65	2,100	46	800	4,000	400	12
	23 to 50	58	128	162	65	2,000	46	800	4,000		12
	51+	58	128	162	65	1,800	46	800	4,000		12
Pregnant						+300	+30	1,000	5,000	400	15
Lactating						+500	+20	1,200	6,000	400	15

[1] The allowances are intended to provide for individual variations among most normal persons as they live in the United States under usual environmental stresses. Diets should be based on a variety of common foods to provide other nutrients for which human requirements have been less well defined.

[2] Kilojoules (KJ) = 4.2 × kcal.

[3] Retinol equivalents.

[4] Assumed to be all as retinol in milk during the first 6 months of life. All subsequent intakes are assumed to be one half as retinol and one half as beta-carotene when calculated from international units. As retinol equivalents, three fourths are as retinol and one fourth as beta-carotene.

	WATER-SOLUBLE VITAMINS						MINERALS					
ASCOR-BIC ACID (MG.)	FOLA-CIN[6] (MCG.)	NIA-CIN[7] (MG.)	RIBO-FLAVIN (MG.)	THIA-MINE (MG.)	VITA-MIN B_6 (MG.)	VITA-MIN B_{12} (MCG.)	CAL-CIUM (MG.)	PHOS-PHORUS (MG.)	IODINE (MCG.)	IRON (MG.)	MAG-NESIUM (MG.)	ZINC (MG.)
35	50	5	0.4	0.3	0.3	0.3	360	240	35	10	60	3
35	50	8	0.6	0.5	0.4	0.3	540	400	45	15	70	5
40	100	9	0.8	0.7	0.6	1.0	800	800	60	15	150	10
40	200	12	1.1	0.9	0.9	1.5	800	800	80	10	200	10
40	300	16	1.2	1.2	1.2	2.0	800	800	110	10	250	10
45	400	18	1.5	1.4	1.6	3.0	1,200	1,200	130	18	350	15
45	400	20	1.8	1.5	1.8	3.0	1,200	1,200	150	18	400	15
45	400	20	1.8	1.5	2.0	3.0	800	800	140	10	350	15
45	400	18	1.6	1.4	2.0	3.0	800	800	130	10	350	15
45	400	16	1.5	1.2	2.0	3.0	800	800	110	10	350	15
45	400	16	1.3	1.2	1.6	3.0	1,200	1,200	115	18	300	15
45	400	14	1.4	1.1	2.0	3.0	1,200	1,200	115	18	300	15
45	400	14	1.4	1.1	2.0	3.0	800	800	100	18	300	15
45	400	13	1.2	1.0	2.0	3.0	800	800	100	18	300	15
45	400	12	1.1	1.0	2.0	3.0	800	800	80	10	300	15
60	800	+2	+0.3	+0.3	2.5	4.0	1,200	1,200	125	18+[8]	450	20
60	600	+4	+0.5	+0.3	2.5	4.0	1,200	1,200	150	18	450	25

[5] Total vitamin E activity, estimated to be 80% as alpha-tocopherol and 20% other tocopherols.

[6] The folacin allowances refer to dietary sources as determined by *Lactobacillus casoi* assay. Pure forms of folacin may be effective in doses less than one fourth of the RDA.

[7] Although allowances are expressed as niacin, it is recognized that on the average 1 mg. of niacin is derived from each 60 mg. of dietary tryptophan.

[8] This increased requirement cannot be met by ordinary diets; therefore the use of supplemental iron is recommended.

F HEIGHT AND WEIGHT TABLES FOR ADULTS

Desirable weights for persons age 25 and over*
Weight in pounds according to frame (with indoor clothing)

HEIGHT (WITH 1-INCH HEELS)		MEN SMALL FRAME (LB.)	MEDIUM FRAME (LB.)	LARGE FRAME (LB.)	HEIGHT (WITH 2-INCH HEELS)		WOMEN† SMALL FRAME (LB.)	MEDIUM FRAME (LB.)	LARGE FRAME (LB.)
(FT.)	(IN.)				(FT.)	(IN.)			
5	2	112-120	118-129	126-141	4	10	92- 98	96-107	104-119
5	3	115-123	121-133	129-144	4	11	94-101	98-110	106-122
5	4	118-126	124-136	132-148	5	0	96-104	101-113	109-125
5	5	121-129	127-139	135-152	5	1	99-107	104-116	112-128
5	6	124-133	130-143	138-156	5	2	102-110	107-119	115-131
5	7	128-137	134-147	142-161	5	3	105-113	110-122	118-134
5	8	132-141	138-152	147-166	5	4	108-116	113-126	121-138
5	9	136-145	142-156	151-170	5	5	111-119	116-130	125-142
5	10	140-150	146-160	155-174	5	6	114-123	120-135	129-146
5	11	144-154	150-165	159-179	5	7	118-127	124-139	133-150
6	0	148-158	154-170	164-184	5	8	122-131	128-143	137-154
6	1	152-162	158-175	168-189	5	9	126-135	132-147	141-158
6	2	156-167	162-180	173-194	5	10	130-140	136-151	145-163
6	3	160-171	167-185	178-199	5	11	134-144	140-155	149-168
6	4	164-175	172-190	182-204	6	0	138-148	144-159	153-173

*Metropolitan Life Insurance Co., New York City.
†For girls between 18 and 25 years, subtract 1 pound for each year under 25.

G AVERAGE HEIGHT AND WEIGHT TABLES FOR CHILDREN

Height-weight tables for girls (juvenile and adolescent ages)*

HEIGHT (IN.)	5 YR.	6 YR.	7 YR.	8 YR.	9 YR.	10 YR.	11 YR.	12 YR.	13 YR.	14 YR.	15 YR.	16 YR.	17 YR.	18 YR.
38	33	33												
39	34	34												
40	36	36	36											
41	37	37	37											
42	39	39	39											
43	41	41	41	41										
44	42	42	42	42										
45	45	45	45	45	45									
46	47	47	47	48	48									
47	49	50	50	50	50	50								
48		52	52	52	52	53	53							
49			54	55	55	56	56							
50			56	57	58	59	61	62						
51			59	60	61	61	63	65						
52			63	64	64	64	65	67						
53			66	67	67	68	68	69	71					
54				69	70	70	71	71	73					
55				72	74	74	74	75	77	78				
56					76	78	78	79	81	83				
57					80	82	82	82	84	88	92			
58						84	86	86	88	93	96	101		
59						87	90	90	92	96	100	103	104	
60						91	95	95	97	101	105	108	109	111
61							99	100	101	105	108	112	113	116
62							104	105	106	109	113	115	117	118
63								110	110	112	116	117	119	120
64								114	115	117	119	120	122	123
65								118	120	121	122	123	125	126
66									124	124	125	128	129	130
67									128	130	131	133	133	135
68									131	133	135	136	138	138
69										135	137	138	140	142
70										136	138	140	142	144
71										138	140	142	144	145

*Prepared by Bird T. Baldwin, Ph.D., and Thomas D. Wood, M.D. Published originally by American Child Health Association.

Continued.

AVERAGE HEIGHT AND WEIGHT TABLES
FOR CHILDREN—cont'd

Height-weight tables for boys (juvenile and adolescent ages)*

HEIGHT (IN.)	5 YR.	6 YR.	7 YR.	8 YR.	9 YR.	10 YR.	11 YR.	12 YR.	13 YR.	14 YR.	15 YR.	16 YR.	17 YR.	18 YR.	19 YR.
38	34	34													
39	35	35													
40	36	36													
41	38	38	38												
42	39	39	39	39											
43	41	41	41	41											
44	44	44	44	44											
45	46	46	46	46	46										
46	47	48	48	48	48										
47	49	50	50	50	50	50									
48		52	53	53	53	53									
49		55	55	55	55	55	55								
50		57	58	58	58	58	58	58							
51			61	61	61	61	61	61							
52			63	64	64	64	64	64	64						
53			66	67	67	67	67	68	68						
54				70	70	70	70	71	71	72					
55				72	72	73	73	74	74	74					
56				75	76	77	77	77	78	78	80				
57					79	80	81	81	82	83	83				
58					83	84	84	85	85	86	87				
59						87	88	89	89	90	90	90			
60						91	92	92	93	94	95	96			
61							95	96	97	99	100	103	106		
62							100	101	102	103	104	107	111	116	
63							105	106	107	108	110	113	118	123	127
64								109	111	113	115	117	121	126	130
65								114	117	118	120	122	127	131	134
66									119	122	125	128	132	136	139
67									124	128	130	134	136	139	142
68										134	134	137	141	143	147
69										137	139	143	146	149	152
70										143	144	145	148	151	155
71										148	150	151	152	154	159
72											153	155	156	158	163
73											157	160	162	164	167
74											160	164	168	170	171

*Prepared by Bird T. Baldwin, Ph.D., and Thomas D. Wood, M.D. Published originally by American Child Health Association.

H RESOURCE AGENCIES FOR NUTRITION EDUCATION MATERIALS

RESOURCE AGENCY	LOCATION
Government agencies	
Government Printing Office	Washington, D. C.
U. S. Department of Agriculture	**Federal Center Building**
Research Service	Hyattsville, Md.
Agricultural Extension Services	State universities
U. S. Department of Health, Education, and Welfare: Children's Bureau, Food and Drug Administration	Washington, D. C.; regional offices
State and local public health departments	State capitals; county seats
Professional organizations	
American Dietetic Association	620 N. Michigan Ave. Chicago, Ill.
American Medical Association Council on Foods and Nutrition	535 N. Dearborn St. Chicago, Ill.
American Home Economics Association	1600 20th St. N. W. Washington, D. C.
American Dental Association	222 E. Superior St. Chicago, Ill.
Society for Nutrition Education	2140 Shattuck Ave. Berkeley, Calif.
Volunteer health organizations	
American Heart Association	44 E. 23rd St. New York, N. Y.
American Diabetes Association	18 E. 48th Street New York, N. Y.
Industry-associated boards and councils	
National Dairy Council	111 N. Canal St. Chicago, Ill.
National Livestock and Meat Board	37 S. Wabash Ave. Chicago, Ill.
American Institute of Baking	400 E. Ontario Chicago, Ill.

Continued.

RESOURCE AGENCIES FOR NUTRITION EDUCATION MATERIALS—cont'd

RESOURCE AGENCY	LOCATION
Commercial agencies (health education services)	
Food Industries	
H. J. Heinz Co.	Pittsburgh, Pa.
Insurance companies	
John Hancock	Boston, Mass.
Metropolitan	New York, N. Y.
Pharmaceutical companies	
Mead Johnson Laboratories	Evansville, Ind.
Parke, Davis & Co.	Detroit, Mich.
Ross Laboratories	Columbus, Ohio
Abbott Laboratories	North Chicago, Ill.
Science foundations	
National Academy of Sciences	2101 Constitution Ave.
National Research Council	Washington, D. C.
Nutrition Foundation	99 Park Ave.
	New York, N. Y.

REFERENCES

The student and the health worker will find a number of references useful in their study of nutrition and in daily encounters with nutritional needs. From these they may want to select several for their personal library and read excerpts from others as they have the opportunity and need. This listing of journals, magazines, and basic texts will provide a recommended cross section of helpful resources.

JOURNALS

American Journal of Clinical Nutrition
American Journal of Public Health
Journal of the American Dietetic Association
Journal of Nutrition Education
Nutrition Today

MAGAZINES (useful references for lay readership and perspective)

Family Health
Today's Health

JOURNALS OF RELATED DISCIPLINES

American Journal of Nursing
Journal of the American Medical Association
Nursing Outlook
Preventive Medicine

BASIC TEXTS

Bogert, L. J., Briggs, G., and Calloway, D.: Nutrition and physical fitness, ed. 9, Philadelphia, 1972, W. B. Saunders Co.

Fomon, S. J.: Infant nutrition, Philadelphia, 1967, W. B. Saunders Co.

Guthrie, H. A.: Introductory nutrition, ed. 2, St. Louis, 1971, The C. V. Mosby Co.

Guyton, A. C.: Function of the human body, Philadelphia, 1971, W. B. Saunders Co.

Howe, P. S.: Basic nutrition in health and disease, ed. 5, Philadelphia, 1971, W. B. Saunders Co.

Lowenberg, M. E., Todhunter, E. N., Wilson, E. D., Feeney, M. C., and Savage, J. R.: Food and man, New York, 1968, John Wiley & Sons, Inc.

Nizel, A. E.: Nutrition in preventive dentistry: science and practice, Philadelphia, 1972, W. B. Saunders Co.

Nizel, A. E.: The science of nutrition and its application in clinical dentistry, Philadelphia, 1966, W. B. Saunders Co.

Shackelton, A. D.: Practical nurse nutrition education, ed. 3, Philadelphia, 1972, W. B. Saunders Co.

Williams, S. R.: Nutrition and diet therapy, ed. 2, St. Louis, 1973, The C. V. Mosby Co.

Williams, S. R.: Nutrition and diet therapy: a learning guide for students, St. Louis, 1973, The C. V. Mosby Co.

REFERENCES FOR BASIC CALCULATIONS

Church, C. F., and Church, H. N.: Food values of portions commonly used, ed. 11, Philadelphia, 1970, J. B. Lippincott Co.

Composition of foods, Agriculture Handbook, No. 8, Agricultural Research Service, U. S. Department of Agriculture, Washington, D. C., 1963, U. S. Government Printing Office.

Recommended dietary allowances, ed. 7, 1968, Washington, D. C., Food and Nutrition Board, National Research Council, National Academy of Sciences.

GENERAL REFERENCES

Arnow, L. E.: Food power, Chicago, 1972, Nelson-Hall Co.

Deutsch, R. M.: The family guide to better food and better health, Des Moines, Iowa, 1971, Meredith Corp.

DiOris, L. P., and Madsen, K. O.: A personalized program educating the patient in the prevention of dental disease, Chicago, 1972, March Publishing Co.

Erikson, E.: Childhood and society, ed. 2, New York, 1963, W. W. Norton & Co.

Garrett, A.: Interviewing: its principles and methods, New York, 1942, Family Service Association of America.

Gifft, H. H., Washbon, M. B., and Harrison, G. G.: Nutrition, behavior, and change, Englewood Cliffs, N. J., 1972, Prentice-Hall, Inc.

Jacobson, M. F.: Eater's digest: the consumer's factbook of food additives, Garden City, N. Y., 1972, Doubleday & Co.

Kotz, N.: Let them eat promises: the politics of hunger in America, Englewood Cliffs, N. J., 1969, Prentice-Hall, Inc.

Lappe, F. M.: Diet for a small planet, New York, 1971, Ballantine Books, Inc.

Latham, M. C., McGandy, R. B., McCann, M. C., and Stare, F. J.: Scope manual on nutrition, Kalamazoo, Mich., 1970, Upjohn Co.

Leverton, R. M.: Food becomes you, Ames, Iowa, 1965, Iowa State University Press.

Mayer, J.: Overweight, Englewood Cliffs, N. J., 1968, Prentice-Hall, Inc.

Mayer, J., Editor: U. S. nutrition policies in the seventies, San Francisco, 1973, W. H. Freeman & Co.

Somers, A. R.: Health care in transition: directions for the future, Chicago, 1971, Hospital Research and Educational Trust.

Stuart, R. B., and Davis, B.: Slim chance in a fat world, Champaign, Ill., 1972 Research Press Co.

Townsend, C.: Old age: the last segregation, New York, 1970, Grossman Publishers.

Turner, J. S.: The chemical feast, New York, 1970, Grossman Publishers.

United States Department of Agriculture Yearbooks: 1959, Food; 1966, Protecting our food; 1969, Food for us all, Washington, D. C., U. S. Government Printing Office.

White, P. L.: Let's talk about food, Chicago, 1967, American Medical Association.

Williams, S. R.: Review of nutrition and diet therapy, St. Louis, 1973, The C. V. Mosby Co.

INDEX